Rheumatology

Editors

SEETHA U. MONRAD
DANIEL F. BATTAFARANO

PRIMARY CARE:
CLINICS IN OFFICE PRACTICE

www.primarycare.theclinics.com

Consulting Editor
JOEL J. HEIDELBAUGH

June 2018 • Volume 45 • Number 2

ELSEVIER

1600 John F. Kennedy Boulevard • Suite 1800 • Philadelphia, Pennsylvania, 19103-2899

http://www.theclinics.com

PRIMARY CARE: CLINICS IN OFFICE PRACTICE Volume 45, Number 2
June 2018 ISSN 0095-4543, ISBN-13: 978-0-323-58415-9

Editor: Jessica McCool
Developmental Editor: Laura Fisher

Primary Care: Clinics in Office Practice (ISSN: 0095-4543) is published quarterly by Elsevier Inc., 360 Park Avenue South, New York, NY 10010-1710. Months of issue are March, June, September, and December. Periodicals postage paid at New York, NY and additional mailing offices. Subscription prices are $237.00 per year (US individuals), $474.00 (US institutions), $100.00 (US students), $289.00 (Canadian individuals), $536.00 (Canadian institutions), $175.00 (Canadian students), $355.00 (international individuals), $536.00 (international institutions), and $175.00 (international students). Foreign air speed delivery is included in all *Clinics* subscription prices. All prices are subject to change without notice. POSTMASTER: Send address changes to *Primary Care: Clinics in Office Practice*, Elsevier Periodicals Customer Service, 11830 Westline Industrial Drive, St. Louis, MO 63146. Customer Service Health Sciences Division, Subscription Customer Service, 3251 Riverport Lane, Maryland Heights, MO 63043. **Customer Service: 1-800-654-2452 (U.S. and Canada); 314-447-8871 (outside U.S. and Canada). Fax: 314-447-8029. E-mail: journalscustomerservice-usa@elsevier.com (for print support); journalsonlinesupport-usa@elsevier.com (for online support).**

Reprints. For copies of 100 or more, of articles in this publication, please contact the Commercial Reprints Department, Elsevier Inc., 360 Park Avenue South, New York, NY 10010-1710. Tel. 212-633-3874; Fax: 212-633-3820; E-mail: reprints@elsevier.com.

Primary Care: Clinics in Office Practice is covered in *MEDLINE/PubMed (Index Medicus)* and *EMBASE/ Excerpta Medica, Current Contents/Clinical Medicine, and ISI/BIOMED.*

Contributors

CONSULTING EDITOR

JOEL J. HEIDELBAUGH, MD, FAAFP, FACG
Clinical Professor, Departments of Family Medicine and Urology, University of Michigan Medical School, Ann Arbor, Michigan, USA

EDITORS

SEETHA U. MONRAD, MD
Clinical Associate Professor of Internal Medicine and Learning Health Sciences, Michigan Medicine Assistant Dean of Evaluation, Assessment, and Quality Improvement, Division of Rheumatology, University of Michigan Medical School, Ann Arbor, Michigan, USA

DANIEL F. BATTAFARANO, DO, MACP, FACR
Program Director, Rheumatology Fellowship, San Antonio Uniformed Services Health Education Consortium, Professor of Medicine, Uniformed Services University of the Health Sciences, San Antonio Military Medical Center, San Antonio, Texas, USA

AUTHORS

DANIEL F. BATTAFARANO, DO, MACP, FACR
Program Director, Rheumatology Fellowship, San Antonio Uniformed Services Health Education Consortium, Professor of Medicine, Uniformed Services University of the Health Sciences, San Antonio Military Medical Center, San Antonio, Texas, USA

MONICA M. BATTAFARANO, PT, DPT, CSOMT
Physical Therapist, Sports Center Physical Therapy, Austin, Texas, USA

ANGELIQUE N. COLLAMER, MD, FACP
Rheumatology Service, Lieutenant Colonel, U.S. Air Force, Medical Corps, Walter Reed National Military Medical Center, Uniformed Services University, Bethesda, Maryland, USA

AYYAPPA S. DUBA, MD, RhMSUS
Dartmouth-Hitchcock Medical Center, Lebanon, New Hampshire, USA

JEFFREY C. EICKHOFF, MD
Rheumatology Service, Lieutenant, U.S. Navy, Medical Corps, Naval Medical Center Portsmouth, Portsmouth, Virginia, USA

ALISON M. GIZINSKI, MD, MS
Assistant Professor, Emory University School of Medicine, Atlanta, Georgia, USA

JAY B. HIGGS, MD
Professor, Uniformed Services University of the Health Sciences, MCHE-ZDM-MDR, Brooke Army Medical Center, JBSA Fort Sam Houston, Texas, USA

BERNARD A. HILDEBRAND, MD, FACP, FACR
Assistant Professor of Medicine, Clinical and Applied Science Education, University of the Incarnate Word School of Osteopathic Medicine, San Antonio, Texas, USA

ERICA HILL, DO
Associate Program Director, Rheumatology, San Antonio Uniformed Services Health Education Consortium, San Antonio, Texas, USA

MATTHEW J. HUBBARD, DO
Fellow, Rheumatology, San Antonio Uniformed Services Health Education Consortium, San Antonio Military Medical Center, San Antonio, Texas, USA

REEM JAN, MBBS, BSc
Assistant Professor, Section of Rheumatology, University of Chicago, Chicago, Illinois, USA

RUBA KADO, MD
Clinical Assistant Professor, Department of Internal Medicine, Division of Rheumatology, University of Michigan, Ann Arbor, Michigan, USA

AMANDA KNOTT, PharmD
Department of Pharmacy, Landstuhl Regional Medical Center, Landstuhl, Germany

EMILY A. LITTLEJOHN, DO
Rheumatologic and Immunologic Diseases, Cleveland Clinic, Orthopaedic & Rheumatologic Institute, Cleveland, Ohio, USA

STEPHANIE D. MATHEW, DO
Dartmouth-Hitchcock Medical Center, Lebanon, New Hampshire, USA

SEETHA U. MONRAD, MD
Division of Rheumatology, University of Michigan Medical School, Ann Arbor, Michigan, USA

LEEZA PATEL, MD
Rheumatology Fellow, University of Arkansas for Medical Sciences, Little Rock, Arkansas, USA

MATHILDE H. PIORO, MDCM, MSc, FRCPC
Staff Physician, Orthopedic & Rheumatologic Institute, Cleveland Clinic Lerner College of Medicine of Case Western Reserve University, Cleveland, Ohio, USA

PANKTI REID, MD
Rheumatology Fellow, Section of Rheumatology, University of Chicago, Chicago, Illinois, USA

THOMAS W. SCHMIDT, MD
Staff Rheumatologist, Department of Rheumatology, David Grant USAF Medical Center, Travis AFB, California, USA

ANTHONY SIDARI, MD
Rheumatology Fellow, San Antonio Uniformed Services Health Education Consortium, San Antonio, Texas, USA

IASZMIN VENTURA, MD
Rheumatology Fellow, Section of Rheumatology, University of Chicago, Chicago, Illinois, USA

IAN M. WARD, MD, FACP
Rheumatology Service, Department of Medicine, Landstuhl Regional Medical Center, Landstuhl, Germany

Contents

Patients with rheumatic disease may present with a myriad of symptoms, from joint pain and rashes to more subtle findings, such as dry eyes and dry mouth. In this article, the authors review in detail the common presenting symptoms of rheumatic disease along with key features in the history and physical examination to help distinguish these from other disease processes.

Rheumatologic laboratory tests are frequently ordered by primary care physicians in patients who complain of joint pain. Clinicians should keep in mind the pretest probability of a rheumatologic disorder before ordering any test because laboratory tests in rheumatology are not diagnostic of any particular disease. Any rheumatologic laboratory test result should be used only to further refine the diagnosis, and it should not replace a thorough history and physical examination. In this article, the authors discuss the diagnostic utility of the commonly ordered rheumatologic laboratory tests based on their sensitivity, specificity, and likelihood ratios.

New and existing rheumatic disease is frequently encountered in the primary care setting. The number of medications used to treat various rheumatic conditions continues to increase. Some medications have very specific indications, whereas others have increasing off-label uses. Regardless of the indication, the medications used in rheumatology have variable dosing recommendations, significant side effects, recommended monitoring parameters, and potential medication interactions. Clinicians need to be aware of the potential uses as well as possible pitfalls associated with medications used in rheumatology.

Gout and pseudogout are crystalline arthropathies commonly seen in primary care. It is important to understand their pathophysiology to facilitate recognition and appropriate treatment. Prompt gouty arthritis treatment relieves short-term suffering. Long-term treatment with urate-lowering therapy prevents recurrent attacks and is generally well-tolerated, although flare risk is increased during treatment initiation. When antiinflammatory medications are prescribed, the flare risk is low. Pseudogout acute treatment is similar to acute gouty arthritis treatment. There is no standard regimen for long-term therapies of pseudogout. This article enhances the recognition and treatment of these diseases in the primary care setting.

Rheumatoid arthritis is the most common inflammatory arthritis and a significant cause of morbidity and mortality. Primary care providers should be able to distinguish the clinical presentation of rheumatoid arthritis from that of osteoarthritis, because the treatment and outcomes differ greatly between these 2 common forms of arthritis. This article provides a current overview of our understanding of rheumatoid arthritis, with an emphasis on early diagnosis and approaches to treatment.

Systemic lupus erythematosus is a chronic autoimmune condition with variable organ system involvement; manifestations can range from mild to potentially life threatening. Early diagnosis is important, as progression of disease can be halted. Diagnosis is made by review of signs and symptoms, imaging, and serology.

The seronegative spondyloarthropathies are a group of five diseases characterized by inflammatory oligoarticular arthritis, enthesitis, and axial involvement. They have an increased incidence of the HLA-B27 gene. They are commonly associated with extraarticular features, including involvement of the skin, eyes, and gastrointestinal tract. Early recognition and referral are key to limit disability, and comanagement with primary care and rheumatology offers the best outcomes.

Soft tissue musculoskeletal pain disorders are common in the primary care setting. Early recognition and diagnosis of these syndromes minimizes patient pain and disability. This article gives a brief overview of the most common soft tissue musculoskeletal pain syndromes. The authors used a regional approach to organize the material, as providers will encounter these syndromes with complaints of pain referring to an anatomic location. The covered disorders include myofascial pain syndrome, rotator cuff tendinopathy, bicipital tendinopathy, subacromial bursitis, olecranon bursitis, epicondylitis, De Quervain disease, trigger finger, trochanteric bursitis, knee bursitis, pes anserine bursitis, Baker cyst, plantar fasciitis, and Achilles tendinopathy.

Mathilde H. Pioro

Polymyalgia rheumatica (PMR) and giant cell arteritis (GCA) are related inflammatory diseases of adults aged 50 years or older. The diagnosis of PMR is based on morning stiffness, proximal shoulder and pelvic girdle pain, and functional impairment. GCA is characterized by headache, jaw claudication, and visual disturbances. Constitutional symptoms and elevated inflammatory markers are common to both conditions. Temporal artery biopsy remains the gold standard for diagnosis of GCA. Glucocorticoids are the cornerstone of therapy, with tapering regimens individualized to the patient. Prompt diagnosis and treatment are essential to avert vision loss in GCA. Tocilizumab increases remission rates in GCA.

Jay B. Higgs

Fibromyalgia is a common disorder and has substantial impact on quality of life. The cause remains unknown, but current evidence points to multifactorial involvement of pain processing. Clinical diagnosis is aided by evidence-based diagnostic criteria with subscores for widespread pain and symptom severity. Nonpharmacologic treatments, including cognitive behavioral therapy, sleep hygiene, and regular aerobic exercise, form the cornerstone of management. Pharmacologic intervention is an important adjunct, but benefit is variable. There is no cure for fibromyalgia at this time, but persistence and patience in management may lead to a satisfactory lifestyle.

Jeffrey C. Eickhoff and Angelique N. Collamer

Musculoskeletal rheumatic syndromes are commonly encountered in the primary care setting. A plethora of commonly encountered and rare infectious agents can produce osteoarticular and soft tissue manifestations. Likewise, malignancies may manifest rheumatic symptoms via direct tumor invasion or paraneoplastic effects. Awareness of these diseases and their clinical risk factors should result in improved screening and earlier recognition and intervention, leading to improved long-term outcomes and overall patient care.

Thomas W. Schmidt

Osteoarthritis is the most common joint disease in the world today. Patients present for evaluation and treatment to primary care providers on a regular basis. A general understanding of its pathogenesis, risk factors, diagnosis, and treatment is imperative. This article provides the primary care provider with a primer on osteoarthritis care and management.

Rheumatology

PRIMARY CARE:
CLINICS IN OFFICE PRACTICE

ISSUE OF RELATED INTEREST

Clinics in Geriatric Medicine, February 2017 (Vol. 33, No. 1)
Rheumatic Diseases in Older Adults
James D. Katz and Brian Walitt, *Editors*
Available at: http://www.geriatric.theclinics.com/

THE CLINICS ARE AVAILABLE ONLINE!
Access your subscription at:
www.theclinics.com

Foreword
A Better Hope

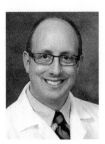

Joel J. Heidelbaugh, MD, FAAFP, FACG
Consulting Editor

In 2010, I wrote in the foreword for our last *Primary Care: Clinics in Office Practice* issue on rheumatologic diseases, "*What cannot be understated here is the increasing need for primary care clinicians to learn the complexities of evaluating and managing rheumatologic diseases, the pharmacokinetics and adverse effects of current and new biologic agents to treat these disorders, and the necessity of a strong and communicative relationship between the rheumatologist and the primary care clinician within the medical home model to promote better outcomes for our patients.*" While this is a rather verbose statement, nearly a decade later, it's even more important and relevant.

Nearly 20 years ago, I met a young African American woman who presented to my practice to establish care. She spent the entire first visit venting that her previous physician told her she has fibromyalgia, and there was no cure. Apparently he also told her that her masklike facial rash was due to her makeup and her joint pain would improve if she lost weight. I had the unfortunate task of creating a detailed rheumatologic workup and ultimately telling her that she has systemic lupus erythematosus and rheumatoid arthritis. She would also be found to have about half a dozen antibodies on her serologic workup that I had never heard of. Ultimately, over the years to follow, she would progress to develop retinal and dermatologic vasculitis.

What complicates this case is that despite multiple rheumatologic consultations, she has largely declined pharmacotherapy save 6 months of intermittent therapy, citing fears that the potential adverse effects from treatment are more unpredictable and toxic that her rheumatologic diseases themselves. In fact, her best friend had lupus and "died from taking the medications." While suffering declining renal function and vision with superimposed chronic pain, she is currently seeking complementary and alternative therapy options.

This issue of the *Primary Care: Clinics in Office Practice* dives deep into the fundamentals of many commonly encountered rheumatologic disorders in primary care. The articles present a very practical and scientific approach that will provide not only a foundation of knowledge for these disorders but will also guide appropriate specialty referrals. I would like to thank Drs Monrad and Battafarano for their dedication in guiding the creation of this important issue of articles on rheumatology. As they noted in their preface, the impending shortage of rheumatologists raises the bar for our diagnostic and therapeutic challenges in primary care.

Joel J. Heidelbaugh, MD, FAAFP, FACG
Departments of Family Medicine and Urology
University of Michigan Medical School
Ann Arbor, MI 48103, USA

Ypsilanti Health Center
200 Arnet, Suite 200
Ypsilanti, MI 48198, USA

E-mail address:
jheidel@umich.edu

Preface

Rheumatic Diseases: Beyond the Musculoskeletal System

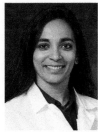

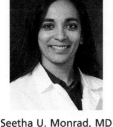

Seetha U. Monrad, MD   Daniel F. Battafarano, DO, MACP, FACR
Editors

Primary care providers do not need statistics to know that the burden of rheumatic diseases is enormous.[1] However, buried within numerous regional musculoskeletal disorders and degenerative joint disease exist disorders of the immune system that manifest with musculoskeletal pain and dysfunction. Identifying these patients with autoimmune rheumatic diseases is critically important, as we now have various medications that are revolutionizing the natural history of autoimmune disease. Early identification and treatment have the potential to radically alter the disease progression and limit the morbidity and mortality associated with these diseases. In addition, as modulating the immune system becomes an increasingly important part of modern medicine, understanding how immune dysfunction manifests in patients will be a useful skillset for all providers.

We had the privilege of leading the most recent workforce study of rheumatologists in the United States,[2] and the results were sobering. Our projections indicate there will not be enough rheumatologists to care for patients with rheumatic disease in the next 20 years. Primary care colleagues are already experiencing challenges in obtaining access to rheumatology subspecialty care for their patients. However, the workforce study identified the imperative need for effective partnerships between rheumatologists and primary care providers, and enhanced education about the rheumatic diseases.

Our hope is that this issue of *Primary Care: Clinics in Office Practice* can serve as one piece of the partnership. We have chosen these topics to encompass a broad range of rheumatologic issues we believe are of relevance to primary care providers. Three articles discuss the approach to evaluating persons with potential rheumatic diseases, key principles regarding the use and interpretation of immunologic labs, and an overview of common rheumatologic medications. Subsequent articles cover core rheumatic diseases: rheumatoid arthritis, systemic lupus erythematosus,

Prim Care Clin Office Pract 45 (2018) xiii–xiv
https://doi.org/10.1016/j.pop.2018.03.001
0095-4543/18/© 2018 Published by Elsevier Inc.

primarycare.theclinics.com

spondyloarthropathies, crystalline arthritis, polymyalgia rheumatica/giant cell arteritis, osteoarthritis, and soft tissue rheumatic syndromes. There is an article on autoimmunity mimics, which must always be considered on the differential. Finally, the rheumatologic perspective on regional rheumatic disorders and fibromyalgia is presented.

We hope you find this issue useful and informative.

Seetha U. Monrad, MD
Division of Rheumatology
Department of Internal Medicine
Department of Learning Health Sciences
University of Michigan
7D08 North Ingalls Building
300 North Ingalls Street
Ann Arbor, MI 48109, USA

Daniel F. Battafarano, DO, MACP, FACR
Rheumatology Fellowship
San Antonio Military Medical Center
Uniformed Services University
of the Health Sciences
3551 Roger Brooke Drive
MCHE-ZDM-R
San Antonio, TX 78234-4504, USA

E-mail addresses:
seetha@med.umich.edu (S.U. Monrad)
daniel.f.battafarano.civ@mail.mil (D.F. Battafarano)

REFERENCES

1. United States Bone and Joint Initiative: the burden of musculoskeletal diseases in the United States (BMUS), 3rd edition. Rosemont (IL): 2014. Available at: http://www.boneandjointburden.org. Accessed October 1, 2017.
2. Battafarano DF, Ditmyer MD, Bolster MB, et al. 2015 American College of Rheumatology Workforce Study: supply and demand projections of adult rheumatology workforce (2015-2030). Arthritis Care Res 2018. [Epub ahead of print].

Approach to Patients with Suspected Rheumatic Disease

Iaszmin Ventura, MD, Pankti Reid, MD, Reem Jan, MBBS, BSc*

KEYWORDS

- Arthralgia • Raynaud • Sicca • Alopecia • Malar rash

KEY POINTS

- Arthralgia is the most frequent presenting symptom of rheumatic disease, and the physician's first step is to make the distinction between inflammatory and noninflammatory joint pain. Thereafter, the pattern of joint involvement, time course, and physical findings will help formulate a narrow differential diagnosis.
- The skin is a frequent target for rheumatic conditions, and familiarity with stereotypical rashes is essential in leading to early diagnosis of systemic disease and appropriate tests and referrals.
- A thorough history and physical examination can lead to a more judicious choice of laboratory tests and in some cases avoid unnecessary serologic testing that can lead to anxiety, expense, and misdiagnoses.

INTRODUCTION

Rheumatic diseases are a fascinating group of conditions that demonstrate the complex role immunology plays in every organ system. The primary care provider can learn to recognize classic presenting symptoms and signs of these diseases, leading to earlier diagnosis and referral to a specialist. It is of paramount importance that a detailed history and physical examination precede any laboratory testing, as many serologic tests are of high sensitivity but low specificity. In this section, the authors describe the characteristic features of common presentations in these diseases, highlighting the aspects most consistent with an autoimmune or inflammatory process.

Arthralgia

Arthralgia is the most common reason for referral to a rheumatology practice. Evaluation of joint pain should always begin with the characterization of type of joint pain as

Disclosure Statement: No disclosures relevant to this work.
Section of Rheumatology, University of Chicago, 5841 South Maryland Avenue, Chicago, IL 60637, USA
* Corresponding author.
E-mail address: rjan@medicine.bsd.uchicago.edu

Prim Care Clin Office Pract 45 (2018) 169–180
https://doi.org/10.1016/j.pop.2018.02.001
0095-4543/18/© 2018 Elsevier Inc. All rights reserved.

primarycare.theclinics.com

inflammatory versus noninflammatory and is followed by attention to the number and pattern of joints involved and the temporal onset and progression of pain.[1] Inflammatory joint pain characteristically peaks in the mornings with 30 minutes or more of morning stiffness (often a couple of hours or more), improves with activity, and does not completely remit with the rest. Types of inflammatory arthritis include autoimmune diseases like rheumatoid arthritis, crystalline arthritis, or infection. Noninflammatory joint pain is usually exacerbated by weight bearing and movement and is typically alleviated by rest. Diseases that lead to noninflammatory joint pain include osteoarthritis and fibromyalgia.

Duration of symptoms and location of the pain also facilitate in deciphering the cause. Symptoms less than 6 weeks are considered acute and may be consistent with viral or postinfectious syndromes, whereas pain lasting more than 6 weeks is categorized as more chronic and raises the index of suspicion for an autoimmune disease. The pattern of small joint disease, for example, in the hands, is very telling. Although rheumatoid arthritis (RA) affects the proximal interphalangeal (PIP) joints, metacarpophalangeal (MCP) joints, and wrist joints, it tends to spare the distal interphalangeal (DIP) joints. Osteoarthritis by contrast affects the DIP and PIP joints and the base of the thumb at the carpometacarpal joint and tends to spare the MCP joints and wrists. Of note, pain and tenderness between joints (between the DIP and PIP joints or between PIP and MCP joints) and into the myofascial planes arouse suspicion for fibromyalgia. Any other organ system involvement, such as the skin, oral mucosa, or simply the presence of profound constitutional symptoms, may indicate an autoimmune process, so a thorough review of systems is always helpful. See **Fig. 1** for clues to the diagnosis of arthropathy given these patterns of joint involvement.

When examining patients, the first step is assessing if the pain is truly in the articular area or if the pain is actually in the periarticular structures. The examiner should "look, feel and move" the joints to assess the true structures involved and any objective stigmata of inflammation or effusion. For example, thickening, sponginess, or soft tissue swelling around a joint implies synovitis, whereas bony or nodal enlargement of a joint is more characteristic of osteoarthritis.

In cases of acute monoarthritis, particularly initial presentations, it is absolutely essential to aspirate the joint and analyze the fluid for cell count, Gram stain, culture, and crystals. This analyzation will help rule in a crystal disease and rule out a septic joint.

Careful history and physical examination will help determine the appropriate laboratory, serologic, and radiographic tests in each setting and lower the likelihood of misleading test results.

INFLAMMATORY BACK PAIN

Back pain is one of the most common complaints in a primary care setting.[2] In fact, chronic lower back pain is a global issue in terms of morbidity, disability, and health care utilization.[3] For the primary care physician, it is important to be able to distinguish mechanical/degenerative back pain from pain that is inflammatory in nature or indicates serious underlying disease. Certain features (so-called red flags) of lower back pain should prompt urgent evaluation for disorders, such as malignancy, vertebral fracture, infection, or cauda equina syndrome. These features include age younger than 20 years or older than 50 years old; acute onset; association with trauma; weakness or sensory disturbance in the limbs; nocturnal pain; saddle anesthesia; urinary incontinence or retention; persistent fever or unexplained weight loss; history of cancer, intravenous drug abuse, or human immunodeficiency virus/AIDS; and osteoporosis.[4,5]

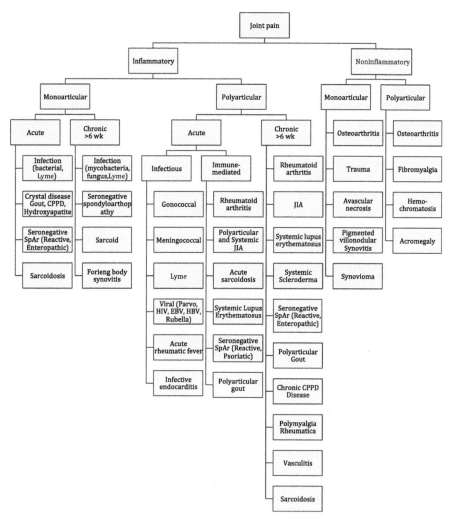

Fig. 1. Arthralgia. EBV, Epstein-Barr virus; HBV, hepatitis B virus; HIV, human immunodeficiency virus; JIA, juvenile idiopathic arthritis.

In addition, it is critical to evaluate patients for inflammatory back pain, as this can fundamentally change options for management. Over the years, there have been different definitions of inflammatory back pain, including the following features[6,7]:

- Age of onset less than 45 years
- Insidious onset and present for greater than 3 months
- Morning back stiffness greater than 30 minutes
- Improvement with exercise without improvement with rest
- Pain at night (particularly the second half of the night)
- Alternating buttock pain (may indicate sacroiliitis)

Together with these characteristic features of inflammatory back pain, the diagnosis of spondyloarthritis can be guided by other systemic features, which are included in the Assessment of SpondyloArthritis International Society's classification criteria for spondyloarthritis.[8] These features include history of uveitis, arthritis, dactylitis, inflammatory bowel disease, enthesitis, good response to nonsteroidal antiinflammatory drugs, and family history for spondyloarthropathy.

If patients are younger than 45 years at the time of the onset of spinal pain and meet the criteria for inflammatory back pain and/or have one other feature that is included in this classification, a referral to a rheumatologist is certainly warranted.

Sicca Syndrome

Sicca syndrome refers to dry eyes and/or dry mouth. In terms of keratoconjunctivitis sicca, patients may describe a feeling of sand or sandpaper in their eyes, inability to produce tears, increased pruritus or conjunctival injection, or need for frequent use of artificial eye drops. Xerostomia may present with constant thirst and frequent need for water intake, difficulty swallowing dry foods like crackers without sipping fluids, and gingivitis that is eventually complicated by tooth decay.

Sicca symptoms are common among the general population, particularly in the elderly. Older adults are more likely to use medications that impair exocrine glandular function, particularly drugs with anticholinergic properties. Age-related atrophy of these glands probably also plays a role.

From the rheumatologic perspective, Sjögren syndrome is characteristically associated with sicca symptoms and must be considered in severe cases, particularly in younger patients when medication side effects are ruled out. Evidence of inflammatory arthritis on history or physical examination in addition to the sicca syndrome may increase suspicion for a rheumatologic cause, given the close association between RA and Sjögren syndrome.

RECURRENT APHTHOUS ULCERS

Recurrent aphthous ulcers are a common complaint among the general population. It is not clear how many episodes are needed to classify these ulcers as recurrent or not[8]; but in clinical practice, episodes occurring more than once monthly may warrant further attention. Aphthous ulcers usually present with single or multiple painful erosions that appear more commonly on unattached oral mucosa of lips, cheeks, and tongue but sometimes also on the gingival and palatal keratinized mucosa. These ulcers vary in size and are characteristically surrounded by an erythematous halo and covered by a fine fibrous coating. These lesions are normally self-limiting and resolve without scarring after a few days. Larger ulcers that last more than 2 weeks are less likely to be idiopathic and are more commonly associated with systemic diseases.

Recurrent aphthae that involves both oral and genital mucosa may be very suggestive of Behçet syndrome, a rare inflammatory disease also associated with vasculitis, inflammatory eye disease, folliculitis, and pustular eruptions. Evaluation by a rheumatologist in this setting is essential, as this remains a clinical diagnosis; biopsy of oral ulcers are rarely helpful unless with the view to exclude an infectious cause.

Raynaud Phenomenon

Raynaud phenomenon (RP) results from vasospasm of the digital arteries in response to cold temperature or stress, resulting in color changes of the digits described as white, blue, or gray (cyanosis) associated with pain and numbness, frequently followed by hyperemia with rewarming. It was first described by its namesake Maurice Raynaud in 1862.[9] Although many individuals may experience digital sensitivity to extreme cold, patients with RP have an exaggerated response to even relatively mild shifts in temperature. In general, symptoms triggered by routine circumstances, such as sitting in air conditioning or reaching into a refrigerator, are suggestive of pathologic process.

RP usually presents symmetrically, though it may not affect all fingers at once, and involves the upper extremity digits preferentially before the lower become symptomatic. It can be a primary condition or secondary, meaning resultant of an underlying disease. It is important to note that patients with characteristics of primary RP can later transition to developing secondary RP; essentially in these cases, Raynaud is the initial presenting symptom of a systemic process but can predate the other findings by some months or years.

Primary RP occurs most commonly in women between 15 years and 30 years old.[10] On physical examination, a rheumatologist may examine the nail fold capillaries with a low-power magnifier, such as an ophthalmoscope. In primary RP this tends to be normal, whereas secondary RP will show enlargement, distortion, or dropout of periungual capillary loops.[11] Primary RP should not progress to digital ulceration, pitting, fissuring, or gangrene. If these symptoms are present, associated autoimmune disease is strongly implied. A 10-year prospective study published in 2006 found that certain features predicted a transition of primary RP to secondary RP, namely, abnormal capillary microscopy, cryoglobulinemia, high antinuclear antibody (ANA) titers ($\geq$1:320), and positivity of specific serologic ANA subsets.[12]

Causes to consider in RP

- Autoimmune diseases (especially scleroderma, mixed connective tissue disease, dermatomyositis, and systemic lupus erythematosus [SLE])
- Use of vibration tools (eg, microtrauma from drill use in construction workers)
- Medications and drugs (propranolol, amphetamines, nicotine)

See **Fig. 2** for an overview of the characteristics that may warrant a workup for a rheumatic disease.

Alopecia

Alopecia, or hair loss, becomes more prevalent with age and can affect up to 50% of the population at some point in their lives. However, it can also be an important symptom in SLE. Gynecologic history is absolutely essential because abnormal menses, history of infertility, hirsutism, virilization, and galactorrhea could all be clues to a diagnosis of possible androgenetic alopecia. After this initial consideration of possible hormonal imbalance as a cause, hair loss is generally categorized into diffuse versus focal and scarring versus nonscarring.

Most focal causes for alopecia are associated with an underlying disorder. Focal scarring alopecia is called cicatricial alopecia, which causes atrophy and scarring of scalp hair with permanent hair loss. The most common cause of cicatricial alopecia is discoid lupus erythematosus,[13] as shown in **Fig. 3**.The differential diagnosis of focal nonscarring alopecia is more extensive and includes alopecia areata, tinea capitis, traction alopecia and trichotillomania.

Causes for diffuse hair loss include female or male pattern baldness, diffuse alopecia areata, telogen effluvium and anagen effluvium along with iron abnormalities, vitamin D deficiency or thyroid pathology. Of these, alopecia areata affects ages less than 20 years, men and women equally, and shows multiple lymphocytes on skin biopsy indicating an autoimmune cause. It is quite common and affects up to 2% of the population.[14] Although the most frequent presentation of alopecia areata is isolated, benign loss of hair, it has been shown to occur in association with autoimmune disorders, such as vitiligo, lichen planus, morphea, lichen sclerosis et

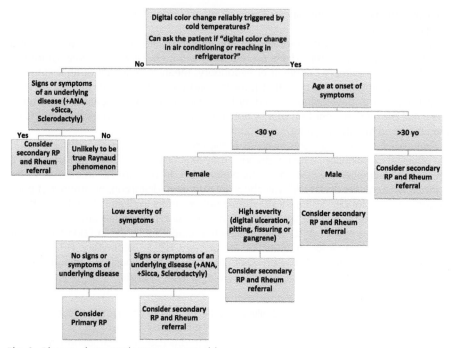

Fig. 2. Rheum, rheumatology; yo, years old.

atrophicus, Hashimoto thyroiditis, SLE, localized scleroderma, ulcerative colitis, and type I diabetes mellitus.[14,15]

To uncover true alopecia, it is helpful to evaluate by the pull test. This test is performed by applying traction or gentle pull of about 40 hairs.[16] The test is considered positive if 6 or more hairs are extracted, whereas the test is considered negative if only 3 or less hairs are extracted. A positive pull test raises concern for a more pathologic underlying cause like alopecia areata or telogen effluvium, whereas a negative pull test indicates the typical presentation of male or female pattern baldness. The typical presentation of male pattern baldness appears as hair thinning and eventual loss in the bitemporal recession, which then progresses to the frontal regions. Female

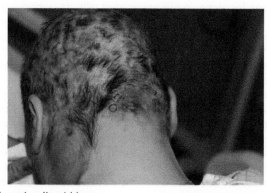

Fig. 3. Scarring alopecia: discoid lupus.

pattern baldness involves hair thinning at the central scalp, which then leads to widening of the midline part. Telogen effluvium usually results from abnormal hair cycling and presents as significant daily shedding of hair follicles. Telogen effluvium is typically caused by medications, emotional stress, vitamin D deficiency, iron deficiency, or active systemic disease like infection or autoimmune disease flare.

When history and physical examination alone do not suffice for a definitive diagnosis of alopecia, referral for further assessment of skin histopathology (via skin scraping or skin biopsy) may be appropriate.

CUTANEOUS MANIFESTATIONS OF RHEUMATIC DISEASE

The skin is a common target of many rheumatologic conditions. Rashes are often the first manifestation of these diseases and the main reason patients seek medical attention. Inspection of the skin is often a crucial element in establishing a differential diagnosis and can help identify a rheumatologic disease right at the first medical encounter.

Lupus Erythematosus and the Skin

Skin manifestations are often an early sign of SLE and one of the most useful clinical clues. The importance of cutaneous aspects of lupus is reflected in the American College of Rheumatology's revised classification criteria of SLE from 1997, in which 3 out of 11 criteria are dermatologic conditions (malar rash, discoid lesions, and photosensitivity) and a minimum of 4 criteria are necessary for the diagnosis.[17] Cutaneous lupus erythematosus (CLE) encompasses a wide range of dermatologic manifestations, which may or may not be associated with systemic disease. CLE is classified in different subtypes, acute CLE (ACLE), subacute CLE (SCLE), and chronic CLE.[18] A definitive diagnosis frequently depends not only on physical examination but also on histology and serologic evaluation. Nevertheless, primary care physicians should be able to identify common characteristic features of these subtypes, which will prompt further investigation.

Photosensitivity refers to the development of rashes secondary to exposure to UV light. This sign is an important characteristic for many dermatoses and is particularly significant in patients with CLE. Exposure to both UVA and UVB triggers the development of many types of lupus rashes, as described later; it can also trigger exacerbations of systemic manifestations, such as mucosal ulcers, constitutional symptoms, cytopenias, and arthralgias. Interestingly, the photosensitive rash can declare itself several days to more than 3 weeks after UV exposure and can take several months to subside. This prolonged gap between exposure and development of symptoms may confuse patients who may not be able to establish an association of causation between these events. Immediate sun reactions, by contrast, may be more consistent with polymorphic light eruptions.

ACLE usually refers to the classic *malar* or butterfly rash, frequently associated with active SLE. Malar rash is the denomination for the erythema over the malar eminences and nasal bridge, sometimes associated with edema and fine desquamation, which spares the nasolabial folds. This type of rash is transient, nonscarring, and classically triggered by sun exposure. ACLE can be also generalized; it presents with erythematous macules and papules, often pruritic. This form of rash can resemble the rash from dermatomyositis (see later discussion), but in contradistinction it spares the interphalangeal and metacarpophalangeal joints and is not associated with periungual involvement.

SCLE is highly photosensitive, occurring more frequently in sun-exposed areas, such as the extensor surfaces of upper extremities, upper back, and chest (**Fig. 4**). It manifests in 2 variants, annular SCLE and papulosquamous SCLE. The former

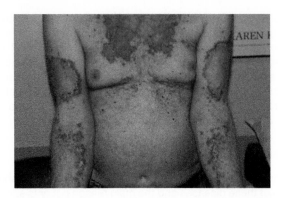

Fig. 4. Scle.

presents with annular erythematous plaques, characteristically coalescent. This rash can be mistaken for tinea corporis; but it typically does not occur below the waistline, a common characteristic of the fungal infection. Papulosquamous SCLE presents with scaly erythematous plaques, sometimes resembling psoriatic plaques or eczema. SCLE usually heals without scarring. Patients with SCLE tend to have mild systemic disease activity, usually with musculoskeletal and mucocutaneous outbreaks. Interestingly, SCLE is the most common cutaneous manifestation of medication-induced lupus; frequent offenders are proton-pump inhibitors, diltiazem, thiazides, terbinafine, tumor necrosis factor inhibitors, and antiepileptic medications.

Discoid lupus is the prototype of chronic cutaneous lupus (see **Fig. 3**). Patients with discoid lupus carry a lower risk of evolution into systemic disease and, therefore, have a more favorable prognosis. Discoid lesions are more commonly restricted to the scalp, face, and ears but can also extend to extensor surfaces of arms and hands and rarely affect mucosal surfaces. Patient with lesions below the neck are thought to be at higher risk of clinically significant systemic disease.[19] These lesions are well-demarcated erythematous and scaly macules and papules, which evolve to annular indurated hyperpigmented and atrophic plaques, with adherent scales. These lesions are characteristically scarring; when they affect the scalp, they cause scarring alopecia, secondary to hair follicle invasion and disruption.

Dermatomyositis

Dermatomyositis is a multisystem inflammatory disease that affects mainly skeletal muscles and skin. Characteristic cutaneous manifestations clinically differentiate this entity from other idiopathic inflammatory myopathies. On occasion, patients can present solely with skin disease and minimal or no muscle weakness. This condition, called dermatomyositis sine myositis or amyopathic dermatomyositis, may have a stronger association with occult malignancy, which underlines the importance of familiarity with these stereotypical rashes.[20]

Gottron papules are pathognomonic of dermatomyositis (**Fig. 5**). These papules are violaceous or wine-colored lesions that occur on the extensor surfaces of interphalangeal joints and less commonly on larger joint surfaces, such as elbows, knees, and medial malleoli, generally in a symmetric distribution. Larger joint involvement is more common in children than adults and is designated as the Gottron sign.

Children are also more vulnerable to calcinosis cutis (painful dystrophic calcification of the skin). A cutaneous vasculitis, manifesting with livedo reticularis and digital microinfarcts/ulcerations, can also be seen in severe cases.

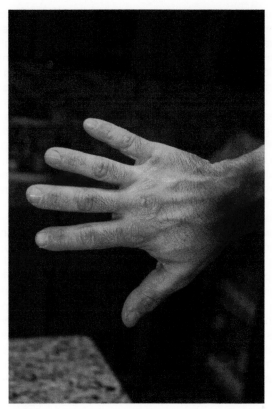

Fig. 5. Gottron papules.

Heliotrope rash describes periorbital edema with violaceous erythema of the upper eyelids. This finding is also pathognomonic. In the resolution stage, atrophy or depigmentation may be apparent.

Shawl and V sign refers to violaceous erythema, sometimes with fine desquamation, of photo-exposed areas, particularly the upper back, neck, and anterior chest. This rash can also be very photosensitive and can be confused with acute lupus erythematosus, as mentioned earlier; but concomitant occurrence of other findings, such as mechanic hands and Gottron papules, help differentiating between these diseases. Moreover, rashes from dermatomyositis are usually more pruritic than those seen in SLE.[21]

Mechanic hands describe rough, scaly hyperkeratotic papules, associated with linear fissures and hyperpigmentation on the lateral and palmar surfaces of the fingers. The cuticles are thickened and distorted; periungual areas are erythematous to the naked eye due to telangiectasias, with prominent dilated and tortuous capillaries and punctiform hemorrhages.

Cutaneous Sclerosis

Cutaneous sclerosis is a generic term that can be used to embrace all diseases characterized by skin thickening and tightening, resulting in a leatherlike appearance. There are many causes, classified as primary cutaneous sclerosis, idiopathic or autoimmune-mediated, and secondary cutaneous sclerosis, due to exposure to medications or toxins, such as bleomycin, polyvinyl chloride, and gadolinium. RP is a marker of vascular involvement and helps identify patients more likely to evolve into systemic sclerosis. In addition, in patients with scleroderma, the tightening starts at the digital tips (causing tapering of digits or sclerodactyly) and extends proximally.

Morphea is an idiopathic inflammatory disease confined to the skin and subcutaneous tissues. Areas of skin tightening and thickening, normally with loss of skin attachment apparatus, such as hair follicles and sweat glands, characterize the disease. Morphea can present in different patterns: as isolated or numerous coalescent plaques, rapidly progressive or indolent and can affect any part of the body, although is more common on the trunk or proximal extremities. The linear pattern, which is more common in children, denotes a band of indurated skin or various sizes. When it involves the scalp or forehead, it is referred to as en coup de sabre and can be associated with seizures when there is involvement of underlying meninges and brain parenchyma. Morphea is not a marker of risk for systemic sclerosis.

Diffuse cutaneous systemic sclerosis is clinically characterized by skin thickening beyond the elbows and involvement of other areas, more commonly the face and trunk, whereas limited disease manifests with puffy digits or sclerodactyly alone. The skin loses its characteristic flexibility and mild redundancy to the point that the examiner cannot pinch the skin between the first and second digits. The skin becomes shiny, and the digits develop flexion contractures over time (claw hand). Nail fold capillary changes are common, with tortuous dilated capillaries and punctate hemorrhages. The extent of these findings tends to correlate with RP severity.

Telangiectasias of varying numbers can be identified on the hands, anterior chest, and face. Skin tightening on the face causes loss of expression lines, thinning of the nose and lips and microstomia, and restriction of mouth opening due to skin induration. Dyspigmentation of the affected skin, featured as hyperpigmented and hypopigmented small macules, commonly occurs in a pattern referred to as "salt and pepper" pattern.[22,23]

CONSTITUTIONAL SYMPTOMS

Nonspecific symptoms, such as fatigue, fever, night sweats, and weight loss, are common manifestations in patients with active rheumatologic diseases. Autoimmune disease may account for 15% to 25% of cases of fever of unknown origin in adults.[24] In these cases, pyrogenic cytokines enter the circulation and adjust the thermoregulatory center in the hypothalamus, ultimately triggering a cascade of phenomena that lead to the increase in body temperature. This systemic inflammatory burden is also suspected to be the reason behind development of fatigue, night sweats, and weight loss. Adult-onset Still disease and temporal arteritis/polymyalgia rheumatica are notorious causes of fever in adults; the former is usually diagnosed in younger adults and classically manifests with a quotidian fever, and the latter may account for up to 15% of cases of fever in the elderly population. In patients with SLE, up to 60% will present with fever during the disease course, as a manifestation of their flares.[25]

Vasculitis is another notorious cause of both fever and weight loss, to the extent that these form part of the diagnostic criteria for polyarteritis nodosa, a seronegative medium vessel vasculitis. Autoinflammatory syndromes, which are usually caused by some sort of genetic error that drives overexpression of inflammatory cytokines, are classic causes of recurrent periodic fever in children and adolescents.

An attentive physician must also keep in mind that acute febrile illnesses of infectious causes may also cause musculoskeletal symptoms and can mimic rheumatologic diseases. Typical examples include mononucleosis syndrome and parvovirus

B19 infection, which can cause rashes, lymphadenopathy, myalgias, and inflammatory arthritis in young adults.

Inflammatory arthritis, such as RA and the spondylarthritides, are less likely to cause fevers; but uncontrolled disease is commonly accompanied by profound fatigue and even weight loss.

Although constitutional symptoms lack specificity for autoimmunity, their presence increases the suspicion for a systemic inflammatory disease and may help the physician distinguish these syndromes from mechanical or central causes of pain.

SUMMARY

Careful history taking remains the cornerstone of effective clinical medicine, and a fundamental knowledge of the characteristic symptoms and signs of rheumatic disease can help avoid common pitfalls in the evaluation of these patients. The physical examination remains an indispensable part of the assessment process and can reveal unexpected clues in the skin, mucosa, joints, and digits that help formulate a differential diagnosis. The laboratory evaluation plays a supportive role to these tools and should only rarely lead the hunt. Early involvement of a rheumatologist is appropriate whenever the primary care physician suspects autoimmune disease.

REFERENCES

1. El-Gabalawy HS, Duray P, Goldbach-Mansky R. Evaluating patients with arthritis of recent onset: studies in pathogenesis and prognosis. JAMA 2000;284(18): 2368–73.
2. Braun J, Baraliakos X, Regel A, et al. Assessment of spinal pain. Best Pract Res Clin Rheumatol 2014;28(6):875–87.
3. Hoy D, March L, Brooks P, et al. The global burden of low back pain: estimates from the global burden of disease 2010 study. Ann Rheum Dis 2014;73(6): 968–74.
4. Petri R, Gimbel R. Evaluation of the patient with spinal trauma and back pain: an evidence based approach. Emerg Med Clin North Am 1999;17(1):25–39, vii–viii.
5. Henschke N, Maher CG, Refshauge KM, et al. Prevalence of and screening for serious spinal pathology in patients presenting to primary care settings with acute low back pain. Arthritis Rheum 2009;60(10):3072–80.
6. Sieper J, van der Heijde D, Landewe R, et al. New criteria for inflammatory back pain in patients with chronic back pain: a real patient exercise by experts from the assessment of SpondyloArthritis International Society (ASAS). Ann Rheum Dis 2009;68(6):784–8.
7. Rudwaleit M, Metter A, Listing J, et al. Inflammatory back pain in ankylosing spondylitis: a reassessment of the clinical history for application as classification and diagnostic criteria. Arthritis Rheum 2006;54(2):569–78.
8. Sieper J, Rudwaleit M, Baraliakos X, et al. The assessment of SpondyloArthritis International Society (ASAS) handbook: a guide to assess spondyloarthritis. Ann Rheum Dis 2009;68(Suppl 2):ii1–44.
9. Slebioda Z, Szponar E, Kowalska A. Etiopathogenesis of recurrent aphthous stomatitis and the role of immunologic aspects: literature review. Arch Immunol Ther Exp 2014;62:205–15.
10. Maurice Raynaud (1834-1881). Raynaud's disease. JAMA 1967;(11):985.
11. Wigley FM, Flavahan NA. Raynaud's phenomenon. N Engl J Med 2016;375(6): 556–65.

12. Lambova SN, Müller-Ladner U. The role of capillaroscopy in differentiation of primary and secondary Raynaud's phenomenon in rheumatic diseases: a review of the literature and two case reports. Rheumatol Int 2009;29(11):1263–71.

13. Hirschl M, Hirschl K, Lenz M, et al. Transition from primary Raynaud's phenomenon to secondary Raynaud's phenomenon identified by diagnosis of an associated disease: results of ten years of prospective surveillance. Arthritis Rheum 2006;54(6):1974–81.

14. Mounsey AL, Reed SW. Diagnosing and treating hair loss. Am Fam Physician 2009;80(4):356–62.

15. Muller SA, Winkelmann RK. Alopecia areata: an evaluation of 736 patients. Arch Dermatol 1963;88:290–7.

16. Thomas EA, Kadyan RS. Alopecia areata and autoimmunity: a clinical study. Indian J Dermatol 2008;53(2):70.

17. Gordon KA, Tosti A. Alopecia: evaluation and treatment. Clin Cosmet Investig Dermatol 2011;4:101–6.

18. Sontheimer RD. Skin manifestations of systemic autoimmune connective tissue disease: diagnostics and therapeutics. Best Pract Res Clin Rheumatol 2004; 18(3):429–62.

19. Okon LG, Werth VP. Cutaneous lupus erythematosus: diagnosis and treatment. Best Pract Res Clin Rheumatol 2013;27(3):391–404.

20. Hejazi EZ, Werth VP. Cutaneous lupus erythematosus: an update on pathogenesis, diagnosis and treatment. Am J Clin Dermatol 2016;17(2):135.

21. Femia A, Vleugels R, Callen J. Cutaneous dermatomyositis: an update review of treatment options and internal associations. Am J Clin Dermatol 2013;14(4): 291–313.

22. Valdez MA, Isamah N, Northway RM. Dermatologic manifestations of systemic diseases. Prim Care 2015;42(4):607–30.

23. Kalus A. Rheumatologic skin disease. Med Clin North Am 2015;99(6):1287–303, xii–xiii.

24. Mourad O, Palda V, Detsky AS. A comprehensive evidence-based approach to fever of unknown origin. Arch Intern Med 2003;163(5):545–51.

25. Beça S, Rodríguez-Pintó I, Alba MA, et al. Development and validation of a risk calculator to differentiate flares from infections in systemic lupus erythematosus patients with fever. Autoimmun Rev 2015;14(7):586–93.

A Primer on Rheumatologic Laboratory Tests

What They Mean and When to Order Them

Leeza Patel, MD[a], Alison M. Gizinski, MD, MS[b],*

KEYWORDS

• ANA • ANCA • CCP • CRP • ESR • RF

KEY POINTS

- Laboratory tests in rheumatology should be interpreted depending on the clinical scenario because they are rarely diagnostic of any particular disease.
- A positive antinuclear antibody can be found in normal individuals and in patients with other inflammatory and autoimmune diseases and is not diagnostic of systemic lupus erythematosus.
- Rheumatoid factor (RF) and anticyclic citrullinated peptide (anti-CCP) antibodies support the diagnosis of rheumatoid arthritis, and anti-CCP is more specific than RF.
- A positive antineutrophilic cytoplasmic antibody test with antiproteinase 3 or antimyeloperoxidase specificity supports the clinical diagnoses of systemic necrotizing vasculitis but is not diagnostic. A biopsy is necessary to confirm the diagnosis.

INTRODUCTION

The diagnosis of a rheumatologic disease is challenging and requires careful integration of a patient's symptoms, physical examination findings, and results of diagnostic tests. A thorough history and physical examination are the best screening tests in the initial evaluation of a rheumatologic disease, and the results of laboratory tests should be used only to further refine the diagnosis. Many tests are now available that may aid in rapid diagnosis, but false positive results may lead to inappropriate therapy and unnecessary health care expenses. Laboratories perform different assays, and this can be a source of discrepancy and is often the reason that some laboratory tests are repeated when people are seen by rheumatologists. Hence, results should be interpreted judiciously based on their test characteristics in the appropriate clinical context.[1]

---

[a] Division of Rheumatology, University of Arkansas for Medical Sciences, 4301 West Markham Street #509, Little Rock, AR 72205-7199, USA; [b] Division of Rheumatology, Emory University School of Medicine, 49 Jesse Hill Jr, Drive, Southeast, Atlanta, GA 30303, USA
* Corresponding author.
E-mail address: amgizinski@gmail.com

Prim Care Clin Office Pract 45 (2018) 181–191
https://doi.org/10.1016/j.pop.2018.02.002
0095-4543/18/© 2018 Elsevier Inc. All rights reserved.

CONSIDERATIONS WHEN INTERPRETING LABORATORY TESTS

Clinicians should have some familiarity with the terms used for interpretation of a test's characteristics (**Table 1**).[1]

The important issue in deciding whether to use a diagnostic test in a particular patient is whether the posttest probability will be significantly different from the pretest probability, given a positive or negative test result.[1] The pretest probability and the posttest probability are the probabilities of the presence of a particular disease before and after ordering a diagnostic test, respectively. The pretest probability is the rough estimate that a clinician makes based on clinical presentation and the prevalence of the disease in question. **Table 2** lists the overall prevalence of selected rheumatologic diseases in the United States.

The sensitivity and specificity of a test are not sufficient to calculate the probability of disease for a given patient. The likelihood ratio (LR) is meant to provide an additional measure that can be of greater value in daily practice. LRs allow the clinician to calculate the posttest probability based upon the pretest probability and the test result. Tests are recommended as being very useful, useful, or not useful based on their associated LRs (**Table 3**).[1]

For example, a 29-year-old African American woman presents with joint swelling, oral ulcers, alopecia, and a facial rash. The clinician thinks her chances of having systemic lupus erythematosus (SLE) are greater than that of the general population and estimates that the patient's pretest probability of SLE is 10%. The clinician wants to order a test (such as an antinuclear antibody [ANA] or related autoantibody test) to confirm this suspicion. If the test has a high positive LR (eg, 10) and the test result is positive, then the posttest probability will be greatly increased. If the LR of the

Table 1
Calculation for sensitivity, specificity, positive predictive value, negative predictive value, and likelihood ratios

Test Result	Disease Present	Disease Absent
Positive	a	b
Negative	c	d
False positive	Positive test result in a patient without the disease	
False negative	Negative test result in a patient with the disease	
Sensitivity	$\dfrac{\text{Number of persons with a positive test with the disease (a)}}{\text{Total number of persons who have the disease (a+c)}}$	
Specificity	$\dfrac{\text{Number of persons with a negative test without the disease (d)}}{\text{Number of persons without the disease (b+d)}}$	

Positive Predictive value
  Probability that subjects with a
    positive screening test truly have
    the disease (depends on prevalence)
	$\dfrac{\text{Number of persons with a positive test with the disease (a)}}{\text{Number of persons with a positive test (a+b)}}$	

Negative predictive value
  Probability that subjects with a
    negative screening test truly do
    not have the disease (depends on
    prevalence)
	$\dfrac{\text{Number of persons with a negative test without the disease (d)}}{\text{Number of persons with a negative test (c+d)}}$	

Positive LR+ (Sensitivity)/(1 – Specificity)	$\dfrac{\text{Probability of an individual } with \text{ the disease having a positive test}}{\text{Probability of an individual } without \text{ the disease having a positive test}}$	
Negative LR– (1 – Sensitivity)/Specificity	$\dfrac{\text{Probability of an individual } with \text{ the disease having a negative test}}{\text{Probability of an individual } without \text{ the disease having a negative test}}$	

Table 2 Prevalence of selected rheumatologic diseases	
Disease	**Prevalence in the United States (per 100,000)**
Giant cell arteritis	278
Polymyalgia rheumatic	739
RA	600
SLE	53.6
Systemic sclerosis	27.6

Data from Helmick CG, Felson DT, Lawrence RC, et al. Estimates of the prevalence of arthritis and other rheumatic conditions in the United States. Part I. Arthritis Rheum 2007;58:15–25; and Lawrence RC, Felson DT, Helmick CG, et al. Estimates of the prevalence of arthritis and other rheumatic conditions in the United States. Part II. Arthritis Rheum 2008;58:26–35.

test were slightly less (eg, 5), there would still be a substantial increase in the posttest probability that could be clinically relevant. However, if the test had a small positive LR (eg, 1.2), then the posttest probability will not differ substantially from the pretest probability, and a positive test result would not help the clinician in making a diagnosis.[1] Hence, obtaining an ANA test with an LR of 2.2 would be a useful test in this patient, because posttest probability would be 20% (**Fig. 1**).

Similarly, in a 71-year-old man presenting with fatigue and joint pain, the pretest probability of SLE would be expected to be only slightly greater than the prevalence of SLE in the general population (approximately 0.1% or less). For this patient, even if the test had a greater positive LR of 5, the posttest probability would not be expected to be significantly different from the pretest probability.[1] Hence obtaining an ANA test would not be useful in this patient because the posttest probability would be only 0.2% (see **Fig. 1**).

Antinuclear Antibodies

The ANA test is one of the most frequently ordered tests to evaluate for autoimmune disease, but it can also be detected in nonrheumatic diseases, infections, malignancies, and healthy persons.[2] More than 32 million persons in the United States have a positive ANA test, and the prevalence is higher in women, older individuals, and African Americans.[3]

Methods

- Indirect Immunofluorescence assays (IIFA)
- Enzyme-linked immunosorbent assays (ELISA)
- Multiplex bead assays

Table 3 Likelihood ratios		
Positive LR	**Negative LR**	**Clinical Implications**
>10	<0.1	Large impact on posttest probability, very useful test
5–10	0.1–0.2	Modest clinical difference, very useful test
2–5	0.2–0.5	Small but relevant clinical difference useful test
<2	>0.5	Rarely any clinical difference, not useful test
1	1	No difference between pretest and posttest probability

Modified from American College of Rheumatology Ad Hoc Committee on Immunologic Testing Guidelines. Guidelines for immunologic laboratory testing in the rheumatic diseases: an introduction. Arthritis Rheum 2002;47:432; with permission.

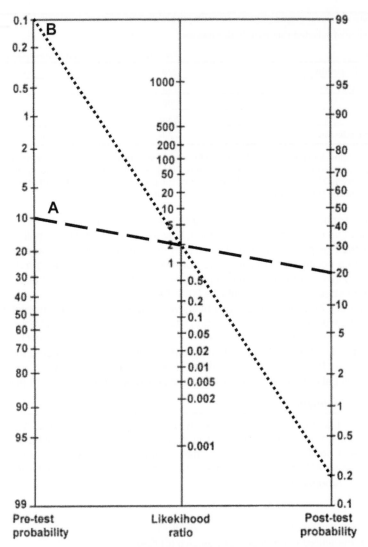

Fig. 1. LR nomogram for patients suspected of having SLE. (*A*) A 29-year-old African American woman with joint swelling, oral ulcers, alopecia, and facial rash. (*B*) A 71-year-old man with fatigue and joint pain. The positive likelihood of SLE in a person with a positive ANA is 2. The 2 examples described in the text are graphed on the nomogram. The estimated pretest probability of case A is 10%. If the woman has a positive ANA, to determine the posttest probability, a line is drawn from the 10% pretest probability through the positive LR of 2. The posttest probability is therefore 20%. For case B with a pretest SLE probability of 0.1%, a positive ANA would translate into a posttest probability of 0.2. (*Modified from* American College of Rheumatology Ad Hoc Committee on Immunologic Testing Guidelines. Guidelines for immunologic laboratory testing in the rheumatic diseases: an introduction. Arthritis Rheum 2002;47:432; with permission.)

IIFA using the HEp-2 cells or variants of this cell line (HEp-2000) is considered the gold-standard technique for the detection of ANA.[2] It involves serial dilutions of positive sera and visual determination of the staining pattern by fluorescent microscopy. The IIFA test is time consuming, is laborious, requires substantial expertise, and lacks specificity.[2] Indeed, depending on demographics, the population being studied, serum dilution, the cutoff used, and other variables of this assay, up to 25% of sera from apparently healthy individuals can be ANA positive.[2] One multicenter study reported that 31.7% of normal individuals were ANA positive at 1:40 dilution, which decreased to 13.3% at 1:80, 5.0% at 1:160 dilution, and 3.3% at 1:320 dilution.[4] Using HEp-2 substrate, titers of 1:80 or higher are usually considered positive.[5] ANA dilution at 1:160 has a sensitivity of 95% in patients with SLE and 87% sensitivity in patients with systemic sclerosis.[4]

Increased demand for ANA testing resulted in the development of novel diagnostic tests, including ELISA and other alternative methods like multiplex bead assays.[2] These tests are ones that are being ordered by primary care physicians (PCPs) more frequently, but one must keep in mind that the false negative and false positive ratios of these methods are different. In addition, several IIFA-positive patients (32.6%) have no detectable autoantibodies using the multiplex ANA screen, thereby suggesting several SLE patients may be ANA negative by this method.[6] Thus, if the clinical suspicion is strong, it is mandatory to perform IIFA.[2]

ANA testing plays an important role in the diagnoses of SLE. It is a part of clinical criteria and is a useful test (LR+ of 2.2) to obtain, if there is high clinical suspicion of SLE (**Table 4**). However, because of the low prevalence of SLE in the general population, most people with positive ANA do not have SLE. A negative ANA by IIFA is a very useful test, because it helps to rule out SLE because of its high sensitivity and negative LR of 0.1.[7] In systemic sclerosis, ANA is not a part of clinical criteria but is a useful test (LR− of 0.27) and should be performed in patients who are suspected of having systemic sclerosis, because a negative result should prompt the consideration of other fibrosing conditions (see **Table 4**).[7]

Other conditions in which ANA can be positive but does not have any proven value for diagnosis, monitoring, or prognosis are rheumatoid arthritis (RA), multiple sclerosis, thyroid disease, infectious diseases, fibromyalgia, and malignancies; thus, it is a not a useful test to order in patients with these conditions.[7]

Recently, the ability to order reflex or cascade testing, in which panels of tests for various other specific ANA-associated autoantibodies like double-stranded DNA (dsDNA), smith (Sm), ribonucleoprotein (nRNP), Ro (SS-A), La (SS-B), anticentromere, Scl-70, and Jo-1 are performed, has become available. Such tests are performed without regard to clinical characteristics, leading to increased costs and erroneous diagnoses.[5] If the ANA is negative by multiplex bead assay, by definition the specific autoantibodies will be negative because it is the same test.

ANA subtypes that can help establish and confirm the diagnosis of SLE include anti-dsDNA and anti-Sm.[5] A positive anti-Sm will likely have a large impact on the pretest

Table 4
Diagnostic utility of antinuclear antibody in autoimmune diseases

Condition	Sensitivity, %	Specificity, %	LR+	Utility	LR−	Utility
SLE	93–100	57	2.2	Useful	0.1	Very useful
SSc	85	54	1.86	Not useful	0.27	Useful
Sjögren syndrome	48	52	0.99	Not useful	1.01	Not useful
Inflammatory myositis	61	63	1.67	Not useful	0.61	Not useful
RA	41	56	0.93	Not useful	1.06	Not useful

Abbreviation: SSc, systemic sclerosis.

Modified from Solomon DH, Kavanaugh AJ, Schur PH. Evidence-based guidelines for the use of immunologic tests: antinuclear antibody testing. Arthritis Rheum 2002;47:437; with permission.

probability, substantially increasing the posttest probability of the diagnosis of SLE; thus, in the setting of some clinical suspicion of SLE, a positive anti-Sm strongly supports the diagnosis and is a very useful test to obtain, but a negative result cannot exclude the diagnoses (**Table 5**).[8]

Anti-dsDNA antibodies are useful to confirm the diagnosis for a patient whose clinical presentation already suggests a reasonable pretest likelihood of SLE being present (5% or more). It is a very useful test (LR+ of 16.3) and will substantially increase the posttest probability.[9] The presence of anti-dsDNA must always be interpreted in the context of the complete clinical picture, and also test characteristic should be taken into consideration because different assays have different characteristics as mentioned earlier. For example, the presence of anti-dsDNA and proteinuria or symptoms should prompt the clinician to investigate the presence of lupus nephritis or active lupus, but in an asymptomatic SLE patient, elevated anti-dsDNA may not indicate active SLE. Tests for antibodies to single-stranded DNA are of no clinical utility and should not be ordered.[5]

Antibodies to ribonucleoproteins, Ro (SS-A) and La (SS-B), are generally associated with SLE and Sjögren syndrome and are not routinely recommended without clinical suspicion. Anti-Ro (SS-A) is detected in approximately 35% to 60% of SLE patients and 40% to 90% in Sjögren syndrome patients and is associated with specific clinical features like photosensitivity, dry eyes and dry mouth, thrombocytopenia, and subacute

Table 5
Diagnostic utility of subserologies based on condition

ANA Subtype	Condition	Sensitivity, %	Specificity, %	LR+	Utility	LR−	Utility
Anti-Sm	SLE vs healthy controls	24	98	>10	Very useful	0.97	Not useful
	SLE vs other rheumatic diseases	30	96	26.5	Very useful	0.48	Useful
Anti-RNP	SLE vs other disease controls	27	82	1.2	Not useful	0.93	Not useful
	MCTD	71–100	84–100	7.14	Very useful	0	Very useful
Anti-dsDNA	SLE vs healthy controls and other diseases	57.3	97.4	16.3	Very useful	0.49	Useful
	Prognosis (overall activity of SLE)	66	66	4.14	Very useful	0.51	Not useful
	Lupus nephritis	65	41	1.7	Not useful	0.76	Not useful
Anti-centromere	SSc vs healthy controls	33	99.9	327	Very useful	0.7	Not useful
	SSc vs other CTDs	31	99.9	12.5	Very useful	0.7	Not useful
	Limited cutaneous (ACR classification)	44	93	6.1	Very useful	0.6	Not useful
Anti-Scl-70	SSc vs normals	20	100	25	Very useful	0.8	Not useful
	SSc vs other CTDs	26	99.5	>15	Very useful	1.5	Not useful
	Diffuse cutaneous involvement	37	82	2.0	Useful	0.8	Not useful
	Predicting pulmonary fibrosis	45	81	2.3	Useful	0.7	Not useful

Abbreviations: CTD, connective tissue disease; MCTD, mixed connective tissue disease.
Data from Refs.[8–10]

cutaneous lupus.[5] A very important correlation with anti-Ro is in neonatal lupus, because maternal immunoglobulin G (IgG) antibodies can cross the placenta. Symptoms in the neonate include rashes, and risk of congenital complete heart block. Hence, women with SLE considering pregnancy should be screened for anti-Ro (SS-A).[5]

Anticentromere and anti-Scl70 antibody testing is very useful in diagnosing systemic sclerosis and will have a large impact on posttest probability because they are rarely found in other connective tissue diseases or in healthy individuals (see **Table 5**).[10] Determination of anticentromere early in course of systemic sclerosis is very useful in predicting limited cutaneous involvement (distal to elbows) (LR+ of 6.1). Anti Scl-70 by immunodiffusion method is useful in predicting development of diffuse cutaneous involvement (LR+ of 2.0) and pulmonary fibrosis (LR+ of 2.3) (see **Table 5**).

Rheumatoid factor RF is any class of immunoglobulin, IgM, IgG, or IgA, that recognizes IgG.[11,12] The IgM-IgG RF subtype is the most widely used serologic marker of RA and is a part of the 2010 American College of Rheumatology/European League against Rheumatism (ACR/EULAR) criteria for the classification of RA.[13]

The prevalence of RF in RA is around 70% to 90%.[14] RF titers have been shown to correlate with both the severity of arthritis and progressive joint destruction.[14] Many studies have shown that the presence of elevated levels of RF precede the symptoms of RA.[12] RF-positive patients are also more likely to develop extra-articular manifestations, including rheumatoid nodules, Felty syndrome, and secondary Sjögren syndrome.[15] Different methods for rheumatoid factor detection include latex agglutination test, nephelometry, and ELISA.[12]

If a patient is presenting with chronic symmetric polyarticular joint swelling, RF is a very useful test (LR+ of 4.42) (**Table 6**) to obtain in order to support the diagnoses of RA. RF titers greater than 50 U/mL are more specific and will substantially increase the posttest probability of RA (LR+ of 20.5).[16] However, RF alone should not be used to make diagnoses of RA because it is present in many other conditions listed in **Table 7**.

Anticitrullinated Cyclic Peptide Antibody

Many novel antibodies are detected in association with RA, including antiperinuclear factor, antikeratin, and antifillagrin antibodies. All of these antibodies target citrullinated peptides. Citrullination is carried out by enzyme peptidylarginine deiminase.[12] Several citrullinated proteins are present in RA; hence, they have been identified as targets of highly RA-specific autoantibodies.[17] Anticyclic citrullinated peptide (anti-CCP) can be detected by ELISA, which is currently being ordered by PCPs.[17]

Table 6
Diagnostic utility of rheumatoid factor and anti-cyclic citrullinated peptide in rheumatoid arthritis

Autoantibodies	Sensitivity	Specificity	LR+	Utility	LR−	Utility
IgMRF (overall)	69%	85%	4.86	Very useful	0.38	Useful
Anti-CCP	67%	95%	12.46	Very useful	0.36	Useful
RF value	>20 U/mL		5.0	Very useful	0.53	Not useful
	>50 U/mL		11.3	Very useful	0.57	Not useful

Data from Nell VP, Machold KP, Stamm TA, et al. Autoantibody profiling as early diagnostic and prognostic tool for rheumatoid arthritis. Ann Rheum Dis 2005;64:1731–6; and Nishimura K, Sugiyama D, Kogata Y, et al. Meta-analysis: diagnostic accuracy of anti-cyclic citrullinated peptide antibody and rheumatoid factor for rheumatoid arthritis. Ann Intern Med 2007;146:797–808.

Table 7
Conditions with positive rheumatoid factor

Condition	Frequency of Occurrence (%)
Rheumatologic conditions	
RA	**60–80**
Juvenile chronic arthritis	15
Psoriatic arthritis	<15
SLE	30
Primary Sjögren syndrome	70
Mixed connective tissue disease	25
Polymyositis/dermatomyositis	20
Infections	
Subacute bacterial endocarditis,	**40**
Tuberculosis	15
Syphilis	8–37
Viral infections (hepatitis A, B, and C)	25
EBV/CMV	20
Coxsackie B	15
Dengue	10
HIV	10–20
Measles	8–15
Rubella	15
Parasitic infections (Chagas)	15–25
Malaria	15–18
Other conditions	
Cryoglobulinemia	**70**
Liver cirrhosis	25
Chronic interstitial lung disease	25

Modified from Dörner T, Egerer K, Fiest E, et al. Rheumatoid factor revisited. Curr Opin Rheumatol 2004;16:251; with permission.

Anti-CCP is a very useful test and is a more specific test to perform, if there is high pretest probability of RA (see **Table 6**).[18] However, anti-CCP can also be detected in many other conditions, including psoriatic arthritis, SLE, Sjögren syndrome, inflammatory myopathy, and active tuberculosis.[16] In patient with undifferentiated arthritis, a positive anti-CCP can indicate that the patient may develop RA and be at higher risk for rapid joint destruction.[17,19] Anti-CCP is also a part of the 2010 ACR/EULAR criteria for the classification of RA.[13]

The positive predictive value of anti-CCP is 95%, if a high-risk population is being tested rather than screening the entire population.[17] Negative test results for both anti-CCP and RF are useful when excluding the diagnosis of RA rather than testing of either antibody alone.[15]

Erythrocyte Sedimentation Rate and C-Reactive Protein

An acute-phase protein is defined as one in which plasma concentration increases or decreases by at least 25% during inflammatory disorders. The changes in concentrations of acute-phase proteins are due largely to changes in their production by hepatocytes through stimulation by cytokines. Conditions that lead to changes in the plasma concentration of acute-phase proteins include infection, trauma, surgery, burns, tissue infarction, rheumatologic diseases, crystal-induced inflammatory conditions, and advanced cancers. Various plasma proteins that increase in concentration during inflammation are complements, fibrinogen, plasminogen, alpha-1 chymotrypsin, ceruloplasmin, haptoglobin, C-reactive protein (CRP), serum amyloid A, fibronectin, fibrinogen, and ferritin. Currently, the most widely used indicators of the response of acute-phase proteins are erythrocyte sedimentation rate (ESR) and plasma CRP.[20]

ESR is a measure of quantity of red blood cells (RBCs) that precipitate in a tube in a defined time and is based on serum protein concentrations and RBC interactions with these proteins and is measured in millimeters per /hour. It depends on the concentration of various plasma proteins like fibrinogen, which increase during inflammation, promoting closer aggregation of RBC. Hence, the ESR is an indirect measure of inflammation.[21] Conditions that increase ESR are anemia, age, female sex, pregnancy, and hypercholesterolemia. ESR can be elevated with increased age, so it is important to adjust for age when interpreting normal range for ESR; in men, it is (age)/2 and in women it is (age + 10)/2.[21] ESR should not be used to make a diagnosis in patients with joint swelling of unclear cause; for example, to make a diagnosis of septic arthritis, ESR is not a useful test because it has LR+ of 0.84 and LR− of 2.4.[22]

Sensitivity of ESR in giant cell arteritis (GCA) is 84%; positive LR is 1.2, and negative LR is 0.35.[23] Hence, in a patient with clinical findings, a very high ESR is most likely due to GCA and justifies initiation of high-dose steroids because of high sensitivity. However, if the clinical evidence of GCA is low, a normal ESR reduces the probability of the disease because the negative LR is 0.35.[21]

CRP was named for its reactivity against C-polysaccharide in the cell wall of *Streptococcus pneumoniae*. Function of CRP is not clear, but it is thought that CRP is an innate immune protein that helps opsonize pathogens for phagocytosis and activates the complement system.[15] Serum CRP is a direct marker of inflammation, and its concentration changes more rapidly than ESR. It is unaffected by serum components and is a stable protein. Therefore, CRP may be a better reflection of current inflammation, but is not diagnostic of any disease.[15]

ANTINEUTROPHIL CYTOPLASMIC ANTIBODIES

Routinely, antineutrophil cytoplasmic antibodies (ANCAs) are detected by IIFA on ethanol-fixed neutrophils, and 2 general immunofluorescent patterns are observed: cytoplasmic (c-ANCA) and perinuclear (p-ANCA). The principal antigens for c-ANCA and p-ANCA are proteinase 3 (PR3) and myeloperoxidase (MPO), respectively, and are present in azurophilic granules of neutrophils. PR3/c-ANCA is strongly associated with granulomatous polyangiitis, with a sensitivity of 65% and specificity of 95% by IIFA method. ANCAs are detected in about 50% to 75% of patients with microscopic polyangiitis (MPA) with a predominant pattern of p-ANCA/MPO, and c-ANCA can also be detected in 25% of MPA patients. ANCA is found in 40% to 60% of patients with eosinophilic granulomatosis with polyangiitis, where both patterns can be found, although p-ANCA is more common. ANCA can also be seen in inflammatory bowel disease, primary biliary cirrhosis, SLE, RA, and juvenile inflammatory arthritis.[24]

Although a positive ANCA supports the diagnoses of vasculitis, physicians should keep in mind that vasculitis is very rare, and the probability that a patient with a positive ANCA test has the disease in question (posttest probability) depends on the patient's clinical manifestations. Tissue biopsy remains the gold standard to diagnose vasculitis given the high toxicity of treatment regimens used in vasculitis.[24]

SUMMARY

Clinicians should not rely on rheumatologic tests to make a diagnosis of a rheumatologic disease but rather take into consideration the prevalence and the posttest probability of a given disease in the right clinical settings.

REFERENCES

1. American College of Rheumatology Ad Hoc Committee on Immunologic Testing Guidelines. Guidelines for immunologic laboratory testing in the rheumatic diseases: an introduction. Arthritis Rheum 2002;47:429–33.
2. Agmon-Levin N, Damoiseaux J, Kallenberg C, et al. International recommendations for the assessment of autoantibodies to cellular antigens referred to as anti-nuclear antibodies. Ann Rheum Dis 2014;73:17–23.
3. Satoh M, Chan EKL, Ho LA, et al. Prevalence and sociodemographic correlates of antinuclear antibodies in the United States. Arthritis Rheum 2012;64:2319–27.
4. Tan EM, Feltkamp TEW, Smolen JS, et al. Range of antinuclear antibodies in "healthy" individuals. Arthritis Rheum 1997;40:1601–11.
5. Kavanaugh A, Tomar R, Reveille J, et al. Guidelines for clinical use of the antinuclear antibody test and tests for specific autoantibodies to nuclear antigens. Arch Pathol Lab Med 2000;124:71–81.
6. Bruner BF, Guthridge J, Lu R, et al. Comparison of autoantibody specificities between traditional and bead-based assays in a large, diverse collection of SLE. Arthritis Rheum 2012;64:3677–86.
7. Solomon DH, Kavanaugh AJ, Schur PH. Evidence-based guidelines for the use of immunologic tests: antinuclear antibody testing. Arthritis Rheum 2002;47:434–44.
8. Benito-Garcia E, Schur P, Lahita R. Guidelines for immunologic laboratory testing in the rheumatic diseases: anti-Sm and anti-RNP antibody tests. Arthritis Rheum 2004;51(No. 6):1030–44.
9. Kavanaugh AF, Solomon DH. Guidelines for immunologic laboratory testing in the rheumatic diseases: anti-DNA antibody tests. Arthritis Rheum 2002;47:546–55.
10. Reveille JD, Solomon DH. Evidence-based guidelines for the use of immunologic tests: anticentromere, Scl-70, and nucleolar antibodies. Arthritis Rheum 2003;49:399–412.
11. Sutton B, Corper A, Bonagura V, et al. The structure and origin of rheumatoid factors. Immunol Today 2000;21:177–83.
12. Lee AN, Beck CE, Hall M. Rheumatoid factor and anti-CCP autoantibodies in rheumatoid arthritis: a review. Clin Lab Sci 2008;21:15–8.
13. Tuhina N, Aletaha D, Silman AJ, et al. The 2010 American College of Rheumatology/European League against Rheumatism classification criteria for rheumatoid arthritis: phase 2 methodological report. Arthritis Rheum 2010;62:2582–91.
14. Jansen LMA, van der Horst-Bruinsma IE, van Schaardenburg D, et al. Predictors of radiographic joint damage with early rheumatoid arthritis. Ann Rheum Dis 2001;60:924–7.
15. Castro C, Gourley M. Diagnostic testing and interpretation of tests for autoimmunity. J Allergy Clin Immunol 2010;125(2 Suppl 2):S238–47.
16. Nell VP, Machold KP, Stamm TA, et al. Autoantibody profiling as early diagnostic and prognostic tool for rheumatoid arthritis. Ann Rheum Dis 2005;64:1731–6.
17. Aggarwal R, Liao K, Nair R, et al. Anti-citrullinated peptide antibody assays and their role in the diagnosis of rheumatoid arthritis. Arthritis Rheum 2009;61:1472–83.

18. Nishimura K, Sugiyama D, Kogata Y, et al. Meta-analysis: diagnostic accuracy of anti-cyclic citrullinated peptide antibody and rheumatoid factor for rheumatoid arthritis. Ann Intern Med 2007;146:797–808.
19. Gaalen FA, Linn-Rasker SP, van Venrooji WJ, et al. Autoantibodies to cyclic citrullinated peptides predict progression to rheumatoid arthritis in patients with undifferentiated arthritis: a prospective cohort study. Arthritis Rheum 2004;50:709–15.
20. Gabay C, Kushner I. Acute-phase proteins and other systemic responses to inflammation. N Engl J Med 1999;340:448–53.
21. Sox H, Liang MH. The erythrocyte sedimentation rate. Guidelines for rational use. Ann Intern Med 1986;104:515–23.
22. Li SF, Cassidy C, Gharib S, et al. Diagnostic utility of laboratory tests in septic arthritis. Emerg Med J 2007;24:75–7.
23. Smetana GW, Shmerling RH. Does this patient have temporal arteritis? JAMA 2002;287:92–101.
24. Vassilopoulos D, Hoffman G. Clinical utility of testing for antineutrophil cytoplasmic antibodies. Clin Diagn Lab Immunol 1999;6:645–51.

Practical Pearls About Current Rheumatic Medications

Ian M. Ward, MD[a],*, Amanda Knott, PharmD[b]

KEYWORDS

- Rheumatic disease • Medications • Pearls and pitfalls

KEY POINTS

- Although commonly used for a variety of musculoskeletal conditions and rheumatic disease, nonsteroidal anti-inflammatory drugs pose cardiac and gastrointestinal risk in both acute and chronic use, necessitating patient education on appropriate use.
- Tuberculosis and viral hepatitis screening, routine vaccinations, and routine laboratory test monitoring are recommended in patients receiving disease-modifying antirheumatic drugs, antimetabolite medications, and biologic agents.
- At the discretion of the surgeon, disease-modifying antirheumatic drugs can be continued perioperatively; however, biologic agents should be held for at least one cycle before surgery.
- Nonsteroidal anti-inflammatory drugs, corticosteroids, hydroxychloroquine, azathioprine, and tumor necrosis factor-α inhibitors have been deemed appropriate for use in pregnancy. The remaining disease-modifying antirheumatic drugs, antimetabolites, and biologic agents are not safe during pregnancy or lactation.

INTRODUCTION

Primary care physicians provide an integral role in the evaluation and management of patients with rheumatic and musculoskeletal diseases. In the United States alone, more than 21% of adults have some form of arthritis.[1] Osteoarthritis affects over 27

Conflict of Interest: None of the authors have any conflict of interest to disclose.

Funding Source: No funding was provided to conduct this study or the preparation of this article.

Disclaimer: The views expressed herein are those of the authors and do not reflect the official policy or position of Landstuhl Regional Medical Center, the US Army Medical Department, the US Army Office of the Surgeon General, the Department of the Army or the Department of Defense, or the US Government. The authors are employees of the US government. This work was prepared as part of their official duties and, as such, there is no copyright to be transferred.

[a] Rheumatology Service, Department of Medicine, Landstuhl Regional Medical Center, Landstuhl, Germany; [b] Department of Pharmacy, Landstuhl Regional Medical Center, Landstuhl, Germany

* Corresponding author. Rheumatology Service, Landstuhl Regional Medical Center, CMR 402, Box 2107, APO, AE 09180-0022.

E-mail address: ian.m.ward.mil@mail.mil

million adults with projections indicating that number growing over the next 25 years.[2] Meanwhile, nearly 1% of the adult population has rheumatoid arthritis (RA) and between 0.3% and 1.3% of adults are afflicted by a seronegative spondyloarthropathy.[1] Primary care providers are likely to encounter patients on a daily basis with a rheumatic disease.

Primary care providers need to be aware of the characteristics and potential issues surrounding the growing number of medications used in rheumatology. For example, 3.8 million combined prescriptions for adalimumab and etanercept were provided between April 2014 and March 2015, placing both of those medications in the top 75 most commonly prescribed medications in the United States.[3] Such medications are not benign, and physicians need to be aware of the properties of these medications even if they are not the one prescribing them. The intent of this article is to provide a broad review of the pharmacotherapy used in musculoskeletal and rheumatic conditions. Understanding drug indications, dosing, drug interactions, adverse effects, and use in special circumstances will allow the primary provider to better counsel and care for their patients with rheumatic conditions.

NONSTEROIDAL ANTI-INFLAMMATORY DRUGS

Nonsteroidal anti-inflammatory drugs (NSAIDs) provide an analgesic effect through the inhibition of cyclooxygenase-1 and cyclooxygenase-2, thereby preventing formation of prostaglandin and thromboxane. Hyperemia, pyrexia, increased vascular permeability, and hyperalgesia are reduced, thereby decreasing inflammation.[4] **Table 1** lists commonly prescribed NSAIDs available in the United States.

The American College of Rheumatology (ACR) specifically endorses NSAID use in the treatment of hand, hip, and knee osteoarthritis, axial spondyloarthritis, and peripheral manifestations of the spondyloarthropathies, such as enthesitis and dactylitis.[5–8] Individually, naproxen, indomethacin, and sulindac are recommended in the acute treatment of gouty arthritis and calcium pyrophosphate dehydrogenase arthropathy.[9,10] Low-dose NSAIDs are also recommended for prophylactic therapy when initiating urate-lowering therapy (ULT) for gout.[9]

Chronic NSAID use confers multiple risks. The gastrointestinal side effects can range from mild dyspepsia to life-threatening bleeding from gastric or intestinal ulcerations.[11] Use of cyclooxygenase-2 selective agents and coadministration of proton pump inhibitors reduce the risk of gastrointestinal toxicity.[12,13] Cardiovascular events,

Table 1 Nonsteroidal anti-inflammatory drugs			
Medication	**Dose (mg)**	**Dosing Frequency**	**Maximum Daily Dose (mg)**
Ibuprofen	200–800	q6–8h	3200
Ketoprofen	25–75	q6–8h	300
Diclofenac	25–50	q6–12h	150
Indomethacin	25–75	q8–12h	150
Sulindac	150–200	q12h	400
Naproxen	250–500	q12h	1250
Celecoxib	100–200	q12–24h	400
Nabumetone	500–1000	q12–24h	2000
Piroxicam	10–20	Daily	20
Meloxicam	7.5–15	Daily	15

such as myocardial infarction, stroke, and decompensated heart failure, increase with chronic NSAID use.[14,15] NSAID use increases morbidity among patients with a recent cardiac event, so it is recommended to avoid NSAIDs within 3 to 6 months of such an event.[16]

Despite the well-known risks, patients continue to use NSAIDs inappropriately. Excessive dosing and concomitant dual NSAIDs are frequently reported in surveys.[17] Patient education should continue to focus on appropriate use as well as the hazards associated with NSAID use.

GLUCOCORTICOIDS

Used in a wide range of diseases, glucocorticoids are frequently prescribed in many medical specialties. Glucocorticoids provide an effective, rapid, anti-inflammatory effect by regulating the DNA transcription and synthesis of proinflammatory proteins.[18] **Table 2** demonstrates the relative potency of various oral corticosteroids typically used in clinical practice. However, because of numerous side effects (**Table 3**),[19,20] a frequent tenet when prescribing glucocorticoids for rheumatic disease is to use the lowest effective dose for the shortest time possible.[21] In a dose-dependent manner, steroid use increases the risk of serious bacterial infections and opportunistic infections, such as *Pneumocystis jiroveci*, herpes zoster, and tuberculosis.[22] Glucocorticoid use significantly increases the risk of cardiovascular events, specifically heart failure, regardless of the indication for therapy.[23]

Glucocorticoid-induced osteoporosis (GIOP) is a concern, especially in postmenopausal women and men over the age of 50. Bisphosphonate therapy decreases the risk of fragility fractures and bone density loss in patients receiving chronic steroid therapy.[24] In patients at moderate to high risk for osteoporotic fracture, recent ACR guidelines preferentially recommend the use of oral bisphosphonates such as alendronate or risedronate for prevention of GIOP.[25]

COLCHICINE

Best known for its use in the treatment of acute gouty arthritis, colchicine has also been shown to be effective in the treatment of several other rheumatic disorders, such as familial Mediterranean fever (FMF).[9,10,26] Colchicine is also recommended as prophylactic therapy when initiating ULT.[9]

For the crystalline arthropathies, colchicine is dosed up to 1.2 to 1.8 mg per day in divided doses for acute attacks as well as for chronic prophylactic therapy.[9] Doses up to 3 g per day may be needed for the treatment of FMF.[26] Colchicine has a narrow therapeutic window, which can lead to adverse reactions, such as abdominal pain,

Table 2 Glucocorticoid potency			
Medication	Equivalent Glucocorticoid Dose (mg)	Relative Glucocorticoid Activity	Duration of Action
Hydrocortisone	25	1	Short
Prednisone	6	4	Intermediate
Methylprednisolone	5	5	Intermediate
Triamcinolone	5	5	Intermediate
Betamethasone	1	25	Long
Dexamethasone	1	25	Long

Table 3
Common glucocorticoid adverse effects

Endocrine	Cardiovascular	Musculoskeletal	Ocular	Psychiatric
Diabetes mellitus	Hypertension	Myopathy	Glaucoma	Anxiety
Adrenal insufficiency	Hyperlipidemia	Osteoporosis	Cataracts	Depression
Cushing Syndrome	Cardiovascular disease	Avascular necrosis		Psychosis
Weight gain				Delirium
				Cognitive deficits
				Insomnia

diarrhea, nausea, vomiting, and rarely, cytopenias. When coadministered with medications that modulate CYP3A4, or in patients with renal or hepatic impairment, colchicine has an increased risk of causing myopathy or rhabdomyolysis.[27] In chronic use, particularly in patients with FMF, routine monitoring of complete blood counts, renal, and liver function is recommended.[26]

URATE-LOWERING THERAPY

Several ULTs are available for the treatment of chronic gout. Dosing and side effects for these medications are demonstrated in **Table 4**.[28–31] Per recommendations by the ACR and the American College of Physicians, allopurinol and febuxostat are appropriate first-line medications to lower serum uric acid levels.[28,29] Allopurinol is much less expensive and is usually used first. Probenecid and lesinurad are considered add-on therapies to either allopurinol or febuxostat when an inadequate response to monotherapy occurs.[30,32,33] In cases of refractory tophaceous gout despite oral ULT, rheumatologists consider using pegloticase as a second-line agent.[32,34]

Allopurinol is usually a well-tolerated medication, with less than 5% of patients stopping the medication because of adverse effects.[35] The most feared complication is allopurinol hypersensitivity syndrome (AHS), which is characterized by renal and hepatic injury, severe rash, fever, eosinophilia, and leukocytosis.[36] Although rare and typically occurring at onset of allopurinol use, AHS has high mortalities.[28,32,36] Risk factors for its development include baseline renal impairment, diuretic use, HLA-B*5801 status, and high starting doses of allopurinol.[36] To mitigate the

Table 4
Prescribing information for urate-lowering therapies

Medication	Dose (mg)	Route	Frequency	Common Side Effects
Allopurinol	50–800	PO	Daily	Liver function abnormalities, pruritus, rash, allopurinol hypersensitivity syndrome, gout flares, nausea, diarrhea
Febuxostat	40–80	PO	Daily	Liver function abnormalities, arthralgias, rash, nausea, headache, gout flares
Lesinurad	200	PO	Daily	Elevated serum creatinine, nephrolithiasis, headache, gastroesophageal reflux, influenza infections, gout flares
Probenecid	250–1000	PO	Twice a day	Rash, gout flares, dizziness, headaches, myalgias, nausea, emesis, nephrolithiasis
Pegloticase	8	IV	Every 2 wk	Anaphylaxis, infusion reactions, gout flares, ecchymosis, nasopharyngitis, nausea, emesis, constipation

development of AHS, the ACR recommends starting allopurinol at low doses and slowly titrating the medication to the target serum urate level, especially in the setting of renal impairment.[32]

Allopurinol can be safely increased to doses greater than 300 mg daily in patients with renal insufficiency if titrated by 50-mg increments on a monthly basis.[37] Patients who develop AHS can still receive ULT in the form of febuxostat. A small risk for recurrence of hypersensitivity syndrome with febuxostat exists, so close monitoring is required when changing to febuxostat after an episode of AHS.[38] Although AHS does not occur with pegloticase, anaphylaxis or infusion reactions can occur, usually within 2 hours of the infusion. Preinfusion serum uric acid levels greater than 6 mg/dL predict infusion reactions.[39]

Allopurinol and febuxostat have several important drug-drug interactions. Both allopurinol and febuxostat increase levels of azathioprine, 6-mercaptopurine, theophylline, and didanosine to toxic levels and should not be coadministered. Allopurinol may also increase the anticoagulant effect of warfarin.[28]

GENERAL CONSIDERATIONS FOR IMMUNOSUPPRESSIVE AGENTS

Before the initiation of immunosuppressive medications, certain screening parameters and vaccinations need to be considered. Hepatitis B and C screening is routinely performed, and screening for latent tuberculosis is included before starting a biologic agent.[40–43] Patients with a history of hepatitis B virus (HBV) infection should be treated with prophylactic antiviral therapy before starting an immunosuppressant. Routine HBV DNA monitoring should occur in patients with hepatitis B surface antigen but negative HBV DNA while on immunosuppressants.[43] Treatment of latent tuberculosis for at least 1 month is also recommended before starting biologics.[40]

Vaccines are important in patients who will become immunosuppressed (**Table 5**). At a minimum, the pneumococcal (pneumococcal conjugate vaccine 13 and pneumococcal polysaccharide vaccine 23), influenza, and hepatitis B vaccines should be provided before the initiation of immunosuppressants.[40] Both live-attenuated and inactive vaccines are recommended to be administered at least 2 weeks before starting an immunosuppressant. Once started on an immunosuppressive regimen, patients may have a reduced response to inactivated vaccines.[40,41,44] Live-attenuated vaccines may still be provided to patients receiving nonbiologic immunosuppressants; however, they are contraindicated in patients on biologic agents.[40,44] Patients

Table 5
Vaccinations and biologic therapy

Contraindicated Live Vaccines	Recommended Inactivated Vaccines
Varicella vaccine[a]	Annual influenza vaccine
Herpes zoster vaccine[a]	Pneumococcal vaccine (administer before initiation of
Yellow fever vaccine[a]	biologic therapy)
MMR (measles, mumps, rubella) vaccine[a]	Tetanus diphtheria acellular pertussis (Tdap)/Tetanus diphtheria (Td) vaccines
BCG (Bacillus Calmette–Guérin) vaccine	Hepatitis B vaccine (if needed)
	Hepatitis A vaccine (if needed)
	Meningococcal vaccine (if needed)
	Typhoid fever vaccine (if needed)
	Human papillomavirus (if needed)
	Haemophilus influenzae type b vaccine (if needed)

[a] Wait at least 3 wk after administration of a live vaccine before initiating biologic therapy.

receiving corticosteroids in doses greater than 2 mg/kg/d or 20 mg/d continuously for more than 14 days are considered immunosuppressed and have the same restrictions for vaccination. Live-attenuated vaccines may be administered 1 month after discontinuation of steroids, and 3 months after discontinuation of biologics. In patients receiving B-cell–depleting therapy such as rituximab, all vaccines should be held for at least 6 months.[44] If a patient develops a bacterial or severe viral infection, noncorticosteroid immunosuppressants should be withheld until complete resolution of infection and at least 8 days after discontinuation of antibiotics.[41,42]

ORAL DISEASE-MODIFYING ANTIRHEUMATIC DRUGS

The oral disease-modifying antirheumatic drugs (DMARDs) most commonly used in rheumatic disease include hydroxychloroquine, sulfasalazine, leflunomide, and methotrexate. The DMARDs modulate aberrant immune system activity seen in autoimmune disease through a variety of pathways. Oral DMARDs are used in a wide range of rheumatic conditions (**Table 6**). DMARDs can be used in combination with other DMARDs or with biologic agents. Methotrexate in particular is frequently used in combination therapy, which has been shown to be more effective in controlling disease activity than monotherapy.[45]

Common side effects are listed in **Table 7**.[46–50] Because of the risk of bone marrow toxicity, nephrotoxicity, and hepatotoxicity, routine monitoring of the complete blood count, liver-associated enzymes, and serum creatinine is recommended at a minimum of every 3 months.[40] Methotrexate and leflunomide side effects can be significant in some cases; however, most side effects due to sulfasalazine and hydroxychloroquine are transient and dissipate over the first 3 months of therapy. Folic or folinic acid supplementation reduces the methotrexate-associated gastrointestinal, hepatic, and mucositis side effects but not hematologic toxicity.[51] Significant drug-drug interactions between DMARDs and nonrheumatic medications are found in **Table 8**.[52]

The highest profile risk of antimalarial use is retinal toxicity. Duration of use for more than 5 years and higher doses both increase the risk of developing an irreversible retinopathy. Additional risk factors include renal insufficiency, concurrent tamoxifen use, and preexisting retinal or macular disease. The American Academy of Ophthalmology recommends daily doses less than 5 mg/kg actual body weight for hydroxychloroquine and less than 2.3 mg/kg actual body weight for chloroquine to prevent the formation of retinopathy. Patients should undergo an initial fundus examination within the first year of use and then annually after 5 years of use or earlier if concomitant risk factors are present.[53]

CALCINEURIN INHIBITORS

The calcineurin inhibitors (CNI) cyclosporine A (CsA) and tacrolimus prevent interleukin-2 production and T-cell activation, limiting the adaptive immune response. Tacrolimus is generally accepted to be about 100 times more potent than CsA.[54] **Table 6** lists clinical settings in which CsA and tacrolimus are prescribed as well as typical dosing regimens.[55–60] When used for a rheumatic condition, CsA and tacrolimus plasma concentrations are not typically monitored because of the lower doses used compared with transplant medicine.[55]

Common side effects from CNI use include hypertension, hyperglycemia, gastrointestinal intolerance, tremors, and electrolyte abnormalities.[55,57,58] Other than hyperglycemia, side effects are less common overall for tacrolimus.[61,62] Although significant, CNI-induced nephrotoxicity is less common in rheumatic disease

Table 6
Oral disease-modifying antirheumatic drug and calcineurin inhibitors characteristics

Medication	Indication	Dose	Dosing Frequency
Hydroxychloroquine	Rheumatoid arthritis Cutaneous lupus Systemic lupus erythematosus Dermatomyositis	<5.0 mg/kg/d	Daily or divided dose bid
Sulfasalazine	Rheumatoid arthritis Peripheral arthritis related to spondyloarthropathy	500–1500	bid
Methotrexate	Rheumatoid arthritis Systemic sclerosis Takayasu arteritis Granulomatosis with polyangiitis Giant cell arteritis Polymyalgia rheumatica Peripheral arthritis related to spondyloarthropathy Systemic lupus erythematosus Noninfectious uveitis Inflammatory myositis	7.5–25 mg	Once a week
Leflunomide	Rheumatoid arthritis Systemic lupus erythematosus Psoriatic arthritis	10–20 mg	Daily
Tacrolimus	Systemic lupus erythematosus Connective tissue disease–related interstitial lung disease (ILD) Inflammatory myositis Ocular Behcet disease	0.075 mg/kg/d or 1–3 mg/d[a]	Divided dose bid
Cyclosporine A	Rheumatoid arthritis Systemic lupus erythematosus Macrophage activation syndrome Psoriatic arthritis Ocular Behcet disease	2.5–4 mg/kg/d	Divided dose bid

[a] Dose adjusted to trough level between 5 and 20 ng/mL.

compared with transplant medicine, and tacrolimus has less risk than CsA.[63] Transient increases in the serum creatinine may occur; however, these typically resolve with dose reduction or medication cessation.[57,58]

ANTIMETABOLITES

The antimetabolites, azathioprine, mycophenolate, and cyclophosphamide, work by inhibiting proliferating B cells and T cells, thereby preventing their cytotoxic effects. Common indications, side effects, drug-drug interactions, and laboratory monitoring recommendations are found in **Table 9**.[64–69] In particular, an important drug-drug interaction to remember occurs between xanthine oxidase inhibitors and azathioprine. Allopurinol and febuxostat increase azathioprine metabolites and should be avoided with azathioprine. If xanthine oxidase inhibitors cannot be avoided, the dose of azathioprine should be reduced by 50% to 75%.[64]

Mycophenolate can cause significant gastrointestinal intolerance, which is considered dose related. It may lead to colonic damage and persistent diarrhea.[67] Dividing

Table 7
Common disease-modifying antirheumatic drugs side effects

Side Effect	Hydroxychloroquine	Sulfasalazine	Methotrexate	Leflunomide
Headache	–	+	+	+
Mucositis	–	–	+	+
Rash	+	+	+	+
Alopecia	–	–	+	+
Hepatotoxicity	–	+	+	+
Gastrointestinal toxicity	+	+	+	+
Pneumonitis	–	Rare	+	Rare
Myelosuppression	–	Rare	+	Rare
Hypertension	–	–	–	+
Other	Cardiomyopathy, myositis	Azoospermia	Flulike symptoms	Weight loss

doses or switching to enteric-coated mycophenolate may help with gastrointestinal adverse effects.[70]

Cyclophosphamide may be administered orally or intravenously (IV) with similar efficacy. However, IV administration is associated with fewer adverse effects.[68,69] Increased hydration, routine voiding of the bladder, and mesna are recommended to prevent bladder toxicity, such as hemorrhagic cystitis.[68,69] Laboratory monitoring should include baseline and periodic complete blood count and renal function and urinalysis to monitor for hematuria.[68] The toxicity and narrow therapeutic index of cyclophosphamide often prevents its use for long-term maintenance. Typically given as induction therapy, cyclophosphamide is usually switched to another less toxic immunosuppressant, such as azathioprine, methotrexate, or mycophenolate, after remission has been achieved.[68]

BIOLOGICS

Numerous biologic agents have been developed to treat rheumatologic disease. These agents target cytokines or specific immune cells (**Table 10**).[41,71–79] Most

Table 8
Disease-modifying antirheumatic drugs drug-drug interactions

DMARD	Medication
Hydroxychloroquine	Cimetidine
Sulfasalazine	Digoxin Isoniazid Ampicillin Rifampicin
Methotrexate	Acitretin Trimethoprim Isoniazid Probenecid
Leflunomide	Warfarin Itraconazole Rifampicin

Table 9
Antimetabolite therapy

	Azathioprine	Mycophenolate	Cyclophosphamide
Indications	Systemic lupus erythematosus Inflammatory myopathy Inflammatory eye disease Behcet disease Small vessel vasculitis Connective tissue disease–related ILD Rheumatoid arthritis	Systemic sclerosis Systemic lupus erythematosus Small vessel vasculitis Inflammatory myopathy Connective tissue disease–related ILD	Systemic vasculitis Connective tissue disease–related ILD Inflammatory eye disease Systemic lupus erythematosus Severe organ threatening manifestations of systemic autoimmune diseases
Adverse effects	Infection Bone marrow toxicity (leukopenia, thrombocytopenia) Gastrointestinal intolerance Pancreatitis Hepatotoxicity	Gastrointestinal intolerance (nausea, vomiting, diarrhea, abdominal pain/cramping) Infection Bone marrow toxicity	Infection Bone marrow suppression Nausea/vomiting Infertility (decreased sperm count and premature ovarian failure) Nephrotoxicity Hemorrhagic cystitis
Drug-drug and drug-food interactions	Allopurinol Febuxostat Cimetidine	Digoxin Isoniazid Ampicillin Rifampicin	Allopurinol Hydrochlorothiazide Sulfonylurea Benzodiazepines Dexamethasone Quinolone antibiotics Digoxin Azole antifungals Grapefruit

biologic agents were initially developed for either RA or psoriatic arthritis; however, the indications have increased over time (**Table 11**). Biologics are indicated as monotherapy or in combination with other oral DMARDs; however, they cannot be used in conjunction with other biologic agents.

Table 10
Mechanism of action of biologic agents

Medication	Mechanism of Action
TNFi[a]	Binds and neutralizes TNF
Anakinra	Binds and neutralizes interleukin 1 receptors
Abatacept	Binds to CD80/86, preventing T-cell costimulation
Tocilizumab	Binds and neutralizes interleukin 6 receptors
Rituximab	Binds to CD20 on B cells activating complement-dependent cytotoxicity
Tofacitinib	Inhibits JAK enzymes preventing immune cell functions
Secukinumab	Binds and inhibits interleukin 17A
Ustekinumab	Binds and inhibits interleukin 12 and 23

[a] Etanercept, adalimumab, infliximab, golimumab, certolizumab pegol.

Table 11 Indications for biologic agents	
Medication	**Indication**
TNFi	Rheumatoid arthritis
	Psoriatic arthritis
	Ankylosing spondylitis
	Behcet disease
Anakinra	Refractory rheumatoid arthritis
	Gout
	Pseudogout
	Adult-onset Still disease
	Periodic fever syndromes
Abatacept	Rheumatoid arthritis
	Juvenile idiopathic arthritis
Tocilizumab	Rheumatoid arthritis
	Juvenile idiopathic arthritis
	Giant cell arteritis
	Polymyalgia rheumatica
Rituximab	Rheumatoid arthritis
	Systemic lupus erythematosus
	ANCA-associated vasculitis
	Cryoglobulinemic vasculitis
	Inflammatory myositis
Tofacitinib	Rheumatoid arthritis
	Psoriatic arthritis
Secukinumab	Psoriatic arthritis
	Plaque psoriasis
	Ankylosing spondylitis
Ustekinumab	Psoriatic arthritis
	Plaque psoriasis
Belimumab	Systemic lupus erythematosus

Patients may have immediate or delayed reactions to IV biologics. Immediate reactions occur during the infusion or within 2 hours after and include symptoms such as fever, chills, nausea, headache, pruritus, chest pain, palpitations, dyspnea, and hypotension. Patients with mild immediate reactions may be treated with antihistamines and/or steroids. Rare delayed reactions may occur 3 to 12 days after treatment and may include myalgia, fever, skin rash, and edema. Severe reactions are rare and require permanent discontinuation.[41,72] Pretreatment with acetaminophen and glucocorticoids reduces the risk of infusion reactions.

Tumor Necrosis Factor-α Inhibitors

Tumor necrosis factor-α inhibitors (TNFi) include etanercept, adalimumab, infliximab, golimumab, and certolizumab pegol. Medication indications are found in **Table 11**.

Concerns exist regarding malignancy risk and TNFi use. Melanoma and skin cancer have been reported to occur more often in patients treated with TNFi. Baseline and periodic skin assessments are recommended for patients taking TNFi.[41,80] Conflicting data regarding lymphoproliferative malignancies and TNFi exist; however, recent studies suggest that TNFi do not increase rates of lymphoma.[81] Although TNFi do not increase lymphoma risks, other DMARDs or biologics are preferentially recommended instead of TNFi in patients previously treated for a lymphoproliferative disorder.[40]

TNFi should be avoided in interstitial lung disease and demyelinating disorders.[41] Heart failure may worsen with TNFi use. TNFi should not be used in patients with New York Heart Association (NYHA) class III or greater heart failure or ejection fraction of 50% or less.[41,82,83] TNFi can be used in patients with mild congestive heart failure (NYHA class I or II) with routine ejection fraction monitoring.[41,83]

TNFi have been associated with paradoxic reactions, including psoriasiform skin lesion and drug-induced lupus. Psoriatic lesions may occur weeks or years after initiation of TNFi and may require evaluation by dermatology. Patients with mild psoriasiform lesions may continue TNFi therapy with addition of topical treatment, phototherapy, or methotrexate for skin inflammation. Severe psoriasis requires discontinuation of the TNFi and initiation of topical therapies. Drug-induced lupus generally resolves after discontinuation of TNFi therapy. Symptoms may include antinuclear antibodies, double-stranded DNA, rash, photosensitivity, arthritis, and hematologic abnormalities, but does not typically cause significant organ manifestations such as nephritis.[84]

Other Biologic Agents

Multiple other cytokines, intracellular signaling pathways, and specific immune cells besides TNF are targeted by biologic agents as listed in **Table 10**. Indications for these agents are found in **Table 11**. Some of these agents have special considerations.

Abatacept may exacerbate chronic obstructive pulmonary disease and should be avoided in moderate to severe pulmonary obstruction.[42] Tocilizumab may cause mild to moderate transient elevations in serum liver transaminases. Liver function tests should be monitored every 4 to 8 weeks for the first 6 months of tocilizumab therapy and then lengthened to every 3 months if no liver impairment is detected. Cholesterol may increase with tocilizumab and can be treated with statin therapy if needed. Lower intestinal perforations have also occurred with tocilizumab, and its use is contraindicated in patients with increased risk or previous perforation.[85,86] Tocilizumab alters the therapeutic effects of benzodiazepines, warfarin, atorvastatin, calcium channel inhibitors, cyclosporine, phenytoin, and theophylline.[85]

Although only approved for use in RA and antineutrophil cytoplasmic antibody (ANCA) -associated vasculitis, rituximab has multiple off-label uses as demonstrated in Table 11. Common adverse effects with rituximab include infusion reactions, hypotension, delayed or late onset neutropenia, and leukopenia.[71] Long-term rituximab treatment has been associated with hypogammaglobulinemia, which increases the risk of infection.[71,87,88] Immunoglobulin replacement therapy may be initiated for patients with hypogammaglobulinemia secondary to rituximab and a history of frequent severe infections.[88]

Demyelinating complications have been reported with rituximab, including progressive multifocal leukoencephalopathy (PML) and Guillain-Barre syndrome.[71,89,90] PML is a viral opportunistic infection that leads to progressive inflammation and demyelination. Symptoms include altered mental status, motor deficits, gait ataxia, and visual changes.[89] Although demyelinating disorders are rare with rituximab (<1 in 20,000), patients should be monitored for new neurologic symptoms.[89,90]

Tofacitinib is the only oral biologic agent currently used in rheumatic disease. The most common adverse effects are headache, infection, and nausea.[74] Additional adverse effects include increased liver function test levels and cytopenias, which are usually transient.[74,75]

Finally, belimumab was the first medication specifically approved for the treatment of systemic lupus erythematosus (SLE) in the last 50 years. Belimumab is used in adults with SLE on standard therapy, such as corticosteroids, antimalarials, immunosuppressives, and NSAIDs.[91,92] Limited drug-drug interaction data are available for belimumab; however, it is safe when used in combination with standard medications used in the treatment of SLE.[93] Common adverse effects with belimumab include headache, infection, arthralgia, diarrhea, nausea, hypotension, and fatigue. Depression and suicidality are rare adverse effects associated with belimumab.[91,92]

APREMILAST

Apremilast is indicated in plaque psoriasis and psoriatic arthritis as monotherapy or with oral DMARDs.[94] Through inhibition of phosphodiesterase 4, proinflammatory cytokines are downregulated and anti-inflammatory cytokines are upregulated.[95] Typical side effects include diarrhea, nausea, emesis, headaches, upper respiratory tract infections, and nasopharyngitis. Worsening depression and weight loss have also been reported.[94]

PERIOPERATIVE MEDICATION MANAGEMENT

Patients with rheumatic disease have higher rates of surgical site infection.[96] Recently, recommendations composed by the ACR and the American Association of Hip and Knee Surgeons outlined perioperative medication management for anti–rheumatic medications in the setting of hip or knee arthroplasty (**Table 12**).[97] Biologic agents

Table 12
Recommendations on perioperative disease-modifying antirheumatic drugs management (level B evidence)

Medication	Perioperative Cessation	Perioperative Continuation
Hydroxychloroquine	None	Yes
Sulfasalazine	None	Yes
Methotrexate	None	Yes
Leflunomide	None	Yes
Azathioprine	Severe disease: None Nonsevere disease: 7 d	Severe disease: Yes Nonsevere disease: No
Mycophenolate mofetil	Severe disease: None Nonsevere disease: 7 d	Severe disease: Yes Nonsevere disease: No
Tacrolimus	Severe disease: None Nonsevere disease: 7 d	Severe disease: Yes Nonsevere disease: No
Etanercept	2 wk	No
Infliximab	a	No
Adalimumab	3 wk	No
Certolizumab pegol	5 wk	No
Golimumab	5 wk	No
Tocilizumab	Subcutaneous: 3 wk Infusion: 5 wk	No
Abatacept	Subcutaneous: 2 wk Infusion: 5 wk	No
Tofacitinib	7 d	No
Rituximab	6 mo and 1 wk	No
Belimumab	5 wk	No

[a] Infliximab is dosed between every 4 wk and every 8 wk. Medication should be held for a full cycle before the surgery, that is, infliximab dosed every 5 wk should be held and surgery performed at week 6.

should be held for a full cycle with the surgery scheduled the week after the missed dose. For example, a patient receiving IV tocilizumab every 4 weeks would schedule a surgery 5 weeks after the last infusion. Medications should be held until the wound has evidence of adequate healing, until all sutures and staples are removed, and until there is no evidence of surgical site infection.

Patients receiving chronic oral corticosteroids should remain on their outpatient oral dose perioperatively.[97] Increasing the glucocorticoid dose in a hemodynamically stable patient has not been shown to be beneficial. When administered, stress dose steroids were found to increase the risk of postoperative infections.[98,99] IV hydrocortisone is reserved for patients undergoing major surgical procedures and those with volume refractory hypotension.[100]

PREGNANCY AND LACTATION

Many medications used in rheumatic diseases can lead to adverse fetal outcomes, particularly congenital abnormalities. The European League Against Rheumatism provided recommendations regarding medication use during pregnancy as well as safety in lactation (**Table 13**).[101] Of the DMARDs, the US Food and Drug Administration applies cautionary labels to hydroxychloroquine, sulfasalazine, and azathioprine; however, these medications are routinely used during pregnancy without evidence of teratogenicity.[102–105] If the anti-TNF agents are used during pregnancy past 30 weeks' gestation, the newborn should not receive any live virus vaccinations for the first 6 months of life because of concerns for potential immunosuppression.[101]

NSAIDs and corticosteroids can also be used during pregnancy with caution. NSAIDs should not be used after 32 weeks' gestation because of risks of fetal and maternal complications, such as hemorrhage, renal dysfunction, and premature closure of the ductus arteriosus.[106] Fluorinated corticosteroids like betamethasone and dexamethasone should be avoided because they can cross the placenta and cause adverse fetal effects.[107] Corticosteroids can increase the risk for pregnancy

Table 13
Recommendations for medication use in pregnancy and lactation

Medication	Safe in Pregnancy	Safe in Lactation
NSAIDs	Yes, 1st and 2nd trimester only	Yes
Corticosteroids	Yes	Yes
Hydroxychloroquine	Yes	Yes
Sulfasalazine	Yes	Yes
Methotrexate	No	No
Leflunomide	No	No
Azathioprine	Yes	Yes
Mycophenolate Mofetil	No	No
Tacrolimus	Yes	Yes
TNFi	Yes	Yes
Tocilizumab	No	No
Abatacept	No	No
Tofacitinib	No	No
Rituximab	No	No
Belimumab	No	No

complications, so the lowest dose and shortest course possible should be used.[108] Because corticosteroids are secreted into breast milk, waiting 4 hours after the corticosteroid dose to breastfeed reduces the concentration of the steroid in the breast milk and limits exposure to the infant.[109]

Methotrexate, leflunomide, mycophenolate, and cyclophosphamide should be stopped before conception. Methotrexate and pulse therapy with cyclophosphamide should be held 3 months before conception.[110,111] Mycophenolate mofetil should be discontinued at least 6 weeks before conception.[110] Leflunomide has a long half-life, and conception should not be attempted unless serum leflunomide levels are undetectable. In the setting of an unexpected pregnancy, cholestyramine can be used to bind to and remove leflunomide.[112]

SUMMARY

The pharmacology of rheumatology is growing, and current medications are being used for increasing numbers of diseases. Primary care providers interact with patients taking these medications on a daily basis. Knowing common dosing parameters, side effects, and monitoring recommendations helps ensure that patients remain safe while taking these medications.

REFERENCES

1. Helmick C, Felson D, Lawrence R, et al. Estimates of the prevalence of arthritis and other rheumatic conditions in the United States, part I. Arthritis Rheum 2008;58:15–25.
2. Lawrence R, Felson D, Helmick C, et al. Estimates of the prevalence of arthritis and other rheumatic conditions in the United States, part II. Arthritis Rheum 2008;58:26–35.
3. Brown T. 100 best-selling, most prescribed branded drugs through March. Medscape; 2015. Available at: https://www.medscape.com/viewarticle/844317. Accessed March 2, 2018.
4. Patrono C. Nonsteroidal anti-inflammatory drugs. In: Hochberg M, Silman A, Smolen J, et al, editors. Rheumatology. 6th edition. Philadelphia: Mosby; 2015. p. 415–22.
5. Hochberg M, Altman R, April K, et al. American College of Rheumatology 2012 recommendations for the use of nonpharmacologic and pharmacologic therapies in osteoarthritis of the hand, hip and knee. Arthritis Care Res 2012;64: 465–74.
6. Kroon F, van der Burg L, Ramiro S, et al. Nonsteroidal anti-inflammatory drugs for axial spondyloarthritis: a Cochrane Review. J Rheumatol 2016;43:607–17.
7. Ward M, Deodhar A, Akl E, et al. American College of Rheumatology/Spondylitis Association of America/Spondyloarthritis Research and Treatment Network 2015 recommendations for the treatment of ankylosing spondylitis and nonradiographic axial spondyloarthritis. Arthritis Rheumatol 2016;68:282–98.
8. Coates L, Kavanaugh A, Mease P, et al. Group for research and assessment of psoriasis and psoriatic arthritis 2015 treatment recommendations for psoriatic arthritis. Arthritis Rheumatol 2016;68:1060–71.
9. Khanna D, Khanna P, Fitzgerald J, et al. 2012 American College of Rheumatology guidelines for management of gout. Part 2: therapy and anti-inflammatory prophylaxis of acute gouty arthritis. Arthritis Care Res 2012; 64(10):1447–61.

10. Zhang W, Doherty M, Pascual E, et al. EULAR recommendations for calcium pyrophosphate deposition. Part II: management. Ann Rheum Dis 2011;70(4): 571–5.
11. American College of Rheumatology Ad Hoc Group on Use of Selective and Nonselective Nonsteroidal Antiinflammatory Drugs. Recommendations for use of selective and nonselective nonsteroidal anti-inflammatory drugs: an American College of Rheumatology white paper. Arthritis Rheum 2008;59:1058–73.
12. Yuan J, Tsoi K, Yang M, et al. Systematic review with network meta-analysis: comparative effectiveness and safety of strategies for preventing NSAID-associated gastrointestinal toxicity. Aliment Pharmacol Ther 2016;43:1262–75.
13. Yang M, He M, Zhao M, et al. Proton pump inhibitors for preventing non-steroidal anti-inflammatory drug induced gastrointestinal toxicity: a systematic review. Curr Med Res Opin 2017;33(6):973–80.
14. Salvo F, Antoniazzi S, Duong M, et al. Cardiovascular events associated with the long term use of NSAIDs: a review of randomized controlled trials and observational studies. Expert Opin Drug Saf 2014;13:573–85.
15. Arfe A, Scotti L, Varas-Lorenzo C, et al. Non-steroidal anti-inflammatory drugs and risk of heart failure in four European countries: nested case-control study. BMJ 2016;354:i4857.
16. Friedewald V, Bennett J, Christo J, et al. AJC editor's consensus: selective and nonselective nonsteroidal anti-inflammatory drugs and cardiovascular risk. Am J Cardiol 2010;106:873–84.
17. Cryer B, Barnett M, Wagner J, et al. Overuse and misperceptions of nonsteroidal anti-inflammatory drugs in the United States. Am J Med Sci 2016;352(5):472–80.
18. Rhen T, Cidlowski JA. Antiinflammatory action of glucocorticoids - new mechanisms for old drugs. N Engl J Med 2005;353:1711–23.
19. Caplan A, Fett N, Rosenbach M, et al. Prevention and management of glucocorticoid-induced side effects: a comprehensive review; ocular, cardiovascular, muscular, and psychiatric side effects and issues unique to pediatric patients. J Am Acad Dermatol 2017;76:201–7.
20. Caplan A, Fett N, Rosenbach M, et al. Prevention and management of glucocorticoid-induced side effects: a comprehensive review; gastrointestinal and endocrinologic side effects. J Am Acad Dermatol 2017;76:11–6.
21. Palmowski Y, Buttgereit T, Dejaco C, et al. The "official view" on glucocorticoids in rheumatoid arthritis: a systematic review of international guidelines and consensus statements. Arthritis Care Res (Hoboken) 2016. https://doi.org/10.1002/acr.23185.
22. Caplan A, Fett N, Rosenbach M, et al. Prevention and management of glucocorticoid-induced side effects: a comprehensive review; infectious complications and vaccination recommendations. J Am Acad Dermatol 2017;76: 191–8.
23. Souverein P, Berard A, van Staa T, et al. Use of oral glucocorticoids and risk of cardiovascular and cerebrovascular disease in a population based case-control study. Heart 2004;90:859–65.
24. Allen C, Yeung J, Vandermeer B, et al. Bisphosphonates for steroid-induced osteoporosis. Cochrane Database Syst Rev 2016;(10):CD001347.
25. Buckley L, Guyatt G, Fink H, et al. 2017 American College of Rheumatology guideline for the prevention and treatment of glucocorticoid-induced osteoporosis. Arthritis Rheumatol 2017;69:1521–37.
26. Ozen S, Demirkaya E, Erer B, et al. EULAR recommendations for the management of familial Mediterranean fever. Ann Rheum Dis 2016;75:644–51.

27. Leung Y, Hui L, Kraus V. Colchicine—update on mechanisms of action and therapeutic uses. Semin Arthritis Rheum 2015;45:341–50.
28. Keenan RT. Safety of urate-lowering therapies: managing the risks to gain the benefits. Rheum Dis Clin North Am 2012;38:663–80.
29. Takeda Pharmaceuticals America, Inc. Uloric® (febuxostat) tablets prescribing information. Deerfield (IL): 2013.
30. AstraZeneca Pharmaceuticals LP. Zurampic® (lesinurad) tablets prescribing information. Wilmington (DE): 2015.
31. Savient Pharmaceuticals, Inc. Krystexxa® (pegloticase) infusion prescribing information. East Brunswick (NJ): 2012.
32. Khanna D, Fitzgerald J, Khanna P, et al. 2012 American College of Rheumatology guidelines for management of gout part 1: systematic nonpharmacologic and pharmacologic therapeutic approaches to hyperuricemia. Arthritis Care Res 2012;64:1431–46.
33. Bardin T, Keenan R, Khanna P, et al. Lesinurad in combination with allopurinol: a randomized, double-blind, placebo-controlled study in patients with gout with inadequate response to standard of care (the multinational CLEAR 2 study). Ann Rheum Dis 2016. https://doi.org/10.1136/annrheumdis-2016-209213.
34. Qaseem A, Harris R, Forciae M. Management of acute and recurrent gout: a clinical practice guideline from the American College of Physicians. Ann Intern Med 2017;166:58–68.
35. Becker M, Fitz-Patrick D, Choi H, et al. An open-label, 6-month study of allopurinol safety in gout: the LASSO study. Semin Arthritis Rheum 2015;45:174–83.
36. Stamp L, Taylor W, Jones P, et al. Starting dose is a risk factor for allopurinol hypersensitivity syndrome: a proposed safe starting dose of allopurinol. Arthritis Rheum 2012;64:2529–36.
37. Stamp L, O'Donnell J, Zhang M, et al. Using allopurinol above the dose based on creatinine clearance is effective and safe in patients with chronic gout, including those with renal impairment. Arthritis Rheum 2011;63:412–21.
38. Chohan S. Safety and efficacy of febuxostat treatment in subjects with gout and severe allopurinol adverse reactions. J Rheumatol 2011;38:1957–9.
39. Baraf H, Yood R, Ottery F, et al. Infusion-related reactions with pegloticase, a recombinant uricase for the treatment of chronic gout refractory to conventional therapy. J Clin Rheumatol 2014;20:427–32.
40. Singh J, Saag K, Bridges S, et al. 2015 American College of Rheumatology guideline for the treatment of rheumatoid arthritis. Arthritis Rheumatol 2016;68:1–25.
41. Pham T, Bachelez H, Berthelot J-M, et al. TNF alpha antagonist therapy and safety monitoring. Joint Bone Spine 2011;78(suppl 1):15–185.
42. Pham T, Bachelez H, Berthelot J-M, et al. Abatacept therapy and safety management. Joint Bone Spine 2012;79(suppl 1):3–84.
43. Karadağ Ö, Kaşifoğlu T, Özer B, et al. Viral hepatitis screening guideline before biological drug use in rheumatic patients. Eur J Rheumatol 2016;3:25–8.
44. Centers for Disease Control and Prevention. Vaccines and Immunizations. Available at: https://www.cdc.gov/vaccines/hcp/acip-recs/general-recs/immunocompetence.html. Accessed September 22, 2017.
45. Hazlewood GS, Barnabe C, Tomlinson G, et al. Methotrexate monotherapy and methotrexate combination therapy with traditional and biologic disease modifying antirheumatic drugs for rheumatoid arthritis: abridged Cochrane systematic review and network meta-analysis. BMJ 2016;353:i1777.

46. Cutolo M, Bolosiu H, Perdriset G. Efficacy and safety of leflunomide in DMARD-naïve patients with early rheumatoid arthritis: comparison of a loading and a fixed-dose regimen. Rheumatology (Oxford) 2013;52:1132–40.

47. Rainsford KD, Parke AL, Clifford-Rashotte M, et al. Therapy and pharmacological properties of hydroxychloroquine and chloroquine in treatment of systemic lupus erythematosus, rheumatoid arthritis and related diseases. Inflammopharmacology 2015;23:231–69.

48. Kivity S, Zafrir Y, Loebstein R, et al. Clinical characteristics and risk factors for low dose methotrexate toxicity: a cohort of 28 patients. Autoimmun Rev 2014; 13:1109–13.

49. Behrens F, Koehm M, Burkhardt H. Update 2011: leflunomide in rheumatoid arthritis – strengths and weaknesses. Curr Opin Rheumatol 2011;23:282–7.

50. Amos R, Pullar T, Bax D, et al. Sulphasalazine for rheumatoid arthritis: toxicity in 774 patients monitored for one to 11 years. BMJ 1986;293:420–3.

51. Shea B, Swinden M, Tanjong Ghogomu E, et al. Folic acid and folinic acid for reducing side effects in patients receiving methotrexate for rheumatoid arthritis. Cochrane Database Syst Rev 2013;31(5):CD000951.

52. Van Roon E, van den Bemt P, Jansen T, et al. An evidence-based assessment of the clinical significant of drug-drug interactions between disease-modifying antirheumatic drugs and non-antirheumatic drugs according to rheumatologists and pharmacists. Clin Ther 2009;31:1737–46.

53. Marmor M, Kellner U, Lai T, et al. Recommendations on screening for chloroquine and hydroxychloroquine retinopathy (2016 revision). Ophthalmology 2016;123:1386–94.

54. Denton M, Magee C, Sayegh M. Immunosuppressive strategies in transplantation. Lancet 1999;353:1083–91.

55. Chighizola C, Ong V, Meroni P. The use of cyclosporine A in rheumatology: a 2016 comprehensive review. Clin Rev Allergy Immunol 2016. https://doi.org/10.1007/s12016-016-8582-3.

56. Kurita T, Yasuda S, Amengual O, et al. The efficacy of calcineurin inhibitors for the treatment of interstitial lung disease associated with polymyositis/dermatomyositis. Lupus 2015;24:3–9.

57. Ge Y, Zhou H, Shi J, et al. The efficacy of tacrolimus in patients with refractory dermatomyositis/polymyositis: a systematic review. Clin Rheumatol 2015;34:2097–103.

58. Hannah J, Casian A, D'Cruz D. Tacrolimus use in lupus nephritis: a systematic review and meta-analysis. Autoimmun Rev 2016;15:93–101.

59. Ozyazgan Y, Yurdakul S, Yazici H, et al. Low dose cyclosporine A versus pulsed cyclophosphamide in Behçet's syndrome: a single masked trial. Br J Ophthalmol 1992;76(4):241–3.

60. Murphy CC, Greiner K, Plskova J, et al. Cyclosporine vs tacrolimus therapy for posterior and intermediate uveitis. Arch Ophthalmol 2005;1213(5):634–41.

61. Webster A, Woodroffe R, Taylor R, et al. Tacrolimus versus cyclosporine as primary immunosuppression for kidney transplant recipients. Cochrane Database Syst Rev 2005;(4):CD003961.

62. Muduma G, Saunders R, Odeyemi I, et al. Systematic review and meta-analysis of tacrolimus versus ciclosporin as primary immunosuppression after liver transplant. PLoS One 2016;11(11):e0160421.

63. Nankivell B, Chow H, O'Connell P, et al. Calcineurin inhibitor nephrotoxicity through the lens of longitudinal histology: comparison of cyclosporine and tacrolimus eras. Transplantation 2016;100:1723–31.

64. Prometheus Laboratories Inc. Imuran® (azathioprine) tablets prescribing information. Hunt Valley (MD): 2014.

65. Genentech USA, Inc. CellCept® (mycophenolate mofetil) tablets prescribing information. South San Francisco (CA): 2015.

66. Baxter Healthcare Corporation. Cyclophosphamide for injection prescribing information. Deerfield (IL): 2017.

67. Al-Absi AI, Cooke CR, Wall BM, et al. Patterns of injury in mycophenolate mofetil-related colitis. Transplant Proc 2010;42:3591–3.

68. Brummaier T, Pohanka E, Studnicka-Benke A, et al. Using cyclophosphamide in inflammatory rheumatic diseases. Eur J Intern Med 2013;24:590–6.

69. Teles KA, Medeiros-Souza P, Lima FAC, et al. Cyclophosphamide administration routine in autoimmune rheumatic diseases: a review. Rev Bras Reumatol 2016. https://doi.org/10.1016/j.rbr.2016.04.009.

70. Mosak J, Furie R. Comparative safety of therapies in systemic lupus erythematosus. Rheum Dis Clin North Am 2012;38:795–807.

71. Genetech, Inc. Rituxin® (Rituximab) prescribing information. South San Francisco (CA): 2016.

72. Singh JA, Wells GA, Christensen R, et al. Adverse effects of biologics: a network meta-analysis and Cochrane overview. Cochrane Database Syst Rev 2011. https://doi.org/10.1002/14651858/CD008794.pub2.

73. Kahlenberg JM. Anti-inflammatory panacea? The expanding therapeutics of interleukin-1 blockade. Curr Opin Rheumatol 2016;28:197–203.

74. Fleischmann R, Kremer J, Tanaka Y, et al. Efficacy and safety of tofacitinib in patients with active rheumatoid arthritis: review of key phase 2 studies. Int J Rheum Dis 2016;19(12):1216–25.

75. Schulze-Koops H, Strand V, Nduaka C, et al. Analysis of haematological changes in tofacitinib-treated patients with rheumatoid arthritis across phase 3 and long-term extension studies. Rheumatology (Oxford) 2017. https://doi.org/10.1093/rheumatology/kew329.

76. Koenders MI, van den Berg WB. Secukinumab for rheumatology: development and its potential place in therapy. Drug Des Devel Ther 2016;10:2069–80.

77. Paine A, Ritchlin CT. Targeting the interleukin-23/17 axis in axial spondyloarthritis. Curr Opin Rheumatol 2016;28:359–67.

78. Wei M, Duan D. Efficacy and safety of monoclonal antibodies targeting interleukin-17 pathway for inflammatory arthritis: a meta-analysis of randomized controlled trials. Drug Des Devel Ther 2016;10:2771–7.

79. Teng MWL, Bowman EP, McElwee JJ, et al. IL-12 and IL-23 cytokines: from discovery to targeted therapies for immune-mediated inflammatory diseases. Nat Med 2015;21(7):719–29.

80. Cush JJ, Dao KH. Malignancy risks with biologic therapies. Rheum Dis Clin North Am 2012;38:761–70.

81. Mercer LK, Galloway JB, Lunt M, et al. Risk of lymphoma in patients exposed to antitumor necrosis factor therapy: results from the British Society for Rheumatology Biologics register for rheumatoid arthritis. Ann Rheum Dis 2017;76:497–503.

82. Makol A, Wright K, Matteson EL. Safe use of antirheumatic agents in patients with cormorbidities. Rheum Dis Clin North Am 2012;38:771–93.

83. Cush JJ, Dao KH, Orozco C. TNF inhibitors and heart failure. American College of Rheumatology Drug Safety Quarterly 2013;5:1–2.

84. Daver N, Ritchlin C. Paradoxical adverse events associated with anti-TNF agents. American College of Rheumatology Drug Safety Quarterly 2013;4(2): 1–2.
85. Pham T, Claudepierre P, Constantin A, et al. Tocilizumab: therapy and safety management. Joint Bone Spine 2010;77(suppl 1):S3–100.
86. Strangfeld A, Richter A, Siegmund B, et al. Risk for lower intestinal perforations in patients with rheumatoid arthritis treated with tocilizumab in comparison to treatment with other biologic or conventional synthetic DMARDs. Ann Rheum Dis 2017;76:504–10.
87. Christou E, Giardino G, Worth A, et al. Risk factors predisposing to the development of hypogammaglobulinemia and infections post-rituximab. Int Rev Immunol 2017;11:1–8.
88. Kado R, Sanders G, McCune WJ. Diagnostic and therapeutic considerations in patients with hypogammaglobulinemia after rituximab therapy. Curr Opin Rheumatol 2017;29:228–33.
89. Valenzuela A, Chung L. Demyelinating complications associated with rituximab and other non-tumor necrosis factor-α inhibitor biologics. American College of Rheumatology Drug Safety Quarterly 2014;5:1–4.
90. Molloy ES, Calabrese CM, Calabrese LH. The risk of progressive multifocal leukoencephalopathy in the biologic era. Rheum Dis Clin North Am 2017;43: 95–109.
91. Manzi S, Sánchez-Guerrero J, Merrill J. Effects of belimumab, a B lymphocyte stimulator-specific inhibitor, on disease activity across multiple organ domains in patients with systemic lupus erythematosus: combined results from two phase III trials. Ann Rheum Dis 2012;71(11):1833–8.
92. Boyce EG, Fusco BE. Belimumab: review of use in systemic lupus erythematosus. Clin Ther 2012;34(5):1006–22.
93. Schwarting A, Dooley MA, Roth DA, et al. Impact of concomitant medication use on belimumab efficacy and safety in patients with systemic lupus erythematosus. Lupus 2016;25:1587–96.
94. Celgene Corporation. Otezla® (apremilast) tablets prescribing information. Summit (NJ): 2014.
95. Schafer P. Apremilast mechanism of action and application to psoriasis and psoriatic arthritis. Biochem Pharmacol 2012;83:1583–90.
96. Miller A, Brause B. Perioperative infection in the patient with rheumatic disease. Curr Rheumatol Rep 2013;15:379.
97. Goodman S, Springer B, Guyatt G, et al. 2017 American College of Rheumatology/American Association of Hip and Knee Surgeons guidelines for the perioperative management of antirheumatic medication in patients with rheumatic diseases undergoing elective total hip or total knee arthroplasty. Arthritis Rheumatol 2017;69(8):1111–24.
98. Dixon W, Abrahamowicz M, Beauchamp M, et al. Immediate and delayed impact of oral glucocorticoid therapy on risk of serious infection in older patients with rheumatoid arthritis: a nested case-control analysis. Ann Rheum Dis 2012; 71(7):1128–33.
99. Somayaji R, Barnabe C, Martin L. Risk factors for infection following total joint arthroplasty in rheumatoid arthritis. Open Rheumatol J 2013;7:119–24.
100. MacKenzie C, Goodman S. Stress dose steroids: myths and perioperative medicine. Curr Rheumatol Rep 2016;18:47.

101. Skorpen C, Hoeltzenbein M, Tincani A, et al. The EULAR points to consider for use of antirheumatic drugs before pregnancy, and during pregnancy and lactation. Ann Rheum Dis 2016;75:795–810.
102. Wallace D, Gudsoorkar V, Weisman M, et al. New insights into mechanisms of therapeutic effects of antimalarial agents in SLE. Nat Rev Rheumatol 2012; 8(9):522–33.
103. Norgard B, Pedersen L, Christensen L, et al. Therapeutic drug use in women with Crohn's disease and birth outcomes: a Danish nationwide cohort study. Am J Gastroenterol 2007;102(7):1406–13.
104. Akbari M, Shah S, Velayos F, et al. Systematic review and meta-analysis on the effects of thiopurines on birth outcomes from female and male patients with inflammatory bowel disease. Inflamm Bowel Dis 2013;19(1):15–22.
105. Viktil K, Engeland A, Furu K. Outcomes after anti-rheumatic drug use before and during pregnancy: a cohort study among 150,000 pregnant women and expectant fathers. Scand J Rheumatol 2012;41(3):196–201.
106. Makol A, Wright K, Amin S. Rheumatoid arthritis and pregnancy: safety considerations in pharmacological management. Drugs 2011;71(15):1973–87.
107. Jain V, Gordon C. Managing pregnancy in inflammatory rheumatological diseases. Arthritis Res Ther 2011;13(1):206.
108. Murphy K, Willan A, Hannah M, et al. Effect of antenatal corticosteroids on fetal growth and gestational age at birth. Obstet Gynecol 2012;119(5):917–23.
109. Noviani M, Wasserman S, Clowse M. Breastfeeding in mothers with systemic lupus erythematosus. Lupus 2016;25(9):973–9.
110. Flint J, Panchal S, Hurrell A, et al. BSR and BHPR guideline on prescribing drugs in pregnancy and breastfeeding—part I: standard and biologic disease modifying anti-rheumatic drugs and corticosteroids. Rheumatology (Oxford) 2016;55(9):1693–7.
111. Harris E. Antirheumatic drugs in pregnancy. Lupus 2002;11(10):683–9.
112. Brent R. Teratogen update: reproductive risks of leflunomide (Arava); a pyrimidine synthesis inhibitor: counseling women taking leflunomide before or during pregnancy and men taking leflunomide who are contemplating fathering a child. Teratology 2001;63(2):106–12.

Diagnosis and Treatment of Gout and Pseudogout for Everyday Practice

Anthony Sidari, MD*, Erica Hill, DO

KEYWORDS

- Crystalline arthropathy • Gout • Arthritis • Pseudogout
- Calcium pyrophosphate deposition disease • Monoarthritis • Polyarthritis
- Urate-lowering therapy

KEY POINTS

- The clinical recognition and differentiation of gout and pseudogout from other causes of inflammatory arthritis is key in rendering appropriate and timely treatment.
- Nonsteroidal antiinflammatory drugs, colchicine, and corticosteroids can control acute gout symptoms; allopurinol and febuxostat are the first-line urate-lowering therapies to definitively treat gout.
- Medication noncompliance is the most common reason for "treatment-resistant" gout.
- Aside from treatment of acute arthritis in pseudogout, there is no proven therapy to prevent recurrence or result in long-term remission.

INTRODUCTION

The crystalline arthropathies, gout and pseudogout, are often successfully managed by the primary care provider. It is essential that primary care clinicians understand the underlying pathophysiology of these diseases, differentiate them from other forms of inflammatory arthritis, know the guidelines for treatment and monitoring, and understand indications for referral to a rheumatologist. A basic knowledge of more advanced medications used in these diseases is important, especially the potential side effects and medication interactions. In this article we present gout and pseudogout from diagnosis to treatment for everyday practice.

Disclosure Statement: The authors have no financial disclosures. The view(s) expressed herein are those of the author(s) and do not reflect the official policy or position of Brooke Army Medical Center, the U.S. Army Medical Department, the U.S. Army Office of the Surgeon General, the Department of the Air Force, the Department of the Army or the Department of Defense or the U.S. Government.
San Antonio Uniformed Services Health Consortium, Department of Rheumatology, 3851 Roger Brooke Drive, San Antonio, TX 78234, USA
* Corresponding author.
E-mail address: Anthony.p.sidari2.mil@mail.mil

Prim Care Clin Office Pract 45 (2018) 213–236
https://doi.org/10.1016/j.pop.2018.02.004
0095-4543/18/Published by Elsevier Inc.

GOUT

Gout incidence is increasing—doubling between the 1970s and 1990s.[1] Hyperuricemia, regardless of the etiology, is the primary cause of this disease. Needle-shaped monosodium urate (MSU) crystals deposit and precipitate within the synovium, ultimately triggering an intense inflammatory response through activation of the innate immune system.

PATHOPHYSIOLOGY
Pathophysiology of Hyperuricemia

Uric acid is a byproduct of purine metabolism. Purines are required for DNA, RNA, adenosine triphosphate, diphosphate, and monophosphate, cyclic adenosine monophosphate, and many other integral molecules. Hyperuricemia results from urate overproduction, underexcretion through the renal tubules, or a combination thereof.

During purine metabolism, uric acid is synthesized via multiple intermediaries, including hypoxanthine and guanine, which converge at the common substrate xanthine (**Fig. 1**). The enzyme xanthine oxidase (XO) then converts xanthine into uric acid. In humans, purine metabolism ends with uric acid. In almost all animals except humans and primates, the enzyme uricase converts uric acid into allantoic acid, a soluble compound that can be degraded into urea and excreted. In addition to de novo synthesis, the purine salvage pathway works through hypoxanthine guanine phosphoribosyl transferase and is responsible for resynthesizing the purines inosine 5'-monophosphate and guanosine monophosphate from hypoxanthine and guanine. The loss of hypoxanthine guanine phosphoribosyl transferase activity results in hyperuricemia. Once serum urate reaches a certain threshold, urate crystals are deposited in synovium. Secondary causes of urate overproduction include increased cell turnover causing increased purine generation (**Box 1**).

Hyperuricemia may also occur as a result of decreased uric acid excretion. Approximately 65% of uric acid is excreted through the renal system.[2] The gastrointestinal tract also excretes uric acid and in chronic kidney disease, may increase its excretion.[3] In the kidneys, uric acid secretion and resorption occur across the proximal tubule epithelium. Important transporters for excretion of uric acid include URAT1, GLUT9, OAT4, and others[4] (**Fig. 2**). URAT1, on the apical tubule surface, transfers tubule lumen urate into the cytosolic environment of the epithelial cell and is the target for some urate lowering therapies. Renal insufficiency and metabolic acidosis, regardless of the cause, promote urate underexcretion, and involve a complex process beginning with a decrease in filtered volume past the glomerulus. Drugs that may promote hyperuricemia include thiazide and loop diuretics and salicylates.

Pathophysiology of Acute and Chronic Gouty Arthritis

Under the appropriate conditions, MSU crystals can activate the NLRP3 inflammasome, a multiprotein cytosolic complex that activates caspase-1.[5] The caspase-1 enzyme cleaves pro-interleukin (IL)-1β to the active IL-1β protein, which is central to the subsequent acute inflammatory response. MSU crystals also induce many other inflammatory cytokines and chemokines, including complement activation. Large amounts of neutrophils are recruited to the joint during an acute gout attack and play a crucial role in the intense inflammation in gout. Neutrophils also release serine proteases that further activate IL-1β, contributing to a positive inflammatory feedback loop.[6]

The tophus is the cardinal feature of chronic gout. A granuloma-like response results in large collections of MSU crystals and inflammatory cells. The tophus produces a persistent inflammatory response in adjacent bone along with reduced osteoblast

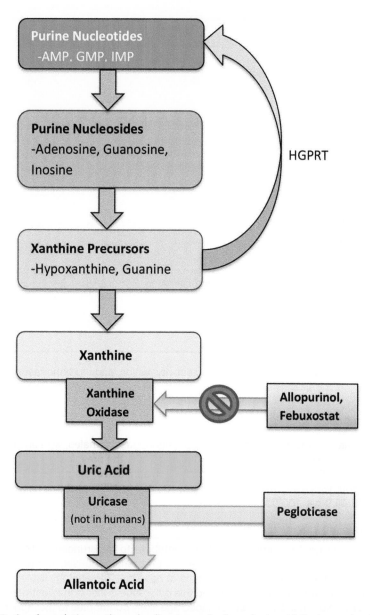

Fig. 1. Purine degradation pathway leading to production of uric acid. Purine nucleotides are degraded into urate precursors, and ultimately into uric acid. The xanthine oxidase inhibitors, allopurinol and febuxostat, inhibit this final step of uric acid production. Pegloticase is recombinant uricase and degrades uric acid into allantoic acid, a soluble metabolite readily excreted by the kidneys. Intermediaries and enzymes not pertinent to the pathophysiology and medications discussed are omitted for simplicity. AMP, adenosine monophosphate; GMP, guanosine monophosphate; HGPRT, hypoxanthine guanine phosphoribosyl transferase; IMP, inosine 5′-monophosphate; XMP, xanthosine 5′-monophosphate.

Box 1
Causes of hyperuricemia

Overproduction
  Acute leukemia and lymphoma
  Tumor lysis syndrome
  Solid organ malignancy
  Hemolytic anemia
  Multiple myeloma, Waldenstrom's macroglobulinemia
  Thalassemia and sickle cell disease
  Myelodysplastic syndrome
  Psoriasis
  Sarcoidosis
  Metabolic and mitochondrial myopathies

Underexcretion
  Renal insufficiency
  Volume depletion
  Medications (diuretics)

Mixed
  Sepsis
  Myocardial infarction and congestive heart failure

Metabolic
  Hypothyroidism and hyperthyroidism
  Hypoparathyroidism and hyperparathyroidism
  Obesity

---

differentiation and increased osteoclastic activity, which leads to bone resorption and erosions.[7]

EPIDEMIOLOGY

Gout is primarily a disease of males and postmenopausal females, with an increasing incidence seen with advancing age. In 2007 and 2008, the prevalence was estimated at 3.9% of all U.S. adults, and upwards of 9.3% in adults over the age of 60.[1] The incidence of gout was estimated to be 20.2 per 100,000 in 1977, and was noted to have doubled to 45.9 per 100,000 in 1995.[8]

Risk Factors

Risk factors for gout include factors that contribute to hyperuricemia. Male gender alone increases risk for gout compared with premenopausal women given a gender-associated 1 mg/dL higher uric acid at baseline. The etiology likely lies in estrogen effects on uric acid clearance, and this difference is lost in the postmenopausal state.[9] Comorbid renal disease in advanced age likely contributes to the higher rate of hyperuricemia seen in the elderly.[9] Ethnic influences on risk include African American ethnicity with higher serum uric acid levels than Caucasians at baseline.[10] Rare X-linked inborn errors of metabolism, such as Lesch-Nyhan syndrome (hypoxanthine guanine phosphoribosyl transferase enzyme deficiency), are associated with hyperuricemia and gout. Metabolic comorbidities, such as obesity, hypertension, hyperlipidemia, and the metabolic syndrome, are also associated with hyperuricemia and gout.[11,12] Endocrine abnormalities including hyperparathyroidism and hypoparathyroidism, and hyperthyroidism and hypothyroidism, are known to influence kidney function, but the effect on serum urate levels and risk of developing clinical gout is less clear.[13]

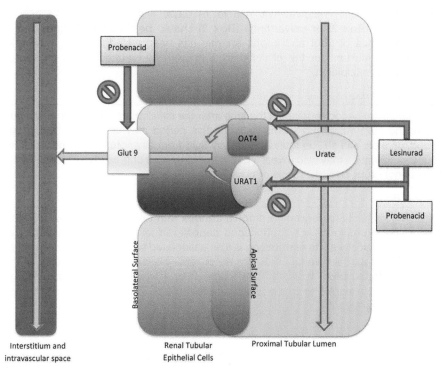

Fig. 2. Renal urate handling. Urate in the renal tubular lumen is ultimately reabsorbed into the intravascular space via action of URAT1 and OAT4/10 on the apical surface, and Glut9 on the basolateral surface of the tubule epithelium. Activity of these transporters is inhibited by the uricosurics probenecid and lesinurad. For simplicity, not all transporters are shown.

Acute Attack Triggers

Repetitive joint microtrauma or severe macrotrauma, purine-rich foods, critical illness, infection, and surgery are associated with attack onset. Medications that increase serum uric acid include diuretics, beta-blockers, low-dose aspirin (<1 g/d) and cyclosporine; initiation or dose changes can precipitate an acute attack.

CLINICAL PRESENTATION

The clinical spectrum of gout spans asymptomatic hyperuricemia to chronic polyarthritis with tophaceous deposits.

Acute Gout

Acute gout typically presents as monoarticular arthritis and is characterized by intense erythema, warmth, swelling, and pain with peak symptoms developing within 24 hours of onset. The most commonly affected joint is the first metatarsophalangeal joint. Other frequently affected joints include the insteps of the feet, heels, ankles, and knees. Less commonly affected joints include the wrists, elbows, and even small joints of the fingers. Acute bursitis, tendinitis, or tenosynovitis can also occur. The hips, shoulders, and spine are almost never affected. Accompanying systemic symptoms are more likely in the setting of polyarticular attacks and may include low-grade fevers, chills, and malaise. If untreated, an acute attack usually resolves within 5 to 14 days. The differential diagnosis of monoarthritis (**Box 2**) or polyarthritis (**Box 3**) should be thoughtfully considered. The coexistence of gout and septic arthritis has been well-described, making it even more important for the clinician to approach the diagnosis with an appropriate level of suspicion.[14]

Intercritical Period

The intercritical period represents the time after the initial attack that is symptom free before the next attack. For some patients, this period may last years. During this period, crystals can still be found in synovial fluid from asymptomatic joints.[15] Ultrasound examination may also reveal a double-contour sign or presence of tophi, which can strongly support a diagnosis of gout.[16]

Chronic Gout

Chronic gout is characterized by chronic arthritis with persistent low-grade inflammation, bone erosions, and tophaceous deposits in joints and soft tissues. This variant is classically a late feature and is also associated with high levels of hyperuricemia as well as concomitant diuretic use or renal disease.[17] From the time of the first gout attack, tophi typically take longer than 10 years to develop, although they may occur earlier in those with more symptomatic disease and decreased creatinine clearance.[17]

DIAGNOSIS

Most patients with hyperuricemia never develop clinical gout.[1] Furthermore, up to 42% of patients may actually have normal serum urate levels during an acute attack.[18] Therefore, the diagnosis of gout should not be based on serum hyperuricemia alone.

Arthrocentesis of the affected joint with visualization of needle-like negatively birefringent MSU crystals remains the gold standard for diagnosis (**Fig. 3**). Because gout is commonly diagnosed by primary care providers in outpatient clinics, arthrocentesis and polarizing light microscopy may not be feasible. The American College of Rheumatology (ACR) and European League Against Rheumatism (EULAR) published clinical classification criteria in 2015 to enable standardized enrollment of individuals with gout into studies[19] (**Table 1**). The criteria were not intended for use in making a diagnosis in a clinical setting. Nonetheless, they can serve as a helpful guide for practitioners who are unable to perform a joint aspiration. In addition to MSU crystals, synovial fluid analysis during an acute gout attack may demonstrate white blood cell counts as high as 50,000 to 100,000. Other useful studies include gram stain and culture, to rule out septic arthritis.

Box 2
Differential diagnosis of acute monoarthritis

Septic arthritis

Hemarthrosis

Trauma

Crystalline arthritis (gout, pseudogout)

Autoimmune disease (spondyloarthropathy, rheumatoid arthritis, sarcoidosis)

Leukemia

Box 3
Differential diagnosis of acute polyarthritis
Crystalline arthritis (gout, pseudogout)
Disseminated *Neisseria* infection
Lyme disease
Autoimmune disease (rheumatoid arthritis, systemic lupus erythematosus, spondyloarthropathy)

Ancillary Studies

Plain radiographs

Radiographic changes indicate chronicity of disease and may not be apparent for 5 to 10 years after the initial gout attack.[20] Chronic tophi in the soft tissues can erode adjacent periarticular bone and produce well-defined erosions with sclerotic borders and a "punched out" appearance with overhanging edges (**Fig. 4**). The joint space is classically preserved until late in the disease.[20,21] The only radiographic changes during an acute gout attack may be nonspecific soft tissue swelling and effusions.

Ultrasound imaging

Musculoskeletal ultrasound imaging is increasingly being used for establishing a diagnosis of gout. In fact, the 2015 ACR-EULAR classification criteria include ultrasound evidence of urate deposition in a joint or bursa.[19] Highly specific ultrasound features of gout include the double-contour sign (**Fig. 5**), a hyperechoic irregular linear density over the surface of the hyaline cartilage, hyperechoic aggregates (**Fig. 6**) within the joint space indicative of tophus, and the "snowstorm" appearance of floating hyperechoic foci suggesting MSU crystals in synovial fluid.[16] There are several generic signs of inflammation associated with gout as well, including synovial hypertrophy, bony erosions, and increased power Doppler signal during acute gout attacks.

Dual-energy computed tomography

Dual-energy computed tomography (DECT) is a new imaging technique used to help diagnose gout. This imaging modality is able to analyze the chemical composition of

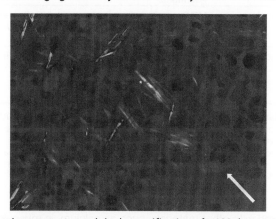

Fig. 3. Polarizing microscopy at an original magnification of x 100 demonstrating negatively birefringent needle-like monosodium urate crystals within milieu of neutrophils consistent with gout (*asterisk*). The polarizer is directed in the upward-left direction as indicated by the white arrow. (*Courtesy of* Jordan M. Hall, MD, Dept of Pathology, BAMC, San Antonio, TX.)

Table 1
The American College of Rheumatology/European League Against Rheumatism gout classification criteria

Criteria	Definitions/Considerations	Score
Entry criterion	Must have ≥1 episode of swelling, pain, or tenderness in a peripheral joint or bursa	Needed for entry into criteria
Sufficient for diagnosis	Tophus or MSU crystals present within symptomatic joint/bursa	Diagnostic of gout If negative, use below criteria
Criteria with scoring (if sufficiency criterion not met above)		
Pattern of joint/bursa involvement during episodes	Distribution of involvement	MTP1: 2 Ankle/midfoot without MTP1: 1 Any other joint: 0
Characteristics of symptomatic episodes	Presence of (1) difficulty with walking or inability to use joint, (2) inability to bear touch/pressure, (3) erythema overlying the affected joint	Three characteristics: 3 Two characteristics: 2 One characteristic: 1 No characteristics: 0
Time course	Typical episode: presence of >2 of the following: time to maximal pain <24 h, resolution ≤14 d, complete resolution between episodes	Recurrent typical episodes: 2 One typical episode: 1 No typical episodes: 0
Clinical evidence of tophus	Present/absent	Present: 4 Absent: 0
Serum urate cut-offs	<4 mg/dL 4–6 mg/dL 6–<8 mg/dL 8–<10 mg/dL ≥10 mg/dL	−4 0 2 3 4
Synovial fluid analysis	MSU negative or not performed (MSU positive is sufficient on its own)	Not performed: 0 MSU negative: −2
Imaging evidence of urate deposition	Ultrasound/DECT presence or absence Presence of gout-related erosions or absence	Present: 4 (either modality) Absent: 0 Present: 4 Absent: 0

A web based calculator can be accessed at http://goutclassificationcalculator.auckland.ac.nz. Synovial fluid positive for monosodium urate crystals immediately classifies a patient as having gout. Otherwise, a score of 8 or higher allows for gout classification.

Adapted from Neogi T, Jansen TL, Dalbeth N, et al. Gout classification criteria: an American College of Rheumatology/European League Against Rheumatism collaborative initiative. Ann Rheum Dis 2015;74(10):1795; with permission.

uric acid compared with other materials, such as calcium, in musculoskeletal tissue. DECT characterizes the composition of the material using different colors.[22] MSU crystals can also be visualized in the tendons, ligaments, and soft tissues using this technique (**Fig. 7**). DECT is especially helpful in cases where there is a high clinical suspicion of gout but aspiration is negative for MSU crystals or in asymptomatic patients during the intercritical period. A recent metaanalysis found DECT to have a high diagnostic accuracy with 84.7% sensitivity and 93.7% specificity.[22] The sensitivity is related to tophaceous burden, with very high sensitivity in joints with tophaceous gout, and lower sensitivity in nontophaceous gout.[22–24] Therefore, false negatives are more likely in patients with recent onset disease.

TREATMENT

If treated properly, gout is a disease from which a patient can enjoy sustained remission. There are published treatment guidelines from multiple organizations including the ACR, American College of Physicians (ACP), and EULAR.[25–27] Although similar in many regards, these guidelines differ in some areas, especially regarding chronic treatment (**Table 2**).

Acute Treatment

The goal of acute gouty arthritis treatment is to quell the intense inflammation. In addition to antiinflammatory medication, all patients should receive appropriate analgesics during this period.

Colchicine

Colchicine is a tricyclic alkaloid that inhibits multiple pathways involved in the inflammatory cascade. In gout, it suppresses the activation of caspase-1, which prevents IL-

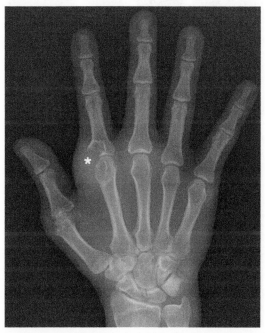

Fig. 4. Plain anteroposterior right hand radiograph demonstrating a punched out lesion with an overhanging edge and sclerosis consistent with gouty erosion (asterisk). Note the presence of adjacent soft tissue swelling.

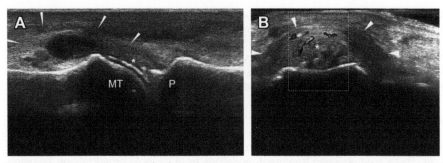

Fig. 5. (A) Ultrasound image of a first metatarsophalangeal joint with double-contour sign (*asterisk*). White arrows outline the synovial lining. MT, metatarsal head; P, phalangeal head. (B) Ultrasound image of a metatarsophalangeal joint in transverse orientation with hyperechoic tophi and increased Doppler signal indicating active inflammation (asterisk). Arrows outline the synovial lining.

1β generation and inflammasome activation. It also prevents neutrophil migration and activity, which causes gout symptoms.[5,28]

Oral colchicine is most effective when given early during the acute flare, that is, within the first 36 hours of symptom onset.[29] The recommended dosing regimen in

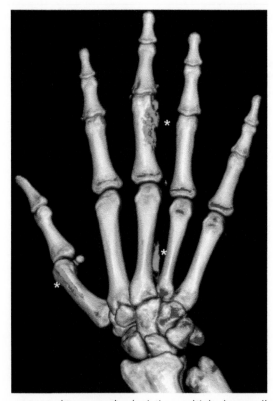

Fig. 6. Dual energy computed tomography depicting multiple dense collections of monosodium urate crystals (*asterisks*) consistent with tophaceous gout. Green is indicative of monosodium urate crystals.

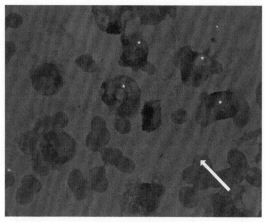

Fig. 7. Polarizing microscopy at an original magnification of x100 demonstrating positively birefringent rhomboid-shaped calcium pyrophosphate crystals present within neutrophils (*asterisks*). Polarizer is directed in the upward-left direction as indicated by the white arrow. (*Courtesy of* Jordan M. Hall, MD, Dept of Pathology, BAMC, San Antonio, TX)

an acute episode is 1.2 mg as a single dose followed 1 hour later by a single 0.6-mg dose.[30] This regimen is typically followed by colchicine 0.6 mg twice daily until symptoms resolve. Gastrointestinal toxicity, including diarrhea and severe nausea, is the most common dose-limiting side effect. Because colchicine is metabolized and eliminated by P-glycoprotein and cytochrome P4503A4, combining it with medications such as clarithromycin, erythromycin, verapamil extended release, diltiazem extended release, and cyclosporine, can result in severe toxicity.[31] The concomitant use of statins increases the risk of myopathy and rhabdomyolysis. Colchicine clearance is decreased in patients with impaired renal function. Low-dose colchicine should be reduced by at least 50% for patients with stage III chronic kidney disease or worse, and the treating clinician should exercise increased caution when considering this treatment in those with more advanced renal disease.[29]

Nonsteroidal Antiinflammatory Drugs

Nonsteroidal antiinflammatory drugs (NSAIDs) inhibit prostaglandin synthesis and reduce inflammation and pain in an acute gout flare. No specific NSAID is recommended over another. Prescribing at the full-strength dose until the acute gout attack has resolved is recommended regardless of the NSAID chosen.[29] Unfortunately, oral NSAID use is limited and complicated by conditions including gastropathy, nephropathy, liver dysfunction, and platelet dysfunction.

A study with initial results made recently available examined the use of naproxen compared with colchicine as the first-choice treatment.[32] Findings from this study suggest that both naproxen and low-dose colchicine are effective in the treatment of acute gout, but there were less side effects with naproxen and possibly greater analgesic effect. This is in line the ACR 2012 guidelines that recommend equally considering an NSAID, oral colchicine, or systemic corticosteroids[29] (**Table 3**).

Systemic Corticosteroids

Corticosteroids reduce the activation, proliferation, and survival of a variety of inflammatory cells. They decrease migration of neutrophils, inhibit prostaglandins and

Table 2
Comparison of the ACR, ACP, and EULAR recommendations for acute and chronic gout management

	ACR	ACP	EULAR
Acute Attack management	Colchicine and NSAIDs as first line, alone or in combination in refractory cases; intraarticular corticosteroid can be considered in cases of 1–2 large joints involved	Steroids first line, can consider colchicine or NSAIDs	Colchicine and/or NSAIDs, oral corticosteroid, or intraarticular corticosteroid
Acute attack management in NPO patient	Intraarticular corticosteroids vs IV/IM methylprednisolone 0.5–2.0 mg/kg	Not addressed	Not addressed
Indication for ULT	Tophi on clinical examination or imaging study, frequency ≥2 attacks per year, CKD stage 2 or worse, past urolithiasis	Not after first attack or <2 attacks per year; use in ≥2 attacks per year or gouty tophi, CKD, or urolithiasis	Recurrent flares, tophi, urate arthropathy and/or renal stones, young age (<40) or very high serum urate (>8 mg/dL) and/or comorbidities (renal disease, HTN, ischemic heart disease, heart failure)
Initial ULT	Allopurinol (starting dose 100 mg/d) or febuxostat 40mg/d	Allopurinol or febuxostat	Allopurinol at 100 mg/d in those with normal renal function, and increase by 100 mg increments every 2–4 wk
Prophylaxis with concomitant ULT	Low-dose NSAID or low-dose colchicine; continue for ≥6 mo; or 3 mo after achieving target serum urate in patients with no tophi or 6 mo after achieving target serum urate in patients with tophi	Low-dose colchicine or low-dose NSAIDs for ≥8 wk while initiating ULT	Prophylaxis with low-dose colchicine for first 6 mo of ULT; if colchicine not tolerated/contraindicated consider low-dose NSAID
Gout flare during ULT	Continue ULT, treat for acute attack	Not addressed	Not addressed
ULT strategy	Treat to target uric acid goal <6 mg/dL at minimum, and in select cases <5 mg/dL; titrate ULT every 2–5 wk to obtain serum urate goal	Treat to avoidance of gout attacks	Goal serum urate <6 mg/dL, or <5 mg/dL in those with severe gout

Abbreviations: ACP, American College of Physicians; ACR, American College of Rheumatology; CKD, chronic kidney disease; EULAR, European League Against Rheumatism; HTN, hypertension; IV/IM, intravenous/intramuscular; NSAID, nonsteroidal antiinflammatory drug; ULT, urate-lowering therapy.
Data from Refs.[26,27,37]

proinflammatory cytokines such as IL-1β.[33] Although there are no placebo-controlled trials examining the efficacy of oral corticosteroids, multiple studies have assessed the effectiveness of corticosteroids against NSAIDs. Both treatment modalities demonstrated similarity in time to symptom resolution and pain reduction, although NSAIDs[34] demonstrated increased gastrointestinal and other NSAID-associated adverse events. A single dose of intramuscular (IM) corticosteroids, such as triamcinolone acetonide or methylprednisolone acetate, is also efficacious in the treatment of acute gout[34,35] (see **Table 3**). Systemic corticosteroids are particularly useful if the acute attack is severe and polyarticular. High doses of corticosteroids are typically required, with starting doses of prednisone typically 0.5 mg to 1 mg/kg tapered over 7 to 14 days.[29]

Intraarticular Steroids

Intraarticular steroid injection is useful in patients with severe attacks involving 1 or 2 joints, especially in large weight-bearing joints. Additionally, this is a useful treatment modality in such patients where NSAIDs and colchicine are contraindicated. One study evaluated intraarticular triamcinolone acetonide 10 mg, which resulted in pain relief within 48 hours in all 19 study patients with no significant side effects or rebound attacks, and no additional treatment needed for the given attack.[36] Dosage of corticosteroid should be adjusted to the size of the joint.

Interleukin-1 Inhibition

IL-1β is activated by the initial inflammasome response to the MSU crystals, and then further propagates the inflammatory reaction. Thus, there are high levels of interest in blocking this pathway with anti–IL-1 agents, including anakinra (IL-1 receptor antagonist) and canakinumab (anti–IL-1β monoclonal antibody). Canakinumab is approved for acute gout in Europe.[37] These agents offer effective treatment for patients in whom first-line acute therapies provided an inadequate response or are contraindicated. Both canakinumab and anakinra are injected subcutaneously at the first sign of an acute gout attack. Current infection is a contraindication to the use of IL-1 blockers.

Table 3 Common dosing and frequency for antiinflammatory medications used in acute gout	
Nonsteroidal Antiinflammatory	**Dosage and Frequency**
Ibuprofen	600–800 mg 3 times daily
Naproxen	500 mg twice daily
Indomethacin	50 mg 3 times daily
Others	
Colchicine	Acute: 1.2 mg followed by 0.6 mg 1 hour later, then 0.6 mg twice daily
Corticosteroids	
IM methylprednisolone	0.5-2.0 mg/kg IV or IM
Prednisone	0.5 mg/kg for 5–10 d then discontinue vs 0.5 mg/kg/day for 2-5 days then taper for 7-10 days
Intraarticular corticosteroid	Dosed based on joint size

Abbreviation: IV/IM, intravenous/intramuscular.
Data from Refs.[27,29,37]

Chronic Urate-Lowering Therapy

The mainstay of treatment in gout is the use of urate-lowering therapy (ULT) to prevent acute flares and ultimately to prevent erosive, destructive, and debilitating joint disease. Aside from obvious functional improvements related to the avoidance of attacks, joint destruction, and tophaceous disease, a recent study found that allopurinol use was associated with decreased acute cardiovascular events in patients with comorbid gout and diabetes.[25] The urate-lowering agents work in various ways to either prevent the production of urate or enhance its excretion.

The treating clinician should consider several factors when deciding whether to initiate long-term ULT. After the initial acute gout attack, the asymptomatic intercritical period may last years in some patients. For this reason, the ACR, EULAR, and ACP guidelines agree that chronic ULT does not need to be started immediately after the first attack in the absence of tophi, nephrolithiasis, chronic kidney disease, or multiple prior attacks ($\geq$2 per year).[29,37] The risk–benefit ratio of starting any lifelong ULT should be discussed individually with a patient. Once initiated, ULT should be continued during any subsequent gout flares and the acute flare should be treated appropriately.

The ACR and EULAR recommend treating to a target serum urate level given that there is decreased uric acid precipitation when serum levels are less than 6 mg/dL.[26] Furthermore, both the ACR and EULAR recognize that for severe disease with tophi, chronic gouty arthritis, or frequent attacks, a lower serum urate target (<5 mg/dL) may be necessary to speed dissolution of crystals. In contrast, the ACP recommends using a "treat to avoid symptoms" approach.[27] This recommendation is based primarily on the relative lack of studies looking specifically at the efficacy of uric acid targets. The primary concern of most rheumatologists is that, even in the absence of acute attacks, MSU crystals continue to deposit in the joints and tissues, and cause cartilage damage and bone erosion.

For many years, it was thought that ULT initiation during an acute episode would prolong the painful gout attack. However, there are 2 high-quality randomized controlled trials that found that initiating allopurinol during an acute gout attack does not adversely affect the resolution of the acute attack, as long as effective acute management has been instituted.[38,39] This finding supports the ACR recommendation that pharmacologic ULT can be started during an acute attack.

Prophylaxis of Acute Gout During Urate-Lowering Therapy

It is well-documented that the initiation of serum ULT is associated with an increased frequency of acute gout flares.[40] Acute gouty attacks during the first months of ULT contribute to decreased adherence.[40,41] All 3 guidelines from the ACR, EULAR, and ACP agree that patients starting ULT should concomitantly receive daily prophylaxis for acute gout. The first-line agents are either low-dose colchicine (0.6 mg twice daily, adjusted for creatinine clearance or drug interactions) or low-dose NSAIDs (naproxen 250 mg twice a day). Prophylaxis should generally be continued for at least 3 months after achieving the target serum urate levels and 6 months after achieving target urate levels in patients with tophi.[26,27,37] For patients who have contraindications to colchicine or NSAIDs, low-dose corticosteroids (prednisone <10 mg) may be considered. There are also data supporting the possibility of using IL-1 inhibitors (anakinra, canakinumab, rilonacept), but none of them are approved for prophylactic treatment yet.[42]

Xanthine Oxidase Inhibition

XO inhibitors are recommended as first-line ULT by the ACR, ACP, and EULAR. XO inhibition is effective regardless of whether the hyperuricemia is due to overproduction or underexcretion. Therefore, it is not necessary to order a 24-hour urine uric acid in all patients before beginning ULT.

Allopurinol

The first XO inhibitor to be used for chronic ULT was allopurinol. The recommended starting dose is 100 mg/d.[26,37] In patients with a glomerular filtration rate of less than 30 mL/min, the initial dose should be no higher than 50 mg/d.[43] Upward titration of the starting dose can occur every 2 to 5 weeks in intervals of 100 mg in normal individuals, and by 50 mg every 2 to 5 weeks in those with a glomerular filtration rate of less than 30 mL/min.[44] Following these guidelines, allopurinol can be safely increased to achieve target serum urate, including in those with a reduced glomerular filtration rate.[44] Most patients will require doses greater than 300 mg/d. The maximum US Food and Drug Administration–approved dose of allopurinol is 800 mg/d.

Allopurinol is generally well-tolerated, although side effects include nausea, diarrhea, and transaminase elevation. The dreaded complication is the allopurinol hypersensitivity syndrome (AHS), characterized by Stevens-Johnson syndrome and toxic epidermal necrolysis, eosinophilia, leukocytosis, fever, hepatitis, and renal failure.[43] The AHS occurs in only 0.1% of patients but it is associated with high mortality and there is no proven treatment, other than allopurinol withdrawal.[44] Risk factors for the AHS include a higher starting dose of allopurinol, increased age, renal impairment, diuretic use, and some ethnic groups. The HLA-B*5801 genotype is associated with an increased risk of AHS.[45,46] The ACR recommends that patients of Han Chinese, Korean, or Thai descent should be screened for the HLA-B*5801 allele and that those with a positive test should not receive allopurinol.[46] It is generally recommended that allopurinol should be stopped at the first sign of a rash. The AHS almost always begins within the first 8 weeks after initiating allopurinol.[45]

Medications to avoid concomitantly with allopurinol include azathioprine, 6-mercaptopurine, and theophylline, because the inhibition of XO can result in severe toxicity of these medications with slowed metabolism and toxic effects.

Febuxostat

Febuxostat is started at a dose of 40 mg/d, and can be increased to 80 mg/d if uric acid does not reach goal after 2 to 4 weeks. Studies have demonstrated that the 40-mg dose of febuxostat is comparable with 300 mg allopurinol dosing for patients with normal renal function. Febuxostat is also safe for use in those with chronic kidney disease stages II and III.[47]

Febuxostat can be used in cases of allopurinol intolerance or inadequate uric acid response to allopurinol. It does not have known cross-reactivity with allopurinol, given that it has a different molecular structure. Because of this, febuxostat is safe to use in patients who have experienced a severe allopurinol adverse reaction, including the AHS.[48] The most common side effects include diarrhea and elevation of liver transaminase enzymes. However, because febuxostat inhibits XO, there are still major potential drug interactions with concomitant use of azathioprine, 6-mercaptopurine, and theophylline.

Treatment of Refractory Gout

Multiple studies have suggested medication nonadherence in gout patients. A systematic review revealed that the proportion of medication-compliant patients with gout is only 10% to 46%.[49] Thus, for those not responding to XO inhibitors, a discussion of mediation compliance and its rationale may provide therapeutic benefits.

Uricosurics

Uricosuric agents increase renal uric acid excretion. The multiple contraindications to uricosuric ULT and drug interactions are the reason they are not considered first-line ULT treatment by any of the major societies. However, they may be useful in cases where XO inhibitors are contraindicated or when an additional urate-lowering effect is needed.

A history of nephrolithiasis presents an important contraindication to uricosurics. Elevated urinary uric acid levels are also a contraindication to uricosuric ULT because this finding indicates uric acid overproduction.[26] Furthermore, they are ineffective in the setting of renal insufficiency with a creatinine clearance of less than 50 mL/min. Uricosurics are also associated with many different drug interactions, resulting in either altered levels of the uricosuric agent or the urinary excretion of other drugs. Medication classes that should be avoided in combination with uricosurics include penicillins, cephalosporins, nitrofurantoin, and NSAIDs, including indomethacin, ketorolac, zidovudine, and methotrexate.

Probenecid

Probenecid is a uricosuric agent that inhibits urate anion reabsorption in the proximal renal tubule (see **Fig. 2**). It is approved for monotherapy but it can also be used in combination with XO inhibitors. Typically, this medication is started at 250 mg twice daily and titrated up to 1000 mg twice daily.

Lesinurad

Lesinurad is another uricosuric agent that decreases uric acid reabsorption in the proximal renal tubule (see **Fig. 2**). A recent double-blind randomized controlled trial found that lesinurad 200 and 400 mg/d in combination with allopurinol 300 mg/d were associated with 52% and 59% of subjects, respectively, achieving a urate level of less than 6 mg/dL at 6 months, as opposed to only 27.9% in the allopurinol-only group.[50] A study is currently underway to evaluate lesinurad as monotherapy (clinicaltrials.gov identifier NCT01508702).

Lowering Urate as a Side Effect

Multiple medications may provide ancillary benefit to traditional ULT. Calcium channel blockers, fenofibrate, and losartan have been found to have modest uricosuric effects and can be added to other ULT.[51]

Uricase

Pegloticase is a recombinant porcine–baboon uricase that converts uric acid to allantoin, which is a more soluble compound that can be easily excreted in the urine (see **Fig. 2**). Pegloticase has been proven to rapidly reduce serum urate levels, which can lead to more rapid resolution of gout attacks and tophi.[52] Severe infusion-related reactions can occur. Preinfusion serum urate levels are monitored, because a loss of response is indicative of drug antibody development. Patients should also be screened for G6PD deficiency before use. This medication is only recommended in severe refractory cases in which other standard treatments are contraindicated.[29,53]

Dietary Modification

Data on the impact of dietary intake generally suggests that purine-rich foods, especially red meat, organ meat, shellfish, high-fructose and glycemic index foods, and alcohol, particularly beers and ales, contribute to hyperuricemia.[54] However, other purine-rich foods such as legumes, fruits, and vegetables do not increase the risk of gout. There is an inverse relationship between increased dairy consumption and serum urate.[55] Additionally, vitamin C may have a mild urate-lowering effect and the consumption of cherries may reduce the risk of recurrent gout attacks.[54] Generally, avoiding excess calorie consumption and decreasing body mass index seems to reduce the risk of gout.[54,56] Although dietary modification and fitness are recommended by both the ACR and EULAR, strict lifestyle modification alone is unlikely to reduce serum urate levels by more than 10% to 18%.[26,53,56] Therefore, most patients will also require pharmacologic ULT.

CALCIUM PYROPHOSPHATE DEPOSITION DISEASE

Pseudogout is clinically similar to gout, but is due to the presence of calcium pyrophosphate (CPP) and not MSU crystals.[57] In this section, we discuss the pathophysiology, epidemiology, clinical presentation and diagnosis, risk factors, and management of pseudogout.

Nomenclature

It is impossible to address "pseudogout" without also addressing the confusing nomenclature. Originally coined as pseudogout, this disease has also been known by several other terms. In 2011, the EULAR recommended a more consistent naming pattern, with the use of CPP crystals to refer to the crystals themselves and CPP deposition (CPPD) as an umbrella term to refer to all occurrences of CPP crystals.[58] The term chondrocalcinosis refers to the radiographic findings consistent with CPPD.

Pathophysiology of Calcium Pyrophosphate Deposition and Inflammation

CPPD is characterized by the deposition of CPP crystals in the articular hyaline and fibrocartilage. The pathogenesis of CPPD is not as clearly defined as gout, but it is known that the first step includes an overproduction of inorganic pyrophosphate anions by chondrocytes. Ultimately, the formation of CPP crystals within the joint cartilage matrix is due to the interaction of the cation, calcium, and the anion, inorganic pyrophosphate.[59] These crystals result in inflammatory-mediated damage by activation of the innate immune system, just as discussed in gout.

Although the articular cartilage is specialized to avoid calcification, the degenerative changes to chondrocytes and cartilage as seen in osteoarthritis, and even normal aging, predisposes to pathologic crystal deposition. Conditions including hyperparathyroidism, hypophosphatasia, hypomagnesemia, and hemochromatosis may predispose to crystal deposition owing to increased inorganic pyrophosphate levels in the synovium.[59–61] Upon generation of CPP crystals, the NLRP3 inflammasome complex is activated, as in gout, to secrete the inflammatory cytokine IL-1β. Additionally, neutrophils are activated and a prolonged neutrophilic inflammatory response is observed in patients with acute CPPD arthritis.[62] Although less well-understood, the long-term presence of these CPP deposits within the synovium results in chronic changes similar to that in osteoarthritis.

Epidemiology and Risk Factors

CPPD is usually found in patients over the age of 60 and there is a strong association with advancing age.[63,64] The prevalence of chondrocalcinosis depends on the joint imaged. Radiographic chondrocalcinosis affects up to 7% to 8% of the middle-aged to elderly adult European and US populations and has been reported in up to 44% of patients over the age of 84 years.[64] However, a definitive diagnosis of CPPD arthritis requires positive identification of CPP crystals on synovial fluid analysis. Radiographic chondrocalcinosis is often asymptomatic and does not always lead to clinical CPPD, making the true estimation of clinical disease uncertain. Conversely, chondrocalcinosis may be difficult to visualize by conventional radiography in some joints despite identification of CPP crystals from the joint. Chondrocalcinosis likely only identifies 40% of those with clinical CPPD disease.[65]

Advancing age is the primary risk factor for developing CPPD. In addition, multiple metabolic conditions increase the risk for development of CPPD, including primary hyperparathyroidism, hemochromatosis, hypomagnesemia, hypophosphatemia, and osteoarthritis in the affected joint[66] (**Table 4**). Acute cases may be associated with trauma or even in acute systemic illness. Of note, there are no particular dietary associations with CPPD development.

Clinical Presentation

Acute arthritis

The most common presentation of acute CPPD arthritis is monoarthritis affecting large joints, most often the knee or wrist, and less frequently the elbow. Analogous to the presentation of acute gout, patients may have severe and sudden inflammation with painful swelling. Attacks typically last as long as 10 days, but unlike typical gout attacks, can linger for weeks. CPPD can cause an oligoarthritis, polyarthritis, or even migratory or additive acute arthritis. In some patients, acute episodes may present similar to rheumatoid arthritis, with inflammation of multiple small joints that can include the metacarpophalangeal joints while also affecting the large joints. In elderly patients, a positive rheumatoid factor may create diagnostic confusion.[60,67] Concomitant fevers and malaise may raise suspicion for septic arthritis given the similarity in presentation and elevated erythrocyte sedimentation rate and C-reactive protein.

Axial disease

CPPD can occur in the axial skeleton, including the atlantoaxial junction, facet and intervertebral joints, and discs. The crowned dens syndrome is due to CPPD at the atlantoaxial junction with calcifications around the dens. Acute attacks may present with severe neck pain, neck rigidity, and fever, and could be misdiagnosed as

Table 4
Comorbidities associated with CPPD and their associated laboratory evaluation

Comorbidity	OR for CPPD[63]	Testing
Hyperparathyroidism	3.35	PTH and calcium increased
Osteoarthritis	2.26	Clinical, radiography
Hemochromatosis	1.87	Ferritin elevated, serum transferrin elevated
Hypomagnesemia	1.23	Low magnesium
Calcium supplementation	1.15	n/a
Chronic kidney disease	1.12	Creatinine, glomerular filtration rate

Abbreviations: CPPD, calcium pyrophosphate deposition; n/a, not applicable; OR, odds ratio; PTH, parathyroid hormone.
From Kleiber Balderrama C, Rosenthal AK, Lans D, et al. Calcium pyrophosphate deposition disease and associated medical co-morbidities: a national cross-sectional study of US veterans. Arthritis Care Res (Hoboken) 2017;69(9):1400–6.

meningitis, polymyalgia rheumatica, or temporal arteritis.[68] Chronic instability of the atlantoaxial joint can result in a severe myelopathy and death.

Chronic Osteoarthritis-Like Calcium Pyrophosphate Deposition

This clinical phenotype resembles osteoarthritis. However, joints such as the shoulder (glenohumoral joint), metacarpophalangeal joints, wrists and elbows, which are not typical of primary osteoarthritis, are often involved. Also, unlike typical osteoarthritis, patients will have flares of inflammatory arthritis.

Diagnosis

CPPD is an underdiagnosed condition. The gold standard lies in obtaining positively birefringent, rhomboid-shaped crystals from synovial fluid of an affected joint (**Fig. 8**). The synovial fluid is typically highly inflammatory with elevated leukocyte counts during an acute attack. Ancillary testing includes radiography with chondrocalcinosis, the radiographic appearance of CPP crystals. CPP crystal deposition appears as heavy rounded calcifications within the fibrocartilage (eg, knee meniscus and triangular fibrocartilage of the wrist), or hyaline (articular) cartilage. Ultrasound examination is a useful tool to detect CPP crystal deposition in cartilage, particularly in the knee.[69] Ultrasound imaging can also distinguish chondrocalcinosis from MSU deposition. CPPD is identified as hyperechoic rounded deposits with in the substance of the cartilage, as opposed to MSU crystals, which appear more linear and deposit on the surface of the cartilage.[70] More advanced imaging modalities include DECT scanning for detection of calcium-containing crystals.

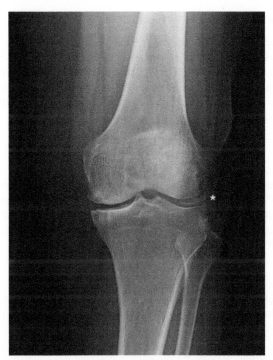

Fig. 8. Weight-bearing knee radiograph depicting chondrocalcinosis within the fibrocartilage (asterisk) and medial compartment joint-space narrowing and subchondral sclerosis (adjacent to asterisk) consistent with concomitant osteoarthritis.

TREATMENT

Acute calcium pyrophosphate deposition arthritis

The acute arthritis owing to CPPD is highly inflammatory and involves activation of the innate immune system and many of the same inflammatory mechanisms as gout. Therefore, the treatment for acute CPPD arthritis is similar to the treatment for acute gouty arthritis. CPPD may respond well to intraarticular corticosteroid injection.[53] However, in patients with a polyarticular flare in which injection of each individual joint is not practical, systemic corticosteroid dosing with prednisone or IM injection of triamcinolone or methylprednisolone can be used.[55] NSAIDs at a full-strength dose and even colchicine, dosed as used in gout, may also relieve inflammation and pain in the acute period.[54]

Chronic calcium pyrophosphate deposition

The approach to chronic CPPD arthritis is problematic given that there is frequently comorbid degenerative joint disease. There are no well-studied, evidence-based chronic suppressive treatment regimens or definitive strategies to lower CPP levels. Rather, there are case reports and small case series reporting the use of colchicine,[71] IL-1 inhibition,[53] and hydroxychloroquine[72] with varying success. A small randomized placebo-controlled trial recently evaluated methotrexate efficacy in chronic or recurrent CPPD arthritis. Unfortunately, the results indicated that methotrexate did not provide a significant benefit.[73] Aside from low-dose colchicine, we would recommend treating only in consultation with a rheumatologist with any of these other DMARD or biologic treatments given the risks and side effect profiles.

REFERRAL TO A RHEUMATOLOGIST FOR GOUT OR PSEUDOGOUT

Ultimately, the time to refer a patient to a rheumatologist relies on a shared decision between the provider and patient. Recalcitrant disease warrants referral for evaluation of other potential etiologies and use of less traditional therapies. Patients with comorbidities that portend a more difficult treatment course owing to contraindications to use of traditional gout medications, such as posttransplant patients taking cyclosporine or azathioprine, warrant specialty consultation.

SUMMARY

Gout and pseudogout represent entities that present commonly to primary care clinics. Upon recognition, gout may be effectively treated in both the acute and chronic stages. Patient medication noncompliance is a common cause of recurrent gout. Pseudogout should be differentiated from gout, because the chronic therapies used in gout will not provide benefit. However, acute CPPD arthritis can be effectively managed using many of the same therapies.

REFERENCES

1. Zhu Y, Pandya BJ, Choi HK. Prevalence of gout and hyperuricemia in the US general population: the National Health and Nutrition Examination Survey 2007-2008. Arthritis Rheum 2011;63(10):3136–41.
2. Levinson DJ, Decker DE, Sorensen LB. Renal handling of uric acid in man. Ann Clin Lab Sci 1982;12(1):73–7.
3. Hatch LL, Sevanian A. Measurement of uric acid, ascorbic acid, and related metabolites in biological fluids. Anal Biochem 1984;138(2):324–8.

4. Hyndman D, Liu S, Miner JN. Urate handling in the human body. Curr Rheumatol Rep 2016;18(6):34.

5. Martinon F, Petrilli V, Mayor A, et al. Gout-associated uric acid crystals activate the NALP3 inflammasome. Nature 2006;440(7081):237–41.

6. Cleophas MC, Crisan TO, Joosten LA. Factors modulating the inflammatory response in acute gouty arthritis. Curr Opin Rheumatol 2017;29(2):163–70.

7. Chhana A, Callon KE, Pool B, et al. Monosodium urate monohydrate crystals inhibit osteoblast viability and function: implications for development of bone erosion in gout. Ann Rheum Dis 2011;70(9):1684–91.

8. Arromdee E, Michet CJ, Crowson CS, et al. Epidemiology of gout: is the incidence rising? J Rheumatol 2002;29(11):2403–6.

9. Hak AE, Choi HK. Menopause, postmenopausal hormone use and serum uric acid levels in US women–the Third National Health and Nutrition Examination Survey. Arthritis Res Ther 2008;10(5):R116.

10. Fang J, Alderman MH. Serum uric acid and cardiovascular mortality the NHANES I epidemiologic follow-up study, 1971-1992. National Health and Nutrition Examination Survey. JAMA 2000;283(18):2404–10.

11. Chen JH, Yeh WT, Chuang SY, et al. Gender-specific risk factors for incident gout: a prospective cohort study. Clin Rheumatol 2012;31(2):239–45.

12. Chen JH, Pan WH, Hsu CC, et al. Impact of obesity and hypertriglyceridemia on gout development with or without hyperuricemia: a prospective study. Arthritis Care Res (Hoboken) 2013;65(1):133–40.

13. Hui JY, Choi JW, Mount DB, et al. The independent association between parathyroid hormone levels and hyperuricemia: a national population study. Arthritis Res Ther 2012;14(2):R56.

14. Lim SY, Lu N, Choi HK. Septic arthritis in gout patients: a population-based cohort study. Rheumatology (Oxford) 2015;54(11):2095–9.

15. Pascual E, Batlle-Gualda E, Martinez A, et al. Synovial fluid analysis for diagnosis of intercritical gout. Ann Intern Med 1999;131(10):756–9.

16. Ogdie A, Taylor WJ, Neogi T, et al. Performance of ultrasound in the diagnosis of gout in a multicenter study: comparison with monosodium urate monohydrate crystal analysis as the gold standard. Arthritis Rheumatol 2017;69(2):429–38.

17. Dalbeth N, House ME, Horne A, et al. Reduced creatinine clearance is associated with early development of subcutaneous tophi in people with gout. BMC Musculoskelet Disord 2013;14:363.

18. Schlesinger N. Diagnosis of gout: clinical, laboratory, and radiologic findings. Am J Manag Care 2005;11(15 Suppl):S443–50 [quiz: S465–8].

19. Neogi T, Jansen TL, Dalbeth N, et al. 2015 Gout classification criteria: an American College of Rheumatology/European League Against Rheumatism collaborative initiative. Ann Rheum Dis 2015;74(10):1789–98.

20. Bloch C, Hermann G, Yu TF. A radiologic reevaluation of gout: a study of 2,000 patients. AJR Am J Roentgenol 1980;134(4):781–7.

21. Omoumi P, Zufferey P, Malghem J, et al. Imaging in gout and other crystal-related arthropathies. Rheum Dis Clin North Am 2016;42(4):621–44.

22. Lee YH, Song GG. Diagnostic accuracy of dual-energy computed tomography in patients with gout: a meta-analysis. Semin Arthritis Rheum 2017;47(1):95–101.

23. Baer AN, Kurano T, Thakur UJ, et al. Dual-energy computed tomography has limited sensitivity for non-tophaceous gout: a comparison study with tophaceous gout. BMC Musculoskelet Disord 2016;17:91.

24. Bongartz T, Glazebrook KN, Kavros SJ, et al. Dual-energy CT for the diagnosis of gout: an accuracy and diagnostic yield study. Ann Rheum Dis 2015;74(6): 1072–7.

25. Singh JA, Ramachandaran R, Yu S, et al. Allopurinol use and the risk of acute cardiovascular events in patients with gout and diabetes. BMC Cardiovasc Disord 2017;17(1):76.

26. Khanna D, Fitzgerald JD, Khanna PP, et al. 2012 American College of Rheumatology guidelines for management of gout. Part 1: systematic nonpharmacologic and pharmacologic therapeutic approaches to hyperuricemia. Arthritis Care Res (Hoboken) 2012;64(10):1431–46.

27. Qaseem A, Harris RP, Forciea MA, Clinical Guidelines Committee of the American College of Physicians, et al. Management of acute and recurrent gout: a clinical practice guideline from the American College of Physicians. Ann Intern Med 2017;166(1):58–68.

28. Slobodnick A, Shah B, Pillinger MH, et al. Colchicine: old and new. Am J Med 2015;128(5):461–70.

29. Khanna D, Khanna PP, Fitzgerald JD, et al. 2012 American College of Rheumatology guidelines for management of gout. Part 2: therapy and antiinflammatory prophylaxis of acute gouty arthritis. Arthritis Care Res (Hoboken) 2012;64(10): 1447–61.

30. Terkeltaub RA, Furst DE, Bennett K, et al. High versus low dosing of oral colchicine for early acute gout flare: twenty-four-hour outcome of the first multicenter, randomized, double-blind, placebo-controlled, parallel-group, dose-comparison colchicine study. Arthritis Rheum 2010;62(4):1060–8.

31. Terkeltaub RA, Furst DE, Digiacinto JL, et al. Novel evidence-based colchicine dose-reduction algorithm to predict and prevent colchicine toxicity in the presence of cytochrome P450 3A4/P-glycoprotein inhibitors. Arthritis Rheum 2011; 63(8):2226–37.

32. Roddy E. Colchicine or naproxen treatment for acute gout: a randomised controlled trial. Raw Data ClinicalTrialsgov Identifier: NCT01994226. 2016.

33. Schlesinger N. Treatment of acute gout. Rheum Dis Clin North Am 2014;40(2): 329–41.

34. Khanna PP, Gladue HS, Singh MK, et al. Treatment of acute gout: a systematic review. Semin Arthritis Rheum 2014;44(1):31–8.

35. Zhang YK, Yang H, Zhang JY, et al. Comparison of intramuscular compound betamethasone and oral diclofenac sodium in the treatment of acute attacks of gout. Int J Clin Pract 2014;68(5):633–8.

36. Fernandez C, Noguera R, Gonzalez JA, et al. Treatment of acute attacks of gout with a small dose of intraarticular triamcinolone acetonide. J Rheumatol 1999; 26(10):2285–6.

37. Richette P, Doherty M, Pascual E, et al. 2016 updated EULAR evidence-based recommendations for the management of gout. Ann Rheum Dis 2017;76(1): 29–42.

38. Hill EM, Sky K, Sit M, et al. Does starting allopurinol prolong acute treated gout? A randomized clinical trial. J Clin Rheumatol 2015;21(3):120–5.

39. Taylor TH, Mecchella JN, Larson RJ, et al. Initiation of allopurinol at first medical contact for acute attacks of gout: a randomized clinical trial. Am J Med 2012; 125(11):1126–34.e7.

40. Becker MA, MacDonald PA, Hunt BJ, et al. Determinants of the clinical outcomes of gout during the first year of urate-lowering therapy. Nucleosides Nucleotides Nucleic Acids 2008;27(6):585–91.

41. Latourte A, Bardin T, Richette P. Prophylaxis for acute gout flares after initiation of urate-lowering therapy. Rheumatology (Oxford) 2014;53(11):1920–6.
42. Terkeltaub RA, Schumacher HR, Carter JD, et al. Rilonacept in the treatment of acute gouty arthritis: a randomized, controlled clinical trial using indomethacin as the active comparator. Arthritis Res Ther 2013;15(1):R25.
43. Stamp LK, Taylor WJ, Jones PB, et al. Starting dose is a risk factor for allopurinol hypersensitivity syndrome: a proposed safe starting dose of allopurinol. Arthritis Rheum 2012;64(8):2529–36.
44. Stamp LK, Chapman PT, Barclay ML, et al. A randomised controlled trial of the efficacy and safety of allopurinol dose escalation to achieve target serum urate in people with gout. Ann Rheum Dis 2017;76(9):1522–8.
45. Stamp LK, Day RO, Yun J. Allopurinol hypersensitivity: investigating the cause and minimizing the risk. Nat Rev Rheumatol 2016;12(4):235–42.
46. Somkrua R, Eickman EE, Saokaew S, et al. Association of HLA-B*5801 allele and allopurinol-induced Stevens Johnson syndrome and toxic epidermal necrolysis: a systematic review and meta-analysis. BMC Med Genet 2011;12:118.
47. Becker MA, Schumacher HR, Espinoza LR, et al. The urate-lowering efficacy and safety of febuxostat in the treatment of the hyperuricemia of gout: the CONFIRMS trial. Arthritis Res Ther 2010;12(2):R63.
48. Chohan S. Safety and efficacy of febuxostat treatment in subjects with gout and severe allopurinol adverse reactions. J Rheumatol 2011;38(9):1957–9.
49. De Vera MA, Marcotte G, Rai S, et al. Medication adherence in gout: a systematic review. Arthritis Care Res (Hoboken) 2014;66(10):1551–9.
50. Saag KG, Fitz-Patrick D, Kopicko J, et al. Lesinurad combined with allopurinol: a randomized, double-blind, placebo-controlled study in gout patients with an inadequate response to standard-of-care allopurinol (a US-based study). Arthritis Rheumatol 2017;69(1):203–12.
51. Choi HK, Soriano LC, Zhang Y, et al. Antihypertensive drugs and risk of incident gout among patients with hypertension: population based case-control study. BMJ 2012;344:d8190.
52. Baraf HS, Becker MA, Gutierrez-Urena SR, et al. Tophus burden reduction with pegloticase: results from phase 3 randomized trials and open-label extension in patients with chronic gout refractory to conventional therapy. Arthritis Res Ther 2013;15(5):R137.
53. Zhang W, Doherty M, Bardin T, et al. EULAR evidence based recommendations for gout. Part II: management. Report of a task force of the EULAR Standing Committee for International Clinical Studies Including Therapeutics (ESCISIT). Ann Rheum Dis 2006;65(10):1312–24.
54. Kolasinski SL. Food, drink, and herbs: alternative therapies and gout. Curr Rheumatol Rep 2014;16(4):409.
55. Choi HK, Liu S, Curhan G. Intake of purine-rich foods, protein, and dairy products and relationship to serum levels of uric acid: the Third National Health and Nutrition Examination Survey. Arthritis Rheum 2005;52(1):283–9.
56. Dessein PH, Shipton EA, Stanwix AE, et al. Beneficial effects of weight loss associated with moderate calorie/carbohydrate restriction, and increased proportional intake of protein and unsaturated fat on serum urate and lipoprotein levels in gout: a pilot study. Ann Rheum Dis 2000;59(7):539–43.
57. Kohn NN, Hughes RE, Mc CD Jr, et al. The significance of calcium phosphate crystals in the synovial fluid of arthritic patients: the "pseudogout syndrome". II. Identification of crystals. Ann Intern Med 1962;56:738–45.

58. Zhang W, Doherty M, Bardin T, et al. European League Against Rheumatism recommendations for calcium pyrophosphate deposition. Part I: terminology and diagnosis. Ann Rheum Dis 2011;70(4):563–70.
59. Rosenthal AK. Pathogenesis of calcium pyrophosphate crystal deposition disease. Curr Rheumatol Rep 2001;3(1):17–23.
60. Rosenthal AK, Ryan LM. Calcium pyrophosphate deposition disease. N Engl J Med 2016;374(26):2575–84.
61. Rho YH, Zhu Y, Zhang Y, et al. Risk factors for pseudogout in the general population. Rheumatology (Oxford) 2012;51(11):2070–4.
62. Pang L, Hayes CP, Buac K, et al. Pseudogout-associated inflammatory calcium pyrophosphate dihydrate microcrystals induce formation of neutrophil extracellular traps. J Immunol 2013;190(12):6488–500.
63. Felson DT, Anderson JJ, Naimark A, et al. The prevalence of chondrocalcinosis in the elderly and its association with knee osteoarthritis: the Framingham Study. J Rheumatol 1989;16(9):1241–5.
64. Neame RL, Carr AJ, Muir K, et al. UK community prevalence of knee chondrocalcinosis: evidence that correlation with osteoarthritis is through a shared association with osteophyte. Ann Rheum Dis 2003;62(6):513–8.
65. Miksanek J, Rosenthal AK. Imaging of calcium pyrophosphate deposition disease. Curr Rheumatol Rep 2015;17(3):20.
66. Kleiber Balderrama C, Rosenthal AK, Lans D, et al. Calcium pyrophosphate deposition disease and associated medical co-morbidities: a national cross-sectional study of US veterans. Arthritis Care Res (Hoboken) 2017;69(9):1400–6.
67. Masuda I, Ishikawa K. Clinical features of pseudogout attack. A survey of 50 cases. Clin Orthop Relat Res 1988;(229):173–81.
68. Oka A, Okazaki K, Takeno A, et al. Crowned dens syndrome: report of three cases and a review of the literature. J Emerg Med 2015;49(1):e9–13.
69. Filippou G, Scire CA, Damjanov N, et al. Definition and reliability assessment of elementary ultrasonographic findings in calcium pyrophosphate deposition disease: a study by the OMERACT calcium pyrophosphate deposition disease ultrasound subtask force. J Rheumatol 2017;44(11):1744–9.
70. Grassi W, Meenagh G, Pascual E, et al. "Crystal clear"-sonographic assessment of gout and calcium pyrophosphate deposition disease. Semin Arthritis Rheum 2006;36(3):197–202.
71. Alvarellos A, Spilberg I. Colchicine prophylaxis in pseudogout. J Rheumatol 1986;13(4):804–5.
72. Rothschild B, Yakubov LE. Prospective 6-month, double-blind trial of hydroxychloroquine treatment of CPDD. Compr Ther 1997;23(5):327–31.
73. Finckh A, Mc Carthy GM, Madigan A, et al. Methotrexate in chronic-recurrent calcium pyrophosphate deposition disease: no significant effect in a randomized crossover trial. Arthritis Res Ther 2014;16(5):458.

Early Diagnosis and Treatment of Rheumatoid Arthritis

Emily A. Littlejohn, DO[a], Seetha U. Monrad, MD[b],*

KEYWORDS

- Rheumatoid arthritis • Synovitis • Extra-articular manifestations • Diagnostic criteria
- Disease-modifying antirheumatic drugs • Biologic agents

KEY POINTS

- Rheumatoid arthritis (RA) is a chronic, systemic, autoimmune disorder that primarily targets synovial joints, resulting in synovitis, synovial hypertrophy, cartilage and bone destruction, autoantibody production, and systemic symptoms.
- RA classically presents as a symmetric inflammatory polyarthritis involving the hands, wrists, and feet; however, there are several important extra-articular manifestations.
- The 2010 diagnostic criteria emphasize early identification of patients with RA to facilitate early treatment, which results in improved outcomes.
- Pharmacologic treatment involves combinations of anti-inflammatory agents, disease-modifying antirheumatic drugs, and biologic therapies.

INTRODUCTION

Rheumatoid arthritis (RA) is a chronic systemic autoimmune disease that primarily targets synovial joints, resulting in pain and functional limitations. It is the most common inflammatory arthritis, and a significant cause of morbidity and mortality. From the primary care perspective, early recognition of this disease, along with its extra-articular manifestations, can lead to faster time to treatment and better health outcomes, in addition to preserved joint functionality.

EPIDEMIOLOGY

Worldwide, the prevalence of RA is believed to range from 0.4% to 1.3%.[1,2] In 2005, an estimated 1.5 million, or 0.6%, of US adults 18 years or older had RA.[3] According to

[a] Rheumatologic and Immunologic Diseases, Cleveland Clinic, Orthopaedic and Rheumatologic Institute, 9500 Euclid Avenue/A50, Cleveland, OH 44195, USA; [b] Division of Rheumatology, Michigan Medicine, 7D08 North Ingalls Building, 300 North Ingalls Street, Ann Arbor, MI 48109, USA
* Corresponding author.
E-mail address: seetha@med.umich.edu

Prim Care Clin Office Pract 45 (2018) 237–255
https://doi.org/10.1016/j.pop.2018.02.010
0095-4543/18/© 2018 Elsevier Inc. All rights reserved.

primarycare.theclinics.com

the most recent data from the Rochester Epidemiology Project,[3] 41 per 100,000 people were diagnosed with RA annually between 1995 and 2007. Although RA can occur in patients at any age, incidence was found to rise with age; among those aged 18 to 34, 8.7 per 100,000 people were affected; in those aged 65 to 74 years, 89 per 100,000 were affected; and in those 85 years or older, 54 per 100,000 were affected. This study cohort estimated the lifetime risk of RA to be 4% among women and 3% among men.[4]

Given increasing life expectancies worldwide, the number of elderly people with RA is growing.[5] This is important, as therapeutic goals differ according to patient age or presence of risk factors for infection,[5] something that both primary care physicians and rheumatologists should be continually monitoring.

From a public health perspective, people with RA have been found to be significantly more likely to have reduced their work hours or stopped working; they are more likely to have lost their job or to have retired early; and are 3 times more likely to have had a reduction in household family income than either individuals with osteoarthritis (OA) or those without arthritis.[6] In this way, the economic effects of RA are staggering and emphasize the importance of early recognition and treatment.

RISK FACTORS

Although the exact cause of RA is unknown, it is generally accepted that multiple factors likely interact in a genetically susceptible host. Studies suggest that heritability is approximately 65%.[7] Genes within the HLA locus, particularly HLA-DRB1, account for just under half of the genetic component of susceptibility,[8] in addition to being associated with increased disease severity.[9] From a gender perspective, women are 2 to 3 times more likely to develop RA than men. It has been postulated this is in part due to the stimulatory effects of estrogen on the immune system.[10,11] Studies have been largely mixed with regard to pregnancy and the risk of RA development, although show a trend toward a protective effect.[12]

Known risk factors for the development of RA include smoking, obesity, and periodontal disease; the gut microbiome and infections also have been implicated. Smoking confers significant risk for the presence of anti-citrullinated protein antibodies (ACPA or anti-CCP), which are important diagnostic and prognostic markers in RA; the risk is amplified in the presence of specific HLA-DRB1 alleles.[13] This is thought to be due to the immunomodulatory effects of smoking, including decreased phagocytic and antibacterial functions of alveolar macrophages, shifts in cytokine production, and oxidative stress.[13] In addition to its effect on susceptibility, cigarette smoking also may be a risk factor for greater disease severity.[14] Although results are mixed, large epidemiologic studies suggest that obesity may be associated with a modestly increased risk for the development of RA.[15] Other studies have shown that obesity is generally associated with worse subjective measures of disease activity, which may be confounded by osteoarthritis, disability, and chronic pain.[15]

The association between oral disease/periodontitis and RA has been recognized since the early 1800s, with the most rudimentary treatment consisting of tooth extraction. Many large epidemiologic studies and smaller case-control and cohort studies have shown an association between periodontal disease and RA with odds ratios ranging 1.8:1 (95% confidence interval [CI] 1.0–3.2, NS) to 8:1 (95% CI 2.9–22.1, P<.001).[16] An emerging body of evidence has outlined periodontal health and its association with RA through the common periodontal microbe Porphyromonas gingivalis. The specific abilities of P gingivalis to citrullinate host peptides can induce autoimmune responses in RA through development of anti-CCP antibodies.[17] The unique interplay between the gut microbiome and functions of the host immune system also has been implicated as having a potential role in the development of RA through multiple molecular mechanisms.[18]

PATHOPHYSIOLOGY

Exposure of the genetically susceptible host to environmental triggers is thought to result in the immune dysregulation (autoimmunity) that underpins RA.[19] The synovium, or cellular lining of joints, is the primary target of autoimmunity in RA, although the vasculature and other organ systems can be affected. Both adaptive and innate immune responses are implicated in the initiation and perpetuation of RA; T cells (particularly of the Th1 and Th17 subset) predominate in involved synovium. Aberrantly stimulated antigen-presenting cells interact with T and B cells in lymph nodes, promoting cytokine and chemokine production, lymphocyte differentiation, and autoantibody formation. T and B lymphocytes migrate to the joints and interact with resident macrophages, dendritic cells, synoviocytes, and osteoclasts, resulting in the recruitment of additional inflammatory cells to the joint space, production of degradative enzymes and inflammatory cytokines (such as tumor necrosis factor [TNF]-alpha, interleukin [IL]-1, and IL-6), neoangiogenesis, and synoviocyte hyperplasia. These interactions result in *synovitis*, which clinically manifests as swollen, warm, and tender joints. Untreated synovitis can result in an inflammatory, destructive *pannus* that destroys cartilage, bone, and other articular structures, resulting in joint deformity and chronic pain (**Fig. 1**). The importance of the immune dysregulation in RA is highlighted by the effectiveness of newer therapeutic agents that target specific inflammatory cytokines and cells.

DIAGNOSIS

The diagnosis of RA relies on a high index of suspicion based on a thorough patient history and physical examination.

In 2010, the American College of Rheumatology (ACR) and the European League Against Rheumatism (EULAR) put forth the most current criteria for the diagnosis of RA.[20] These guidelines are aimed at identifying RA among patients newly presenting with synovitis in at least one joint, the absence of an alternative diagnosis that better explains the synovitis, and the achievement of a total score of at least 6 (of a possible 10) from 4 domains. These include the following: (1) the number and site of involved joints, (2) serologic abnormalities (presence of rheumatoid factor or anti-citrullinated peptide/protein antibody), (3) elevations of inflammatory markers (erythrocyte sedimentation rate and/or C-reactive protein [CRP]), and (4) the duration of symptoms (**Table 1**). The 2010 criteria differ from previous criteria[21] in their ability to identify and diagnose early (rather than established) RA.

Typically, patients with RA present with symmetric polyarticular joint pain and swelling, most pronounced in the metacarpophalangeal (MCP) and proximal interphalangeal (PIP) joints of the hands. Other commonly affected sites in early disease include the wrists, thumbs, and metatarsophalangeal (MTP) joints of the toes. Arthritis of medium/large joints can present early on in the elbows, shoulders, ankles, and knees, and is associated with more severe disease.[22] Although a symmetric small joint polyarthritis is the most common presentation, it is important to recognize some less common presentations of RA. Monoarticular arthritis is an atypical presentation but may occur. Palindromic rheumatism describes episodic sudden-onset joint pain with one to several joint areas being affected for hours to days, typically involving small joints of the hands, and alternating with symptom-free periods; up to two-thirds of patients with this presentation will develop RA.[23] Rarely, patients will present with

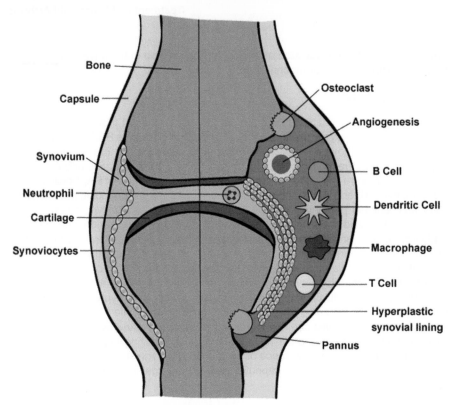

Fig. 1. Pathophysiology of RA. The left half of the picture is of a normal synovial joint; the right half demonstrates key pathophysiologic processes, including synovial hyperplasia, inflammatory cell recruitment, neoangiogenesis, cartilage destruction, and periarticular bony erosions.

Table 1
The 2010 ACR-EULAR rheumatoid arthritis classification criteria

Target population: patients with at least 1 joint with definite clinical synovitis (swelling), and without another cause for the synovitis (eg, other inflammatory arthritis conditions, infection, trauma)

Criteria		Points (need ≥6 total)
Joint involvement	1 large	0
	2–10 large	1
	1–3 small	2
	4–10 small	3
	>10 (at least 1 small)	5
Serology	Negative RF and ACPA	0
	Low positive RF OR low positive ACPA	2
	High positive RF OR high positive ACPA	3
Acute phase reactants	Normal CRP AND normal ESR	0
	Abnormal CRP OR abnormal ESR	1
Duration of symptoms	<6 wk	0
	≥6 wk	1

Abbreviations: ACPA, anti-citrullinated protein antibodies; ACR, American College of Rheumatology; CRP, C-reactive protein; ESR, erythrocyte sedimentation rate; EULAR, European League Against Rheumatism; RF, rheumatoid factor.

Adapted from Aletaha D, Neogi T, Silman AJ, et al. 2010 rheumatoid arthritis classification criteria: an American College of Rheumatology/European League Against Rheumatism collaborative initiative. Arthritis Rheum. 2010;62(9):2574; with permission.

persistent extra-articular symptoms, such as generalized aching/stiffness, bilateral carpal tunnel syndrome, weight loss, failure to thrive, or inflammatory organ involvement (**Fig. 2**).

Arthritis symptoms are typically worse in the morning, and patients usually report more than 30 minutes of morning pain and stiffness, which tends to improve with activity throughout the day. Warm water in the form of a bath or shower typically helps with the pain, as do warm climates; patients often endorse improvement of their pain on tropical or warm weather vacations. Other presenting systemic features of

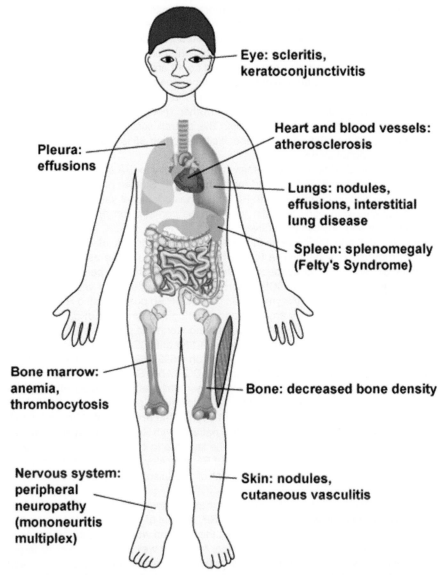

Fig. 2. EAMs of RA. (*Courtesy of* Regents of the University of Michigan; and *Courtesy of* Slide Team.)

RA include fatigue, myalgia, weight loss, low-grade fevers, and, in some instances, depression.

On physical examination, patients will have joint swelling and/or tenderness of affected joints. Range of motion can be limited due to pain or swelling. Large joint involvement can result in detectable joint effusions, particularly in the knee. A commonly used clinical tool is the squeeze test, a maneuver in which the knuckles of the hands or feet are squeezed across the MCP or MTP joints to assess for pain. Although a helpful tool to add to the clinical picture, the squeeze test, on its own, is insufficient to detect early arthritis, and providers should be comfortable with identifying swollen joints in the absence of pain or tenderness.[24]

Once there is clinical suspicion for RA, laboratory tests should be obtained to both help confirm the diagnosis and assess severity of disease. These tests include rheumatoid factor (RF), antibodies to cyclic citrullinated peptides (anti-CCP Abs), inflammatory markers such as the erythrocyte sedimentation rate (ESR) and CRP, and basic laboratory work such as complete blood count and complete metabolic panel. The RF and anti-CCP Abs are the antibodies that define a patient as having "seropositive" RA. RFs are antibodies that bind to the Fc portion of immunoglobulin G, and thus can be seen in conditions other than RA (other rheumatic diseases, infections, malignancies, and in healthy individuals). The overall sensitivity of RF in RA has been reported to be 69%, with the specificity reaching 85%[25] and even higher in young, healthy populations.

The newer anti-CCP test has extremely high specificity for RA at 97%, with a sensitivity of approximately 67% in pooled meta analyses.[26] Studies have found that anti-CCP antibody testing combined with RF testing has additional value over RF testing alone in patients with early arthritis; together the combination of tests has a very high specificity and positive predictive value.[27]

Anti-CCP Abs and their role with respect to the diagnosis of RA and disease severity/prognosis has become a topic of interest. Although the association of RF and anti-CCP Abs and the subsequent development of RA has been well defined, research has shown that anti-CCP Abs may be detectable many years before the RF and before the onset of RA symptoms.[28] Anti-CCP Ab positivity also is associated with the development of bony erosions and radiologic progression of disease, independent of RF presence.[29] Therefore, careful monitoring of patients with few symptoms or atypical inflammatory arthritis and high-titer anti-CCP Abs is recommended.

Important to note is that a significant proportion (15%–25%) of RA can be seronegative, defined by the absence of RF and anti-CCP Abs. Seronegative patients can have significant joint pain and swelling and are generally less likely to develop erosive joint disease than seropositive patients.[30] As described previously, the 2010 ACR guidelines for RA diagnosis still can be met even in the absence of RF or anti-CCP, and some recent data suggest seronegative patients with RA may have higher disease activity on diagnosis,[31] which may reflect the lag time to diagnosis given the lack of seronegativity. Clinical features suggestive of RA, with elevated inflammatory markers and a robust, sustained response to a trial of prednisone, may point toward this diagnosis.

Other laboratory findings that may present at diagnosis and that reflect systemic inflammation include elevated ESR and/or CRP, anemia of chronic disease, thrombocytosis, and/or hypoalbuminemia. However, there are no well-defined cutoff points to indicate disease activity or quiescence. What has been well defined is treat-to-target recommendations; a series of recommendations implementing strategies to reach optimal outcomes of RA based on both evidence and expert opinion. The most current recommendations state the primary target for treatment of RA should be a state of clinical remission, with a suggestion that inflammatory markers be obtained and documented regularly.[32] These markers can be interpreted alone or with RA disease activity tools (such as the Disease Activity Score or DAS28). In this way, obtaining baseline markers of inflammation on diagnosis can be helpful for disease monitoring over time.

OTHER DIAGNOSTIC TOOLS

Arthrocentesis, or joint aspiration, of a medium or large joint effusion can be both therapeutic and diagnostic. Synovial fluid cell count will show an inflammatory pattern, with elevated leukocyte counts in the range of 2000 to 10s of thousands/mm^3, and with greater than 50% neutrophils. In addition to cell count, Gram stain, culture, and crystal analysis always should be performed to rule out infection or crystal arthropathy.

Plain radiographs of commonly affected joints, including hands, wrists, feet, and ankles, may be helpful for diagnosis. Earliest findings include periarticular soft tissue swelling, periarticular osteopenia, and/or joint effusions. Initially, joint spaces in the small joints of the hands may be normal, but with ongoing cartilage destruction, joint spaces will symmetrically narrow. Erosions usually begin at the intracapsular articular margins, an area not covered by cartilage and therefore susceptible to early bony damage. One large study showed that radiographically confirmed erosions were present in 30% of patients at diagnosis, and in 70% 3 years later.[33] When present, erosions are traditionally appreciated in the PIP and MCP joints of the hands, and the MTPs of the feet, particularly the fourth and fifth. Subluxation with ulnar deviation and subsequent fusion can be seen on radiographs in advanced disease.

Ultrasonography, especially with Doppler, is another diagnostic tool with utility for detection of early inflammatory arthritis. When patients present with joint swelling or pain and have questionable synovitis on examination, ultrasonography can visualize synovial hyperemia at the symptomatic sites of disease. This is particularly useful, as many early cases of RA present with isolated soft tissue (nonosseous) abnormalities, and ultrasound can detect early erosions not seen on radiographs.[34]

Computed tomography imaging can be useful for demonstrating bony pathology. MRI has the added ability to visualize synovial or soft tissue involvement and cartilaginous defects. Studies have shown superiority of MRI in the early detection of bone erosions compared with radiographs[35,36]; MRI can detect bone marrow edema, synovial hypertrophy, and pannus formation before the onset of bony erosions, making it a very sensitive measure.[37] Routine use of MRI in diagnosis of RA is limited, however, by cost and difficulty in imaging multiple joints at one time. When available, MR with intravenous gadolinium-based contrast is preferable to noncontrast MR given its value in the detection and characterization of synovitis and in the distinction of inflammatory soft tissue changes.

EXTRA-ARTICULAR MANIFESTATIONS

Although classified as an inflammatory joint disease of symmetric synovial joints, extra-articular involvement in RA is common. One Italian study found extra-articular involvement in as many as 40% of patients with RA at some point the during the course of their disease,[38] which is consistent with other large cohort findings. The extra-articular manifestations (EAMs) of RA can occur at any age after disease onset, and the presence of these manifestations are associated with increased mortality.[39] Extra-articular organ involvement in RA is more frequently seen in patients with severe, active disease and in those with rheumatoid factor/anti-CCP Abs positivity and/or HLA-DR4 positivity.

EAMs encompass involvement of the skin, eye, heart, lung, renal, nervous, and gastrointestinal systems, along with tendons, ligaments, and fascia. It is important to identify EAM because treatment is often aimed at controlling the underlying RA disease (see **Fig. 2**).

One of the most common ocular manifestations is keratoconjunctivitis, inflammation of the cornea and conjunctiva, which presents with burning, itchy eyes, pressure behind the eye, or a feeling of grittiness in the eye. Scleritis is a less common but more aggressive process, characterized by an intensely painful inflammation of the sclera.

Pleuropulmonary involvement is common in RA, and pleural effusions can be found on routine chest radiograph. Patients with pleural effusions may be asymptomatic and do not require treatment, as effusions commonly resolve spontaneously or with treatment of joint disease. Lung nodules also can be found in patients with RA. They typically occur in patients with long-standing RA disease and in patients with coexisting subcutaneous rheumatoid nodules. The prognosis of rheumatoid pulmonary nodules is generally good, but monitoring is warranted for potential neoplasm, especially in those with a smoking history. Another common pulmonary manifestation is interstitial lung disease (ILD), which is also the most serious form of lung involvement in RA. The risk of developing ILD is greatest in patients who are male, older at the time of disease onset, and in those with more severe disease. When suspected in the right clinical setting, workup includes pulmonary function testing, high-resolution computed tomography, and exclusion of infectious or malignant processes before prompt referral to a pulmonologist.

Given the systemic inflammatory nature of RA, the biggest cardiac concern in these patients is atherosclerosis. Studies have found accelerated cardiovascular morbidity in patients with RA; when compared with age-matched and sex-matched controls, patients with RA are at increased risk of cardiovascular death, ischemic heart disease, and heart failure.[40] This same study found that coronary artery tissue from autopsied patients with RA had increased evidence of inflammation and an increased proportion of unstable plaques.[40] In this way, careful consideration must be given to symptoms of chest pain, claudication, or an atypical anginal equivalent.

Osteoporosis in RA arises from an interplay of factors, including systemic and local inflammation, patient immobilization due to joint damage and pain, and the concomitant use of glucocorticoids. These, in addition to primary osteoporosis risk factors, necessitate attention to dual-energy X-ray absorptiometry screening and maintenance of bone health.

Hematologic abnormalities are common in RA, and bone marrow suppression can arise from both disease processes and medical therapy. Clinically this may present as anemia, leukopenia, neutropenia, eosinophilia, thrombocytopenia, or thrombocytosis. Anemia of chronic disease is the most common abnormality, which can present concomitantly with iron deficiency anemia and will tend to get better with good disease control.

Mononeuritis multiplex is an asymmetric sensory and/or motor peripheral neuropathy involving damage to at least 2 separate, seemingly random, nerve areas. Mononeuritis multiplex is common in diabetes but can observed in vasculitic processes, such as RA.

Splenomegaly is another EAM of RA that can present as Felty syndrome or on its own. Felty syndrome is a severe extra-articular feature of RA and is characterized by the triad of arthritis, neutropenia, and splenomegaly. The lifetime risk of Felty syndrome in patients with RA is quite low at less than 1%,[41] and Felty syndrome typically develops after a long course of RA. Therapy in Felty syndrome is anchored in treating underlying RA, and splenectomy is reserved for specific situations.

DIFFERENTIAL DIAGNOSIS

When patients present with persistent joint pain, whether it be polyarticular or oligoarticular, there are many diagnoses to consider, and RA should be primarily differentiated from OA.

OA is a degenerative arthritis, described as "wear and tear" arthritis from repetitive motion, trauma, weight-related strain, and/or age. Patients with OA can have morning stiffness, although it normally lasts less than 30 minutes. Joint pain is worse with use and relieved by rest, which is in marked contradistinction from inflammatory joints. Importantly, the distribution of joint involvement is in a pattern different from RA, although overlap exists (**Fig. 3**). OA most commonly affects the weight-bearing joints of the hips and knees along with the cervical and lower lumbar spine. Distal interphalangeal (DIP), PIP, first carpometacarpal joint, and first MTP joint involvement is very common. Unlike RA, OA manifests with bony joint enlargement rather than synovitis. Heberden and Bouchard nodes are the bony enlargements of the DIP and PIP joints, respectively (**Fig. 4**). This is in contrast to the fusiform swelling of PIP/MCP joints often seen in early RA (**Fig. 5**), and ulnar deviation and MCP subluxation with interosseous muscle atrophy noted late in the course of RA (**Fig. 6**).

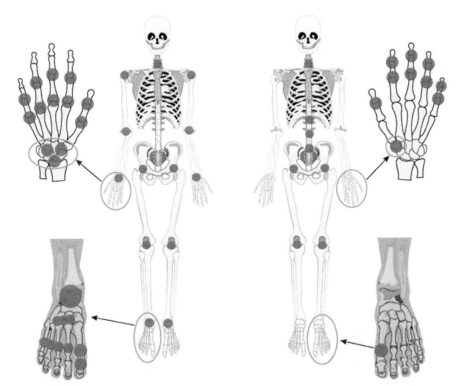

Fig. 3. Distribution of joint involvement in RA versus OA. (*Courtesy of* Regents of the University of Michigan; and *Courtesy of* Slide Team.)

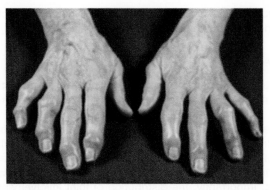

Fig. 4. OA with boney deformities and presence of Heberden and Bouchard nodes. (*From* ACR Image Library, American College of Rheumatology; with permission.)

Psoriatic arthritis should be considered in the presence of seronegative inflammatory arthritis, distal (DIP) arthritis with a history of dactylitis, psoriasis, or low back pain suggestive of sacroiliitis or spondylitis. Nail pitting or onycholysis, separation of the nail from its bed, also may support this diagnosis. Symmetric polyarticular joint pain and swelling in young women should always prompt the consideration of lupus. The presence of mucosal ulcers, photosensitivity, rash, or a history of Raynaud phenomena will help support this diagnosis. Crystalline arthropathy, such as gout or pseudogout, should be considered in polyarticular joint pain. Affected joints are acutely tender, red, and warm in high-risk patients. There should be a high suspicion for acute gout in older male patients on diuretics, who have a history of alcohol consumption, recent surgery, dietary overindulgence, or those with recent medication changes. The presence of tophi can indicate long-standing hyperuricemia, although the gold standard for diagnosis relies on the presence of urate or calcium pyrophosphate crystals found on joint aspiration.

Hemochromatosis can present clinically like RA, with MCP and wrist arthritis; typically the second and third MCPs are affected in early disease. Patients are often younger male individuals, and any suspicion should prompt serum iron studies and HFE genotyping. Infectious arthritis always should be considered in acute-onset monoarthritis. This is especially important to consider in the setting of coexisting

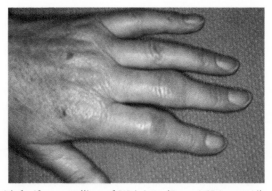

Fig. 5. Early RA, with fusiform swelling of PIP joints. (*From* ACR Image Library, American College of Rheumatology; with permission.)

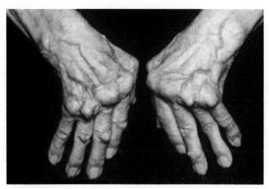

Fig. 6. Advanced RA with ulnar deviation, MCP subluxation, and interosseous muscle atrophy. (*From* ACR Image Library, American College of Rheumatology; with permission.)

comorbidities such as glucocorticoid use, an immunosuppressive state, diabetes, or recent surgery/trauma. Fever and leukocytosis can help differentiate the diagnosis, although these features are nonspecific and may be present in flares of other inflammatory conditions. Arthrocentesis for cell count and culture, along with empiric antibiotics, are usually indicated, as septic arthritis is considered an orthopedic emergency.

TREATMENT

An important paradigm in the management of RA is that disease-modifying treatment should be initiated as soon as possible after diagnosis, with a goal of treating to low disease activity or complete remission.[42] The ACR currently defines early RA as disease duration of less than 6 months, and this is the window wherein treatment should be initiated. Early treatment of RA has been shown to prevent irreversible structural damage and chronic functional impairment,[43] with delays of even a few months altering long-term outcomes. As primary care providers are usually the first point of contact for patients presenting with new arthritis, early identification and referral of RA is critical for achieving the best possible outcomes. However, there are important therapeutic strategies that can be initiated by primary care providers while awaiting subspecialty evaluation.

Nonpharmacologic management includes educating patients about RA. The Arthritis Foundation (www.arthritis.org) is a long-standing, nonprofit advocacy organization that provides educational materials and links to local resources and community programming for patients. Referral to occupational therapy and physical therapy for adjunctive pain management, strengthening, assistive devices, and joint-protection strategies also can make a meaningful impact on pain and functioning.[44,45]

Anti-inflammatory agents, such as nonsteroidal anti-inflammatory drugs (NSAIDs) and glucocorticoids are important adjuncts in early management of pain or inflammation. NSAID use must be carefully monitored, taking into consideration the patient's age, comorbid conditions, and risk of adverse effects, particularly gastrointestinal bleeding and renal insufficiency. Glucocorticoids are extremely potent anti-inflammatory agents, and in addition to controlling inflammatory symptoms, there is evidence that early initiation of low-dose glucocorticoids (ie, ≤10 mg of prednisone equivalent) can delay radiologic progression within the first 6 months.[46] However, the disease-modifying properties of glucocorticoids are minimal, and multisystem metabolic side effects are common. Importantly, the risk of gastrointestinal bleeding is increased with concomitant use of nonselective NSAIDs and glucocorticoids.[47] Thus, current guidelines recommend using the lowest dose of glucocorticoid for the shortest period of time (<3 months).

The current approach to pharmacologic disease-modifying treatment of early RA is presented in **Fig. 7**. Medications in this category are classified as either conventional disease-modifying antirheumatic drugs (DMARDs) or biologic agents (**Table 2**). Conventional DMARDs are typically nonspecific immunomodulatory drugs, contributing to their efficacy in RA. Biologics are much more specific drugs that target cytokines, cell surface markers, and intracellular pathways important in disease pathogenesis and activity. Many of these medications are described in greater detail in another article in this issue.

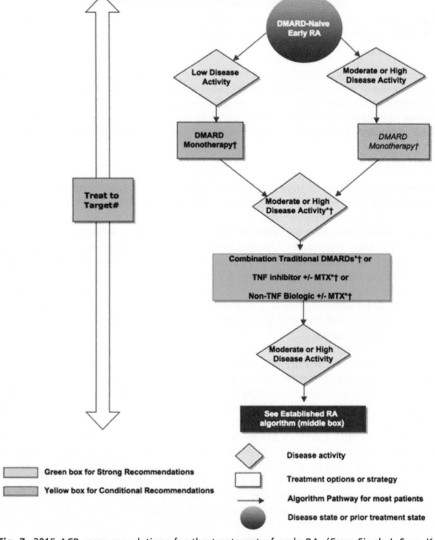

Fig. 7. 2015 ACR recommendations for the treatment of early RA. (*From* Singh J, Saag K, Bridges S, et al. 2015 American College of Rheumatology guideline for the treatment of rheumatoid arthritis. Arthritis & Rheum. 2015;68(1):9; with permission.)

Table 2	
DMARDs and biologic agents used in the treatment of RA	
Conventional DMARDs	**Biologics**
Hydroxychloroquine (Plaquenil)	TNF inhibitors: etanercept (Enbrel), adalimumab (Humira),
Sulfasalazine (Azulfidine)	infliximab (Remicade), certolizumab (Cimzia),
Methotrexate	golimumab (Simponi)
Leflunomide (Arava)	Tocilizumab (Actemra)
	Rituximab (Rituxan, MabThera)
	Abatacept (Orencia)
	Tofacitinib (Xeljanz)

Abbreviations: DMARD, disease-modifying antirheumatic drug; RA, rheumatoid arthritis.
 Data from Singh J, Saag K, Bridges S, et al. 2015 American College of Rheumatology guideline for the treatment of rheumatoid arthritis. Arthritis Rheumatol 2015;68(1):1–26.

DISEASE-MODIFYING ANTIRHEUMATIC DRUG THERAPY

Monotherapy with a DMARD is the first step in treatment. Methotrexate is the most common choice of DMARD as a first-line agent, given its excellent efficacy in achieving remission or low disease activity in 30% to 40% of patients,[48] its well-known safety and toxicity profile, and its relative inexpensiveness. Its mechanism of action in RA is not fully understood; it is a structural analogue of folic acid that impairs DNA synthesis and enhances adenosine release through effects on many different enzymes, resulting in decreased inflammatory responses and lymphocyte proliferation.[49] It is taken as a weekly oral or subcutaneous dose, with typical therapeutic doses ranging from 15 to 20 mg weekly, along with daily folic acid or weekly folinic acid to prevent potential side effects (mucosal ulcers, anemia) attributed to its folate antagonism. Regular monitoring for cytopenias and hepatotoxicity through periodic laboratory work is required, along with creatinine due to its renal clearance. Leflunomide is an alternate first-line DMARD that inhibits dihydroorotate dehydrogenase, also important for DNA synthesis and lymphocyte proliferation.[50] It is administered as a daily oral dose, with similar toxicities and monitoring requirements to methotrexate. Both methotrexate and leflunomide are teratogenic, and women of childbearing age need effective birth control when taking these medications. Leflunomide, due to its prolonged enterohepatic circulation, requires washout with cholestyramine in the event of toxicity or pregnancy.

If patients do not achieve adequate disease control with conventional DMARD monotherapy, one strategy is to add additional nonbiologic DMARDs. Hydroxychloroquine is an antimalarial agent with anti-inflammatory and immunomodulatory properties that make it an important, albeit mild, treatment for inflammatory arthritis.[51] A slow-acting drug that takes months of treatment to achieve full efficacy, hydroxychloroquine is relatively well tolerated, with the most severe side effect being a rare but irreversible, cumulative dose-related retinopathy necessitating regular ophthalmologic evaluation.[51] Sulfasalazine, a drug with salicylate and sulfa antibiotic components whose mechanism of action in RA is not completely understood, can be efficacious in the management of moderate inflammatory arthritis.[52] Triple therapy (methotrexate + sulfasalazine + hydroxychloroquine) was a staple of RA treatment in the prebiologic era; more recently, triple therapy was shown to be noninferior to methotrexate + etanercept (a TNF blocker) in patients who had failed methotrexate monotherapy,[53] in addition to being more cost-effective.[54] Triple therapy is an effective and relatively inexpensive regimen to improve outcomes compared with DMARD monotherapy; however, it requires adherence with taking multiple pills daily (8–16 tablets daily).

BIOLOGIC THERAPY

There are currently 6 classes of biologic agents approved for use in RA. These are more potent immunosuppressive agents than conventional DMARDs that should be initiated and primarily monitored by rheumatology specialists.[55] However, primary care providers should understand the effects of biologic therapies, both generally and class specific, and have a working knowledge of screening and monitoring strategies.

TNF inhibitors are the first-line biologic therapies used in the event of incomplete response or adverse reaction to conventional DMARDs. The 5 drugs in this class differ in structure, half-life, and route/frequency of administration, but all work via blocking the interaction of TNF-alpha with its receptors. TNF-alpha is an important proinflammatory cytokine produced by macrophages and other cells, with myriad actions relevant to the pathogenesis of RA, including stimulation of other proinflammatory cytokine production, expression of endothelial cell adhesion molecules, production of metalloproteinases, and stimulation of osteoclasts.[56] TNF inhibition results in significant improvement of joint inflammation and radiographic damage. Studies have demonstrated that combination therapy of methotrexate and a TNF blocker is more efficacious than either agent alone.[57–59] Side effects can include injection/infusion reactions, which are typically mild and manageable. More serious effects include an increased risk of infections, particularly with higher doses of treatment.[60] Of particular note is the risk of *Mycobacterium tuberculosis* (TB) infection and/or reactivation, given the critical role TNF-alpha plays in granuloma formation and control of TB.[61] Importantly, TB infections in patients on TNF blockers are more likely to present atypically with extrapulmonary and disseminated manifestations;[62] thus, a heightened suspicion and vigilance is necessary.

The other biologic agents work via several mechanisms relevant to the pathophysiology of RA, including targeting other proinflammatory cytokines such as IL-6 (tocilizumab); targeting B cells (rituximab) and T-cell costimulation (abatacept); and inhibiting intracellular JAK-STAT signaling (tofacitinib). These agents also have demonstrated efficacy in controlling the clinical manifestations and achieving remission.[63]

PRIMARY CARE CONSIDERATIONS
Laboratory Monitoring

Patients initiating DMARD or biologic therapy should undergo basic laboratory evaluation, along with screening for hepatitis B, hepatitis C, and tuberculosis; this is typically performed by the prescribing rheumatologist. Presence of viral hepatitis or latent TB does not preclude immunosuppressive use, but requires concomitant antiviral/antimycobacterial treatment, typically initiated at least 1 month before starting biologic therapy.[42]

Current recommendations for monitoring complete blood counts, transaminases, and serum creatinine in patients on conventional DMARDs are listed in **Table 3**. These represent general recommendations from an expert consensus panel; patients with comorbidities or on other medications may require different intervals.

Vaccinations

Before initiating DMARD or biologic therapy, patients ideally should receive the following vaccinations: pneumococcal, influenza, hepatitis B, human papilloma virus,

Table 3
Intervals for monitoring of CBC, transaminases, and creatinine while on DMARDs

	Monitoring Interval Based on Duration of Therapy		
DMARD	<3 mo or with dose adjustment	3–6 mo	>6 mo
Hydroxychloroquine	None	None	None
Sulfasalazine	2–4 wk	8–12 wk	12 wk
Methotrexate	2–4 wk	8–12 wk	12 wk
Leflunomide	2–4 wk	8–12 wk	12 wk

Abbreviations: CBC, complete blood count; DMARD, disease-modifying antirheumatic drug.
Adapted from Singh J, Saag K, Bridges S, et al. 2015 American College of Rheumatology guideline for the treatment of rheumatoid arthritis. Arthritis Rheumatol 2015;68(1):14; with permission.

and herpes zoster.[42] Depending on patients' insurances, some of these vaccinations will be covered only if provided through a primary care provider's office. In patients already on treatment, the same immunization recommendations apply, with the exception of the zoster vaccine; being a live attenuated vaccine (as opposed to a killed or recombinant one), it is currently contraindicated in patients receiving biologic therapy, but not DMARDs. Studies are ongoing to assess the safety of administering live vaccines to persons on biologic agents.

Age-Specific Considerations

Polypharmacy continues to be an important issue in geriatric populations. With increasing age-related comorbidities comes more medication and the heightened risk of medication interactions. This is especially important with the use of DMARDs and biologics that come with both immunosuppressive and immunomodulating properties. Important to note is that immunosuppressive therapeutic regimens have an acceptable safety profile in elderly patients; large review analyses have shown that both DMARDs and biologic agents are effective and well tolerated in elderly patients with RA with no increased relative risk of infection.[5]

As discussed previously, patients with RA are at increased risk of ischemic heart disease and heart failure. The risk of cancer also is increased in the RA population, with an established increased risk of lymphoma and lung cancer[64,65] compared with the general population.

Other considerations in this population include screening for cervical spine instability, especially preoperatively, to look for atlantoaxial subluxation. Posterior to anterior and lateral radiographs in flexion and extension views in addition to frontal views of the odontoid are most useful in looking for cervical spine instability. Any indication of instability can affect anesthetic management and may prompt techniques that avoid unprotected manipulations of the neck.

When to Refer

Referral to rheumatology is appropriate in almost all clinical settings in which RA is suspected or confirmed. Given the ever-evolving industry of biologics and targeted treatments, the specifics of medication dosing and monitoring is best managed by rheumatology specialists.

We would urge primary care physicians to adhere to the 2010 ACR/EULAR guidelines in terms of clinical presentation and serologies while navigating an RA workup, and to be diligent in ruling out OA before referral. When a referral to rheumatology is not available or when the referral time is prolonged, these guidelines will elucidate management of early RA to mitigate disease activity and prevent permanent joint damage and disability.

SUMMARY

Patients typically present first to their primary care providers with arthritis, and it is critical that these providers are able to distinguish the presenting features of RA from other causes of joint pain, particularly OA. Early recognition and referral to a rheumatologist will lead to earlier initiation of treatment and improved long-term outcomes. However, primary care providers are also essential partners in the ongoing management of patients with RA on treatment, ranging from facilitating appropriate laboratory monitoring and vaccinations, screening for infections and EAMs, and managing treatment side effects and comorbid conditions. As our understanding of the pathogenesis and subsequent treatment strategies expand, a shared management approach will lead to the best possible care for patients with RA.

REFERENCES

1. Sacks JJ, Luo YH, Helmick CG. Prevalence of specific types of arthritis and other rheumatic conditions in the ambulatory health care system in the United States, 2001-2005. Arthritis Care Res. In: Silman AJ, Hochberg MC, editors. Epidemiology of the rheumatic diseases. 2nd edition. Oxford University Press; 2001.
2. Dieppe P. Epidemiology of the rheumatic diseases. Second edition. AJ Silman, MC Hochberg (eds). Oxford: Oxford university press, 2001, pp. 377. Int J Epidemiol 2002;31(5):1079–80.
3. Myasoedova E, Crowson C, Kremers H, et al. Is the incidence of rheumatoid arthritis rising? Results from Olmsted county, Minnesota, 1955-2007. Arthritis Rheum 2010;62(6):1576–82.
4. Crowson CS, Matteson EL, Myasoedova E, et al. The lifetime risk of adult-onset rheumatoid arthritis and other inflammatory autoimmune rheumatic diseases. Arthritis Rheum 2011;63(3):633–9.
5. Boots A, Maier A, Stinissen P, et al. The influence of ageing on the development and management of rheumatoid arthritis. Nat Rev Rheumatol 2013;9(10):604–13.
6. Gabriel S, Crowson C, Campion M, et al. Indirect and nonmedical costs among people with rheumatoid arthritis and osteoarthritis compared with nonarthritic controls. J Rheumatol 1997;24(1):43–8.
7. Kim K, Bang S, Lee H, et al. Update on the genetic architecture of rheumatoid arthritis. Nat Rev Rheumatol 2016;13(1):13–24.
8. Wordsworth P, Bell J. Polygenic susceptibility in rheumatoid arthritis. Ann Rheum Dis 1991;50(6):343–6.
9. Viatte S, Plant D, Han B, et al. Association of HLA-DRB1 haplotypes with rheumatoid arthritis severity, mortality, and treatment response. JAMA 2015;313(16):1645–56.
10. Ansar Ahmed S, Dauphinee MJ, Talal N. Effects of short-term administration of sex hormones on normal and autoimmune mice. J Immunol 1985;134:204.
11. Roubinian JR, Talal N, Greenspan JS, et al. Effect of castration and sex hormone treatment on survival. Anti-nucleic acid antibodies and glomerulonephritis in NZB x NZW F1 mice. J Exp Med 1978;147:1568.
12. Marder W, Somers EC. Is pregnancy a risk factor for rheumatic autoimmune diseases? Curr Opin Rheumatol 2014;26(3):321–8.
13. Baka Z, Buzás E, Nagy G. Rheumatoid arthritis and smoking: putting the pieces together. Arthritis Res Ther 2009;11(4):238.

14. Saag K, Cerhan J, Kolluri S, et al. Cigarette smoking and rheumatoid arthritis severity. Ann Rheum Dis 1997;56(8):463–9.

15. George M, Baker J. The obesity epidemic and consequences for rheumatoid arthritis care. Curr Rheumatol Rep 2016;18(1):6.

16. Rutger Persson G. Rheumatoid arthritis and periodontitis–inflammatory and infectious connections. Review of the literature. J Oral Microbiol 2012;4:10.

17. McGraw W, Potempa J, Farley D, et al. Purification, characterization, and sequence analysis of a potential virulence factor from *Porphyromonas gingivalis*, peptidylarginine deiminase. Infect Immun 1999;67(7):3248–56.

18. Wu X, He B, Liu J, et al. Molecular insight into gut microbiota and rheumatoid arthritis. Malemud CJ, ed. Int J Mol Sci 2016;17(3):431.

19. McInnes I, Schett G. The pathogenesis of rheumatoid arthritis. N Engl J Med 2011;365(23):2205–19.

20. Aletaha D, Neogi T, Silman A, et al. 2010 rheumatoid arthritis classification criteria: an American College of Rheumatology/European League Against Rheumatism collaborative initiative. Arthritis Rheum 2010;62(9):2569–81.

21. Arnett F, Edworthy S, Bloch D, et al. The American Rheumatism Association 1987 revised criteria for the classification of rheumatoid arthritis. Arthritis Rheum 1988; 31(3):315–24.

22. Linn-Rasker S, der van, Breedveld F, Huizinga T. Arthritis of the large joints - in particular, the knee - at first presentation is predictive for a high level of radiological destruction of the small joints in rheumatoid arthritis. Ann Rheum Dis 2006; 66(5):646–50.

23. Koskinen E, Hannonen P, Sokka T. Palindromic rheumatism: longterm outcomes of 60 patients diagnosed in 1967-84. J Rheumatol 2009;36(9):1873–5.

24. van den Bosch WB, Mangnus L, Reijnierse M, et al. The diagnostic accuracy of the squeeze test to identify arthritis: a cross-sectional cohort study. Ann Rheum Dis 2015;74(10):1886–9.

25. Nishimura K, Sugiyama D, Kogata Y, et al. Meta-analysis: diagnostic accuracy of anti-cyclic citrullinated peptide antibody and rheumatoid factor for rheumatoid arthritis. Ann Intern Med 2007;146:797.

26. Urban A, Danis P. Which serum test is better for confirming suspected rheumatoid arthritis (RA) in an adult: rheumatoid factor (RF) or anti-cyclic citrullinated peptide antibody (ACPA)? Evid Based Pract 2014;17(2):01–2.

27. Ateş A, Karaaslan Y, Aksaray S. Predictive value of antibodies to cyclic citrullinated peptide in patients with early arthritis. Clin Rheumatol 2006;26(4):499–504.

28. Berglin E, Johansson T, Sundin U, et al. Radiological outcome in rheumatoid arthritis is predicted by presence of antibodies against cyclic citrullinated peptide before and at disease onset, and by IgA-RF at disease onset. Ann Rheum Dis 2005;65(4):453–8.

29. Farragher T, Lunt M, Plant D, et al. Benefit of early treatment in inflammatory polyarthritis patients with anti-cyclic citrullinated peptide antibodies versus those without antibodies. Arthritis Care Res 2010;62(5):664–75.

30. Barra L, Pope J, Orav J, et al. Prognosis of seronegative patients in a large prospective cohort of patients with early inflammatory arthritis. J Rheumatol 2014; 41(12):2361–9.

31. Nordberg LB, Lillegraven S, Lie E, et al, and the ARCTIC Working Group. Patients with seronegative RA have more inflammatory activity compared with patients with seropositive RA in an inception cohort of DMARD-naïve patients classified according to the 2010 ACR/EULAR criteria. Ann Rheum Dis 2017;76:341–5.

32. Smolen J, Breedveld F, Burmester G, et al. Treating rheumatoid arthritis to target: 2014 update of the recommendations of an international task force. Ann Rheum Dis 2015;75(1):3–15.

33. Dixey J, Solymossy C, Young A, et al. Is it possible to predict radiological damage in early rheumatoid arthritis (RA)? A report on the occurrence, progression, and prognostic factors of radiological erosions over the first 3 years in 866 patients from the early RA study (ERAS). J Rheumatol 2004;69:48–54.

34. Wakefield RJ, Gibbon WW, Conaghan PG, et al. The value of sonography in the detection of bone erosions in patients with rheumatoid arthritis: a comparison with conventional radiography. Arthritis Rheum 2000;43:2762–70.

35. McQueen FM, Stewart N, Crabbe J, et al. Magnetic resonance imaging of the wrist in early rheumatoid arthritis reveals a high prevalence of erosions at four months after symptom onset. Ann Rheum Dis 1998;57:350.

36. Klarlund M, Ostergaard M, Jensen KE, et al. Magnetic resonance imaging, radiography, and scintigraphy of the finger joints: one year follow up of patients with early arthritis. The TIRA Group. Ann Rheum Dis 2000;59:521.

37. Cohen SB, Potter H, Deodhar A, et al. Extremity magnetic resonance imaging in rheumatoid arthritis: updated literature review. Arthritis Care Res (Hoboken) 2011;63:660.

38. Cojocaru M, Cojocaru IM, Silosi I, et al. Extra-articular manifestations in rheumatoid arthritis. Mædica 2010;5(4):286–91.

39. Turesson C, O'Fallon WM, Crowson CS, et al. Occurrence of extraarticular disease manifestations is associated with excess mortality in a community based cohort of patients with rheumatoid arthritis. J Rheumatol 2002;29(1):62–7.

40. Gabriel SE. Cardiovascular morbidity and mortality in rheumatoid arthritis. Am J Med 2008;121(10 Suppl 1):S9–14.

41. Balint GP, Balint PV. Felty's syndrome. Best Pract Res Clin Rheumatol 2004;18(5): 631–45.

42. Singh J, Saag K, Bridges S, et al. 2015 American College of Rheumatology guideline for the treatment of rheumatoid arthritis. Arthritis Rheumatol 2015; 68(1):1–26.

43. Finckh A, Liang MH, van Herckenrode CM, et al. Long-term impact of early treatment on radiographic progression in rheumatoid arthritis: a meta-analysis. Arthritis Rheum 2006;55(6):864–72.

44. Steultjens E, Dekker J, Bouter L, et al. Occupational therapy for rheumatoid arthritis. Cochrane Database Syst Rev 2004;(1):CD003114.

45. Hurkmans E, van der Giesen FJ, Vliet Vlieland TP, et al. Dynamic exercise programs (aerobic capacity and/or muscle strength training) in patients with rheumatoid arthritis. The Cochrane database Syst Rev 2009;(4):CD006853.

46. van Everdingen AA, Jacobs J, Van S, et al. Low-dose prednisone therapy for patients with early active rheumatoid arthritis: clinical efficacy, disease-modifying properties, and side effects: a randomized, double-blind, placebo-controlled clinical trial. Ann Intern Med 2002;136(1):1–12.

47. Piper JM, Ray WA, Daugherty JR, et al. Corticosteroid use and peptic ulcer disease: role of nonsteroidal anti-inflammatory drugs. Ann Intern Med 1991;114(9): 735–40.

48. Sethi M, O'Dell J. Combination conventional DMARDs compared to biologicals: what is the evidence? Curr Opin Rheumatol 2015;27(2):183–8.

49. Borchers A, Keen C, Cheema G, et al. The use of methotrexate in rheumatoid arthritis. Semin Arthritis Rheum 2004;34(1):465–83.

50. Behrens F, Koehm M, Burkhardt H. Update 2011: leflunomide in rheumatoid arthritis—strengths and weaknesses. Curr Opin Rheumatol 2011;23(3):282–7.
51. Rainsford K, Parke A, Clifford-Rashotte M, et al. Therapy and pharmacological properties of hydroxychloroquine and chloroquine in treatment of systemic lupus erythematosus, rheumatoid arthritis and related diseases. Inflammopharmacology 2015;23(5):231–69.
52. Plosker G, Croom K. Sulfasalazine: a review of its use in the management of rheumatoid arthritis. Drugs 2005;65(13):1825–49.
53. O'Dell J, Mikuls T, Taylor T, et al. Therapies for active rheumatoid arthritis after methotrexate failure. N Engl J Med 2013;369(4):307–18.
54. Jalal H, O'Dell J, Bridges S, et al. Cost-effectiveness of triple therapy versus etanercept plus methotrexate in early aggressive rheumatoid arthritis. Arthritis Care Res 2016;68(12):1751–7.
55. Guideline summary: Rheumatoid arthritis: diagnosis, management and monitoring. National Guideline Clearinghouse (NGC) Agency for Healthcare Research and Quality (AHRQ) website. 2012. Available at: https://www.guideline.gov. Accessed January 31, 2017.
56. Brennan FM, McInnes IB. Evidence that cytokines play a role in rheumatoid arthritis. J Clin Invest 2008;118(11):3537–45.
57. Klareskog L, van der Heijde D, de Jager JP, et al. Therapeutic effect of the combination of etanercept and methotrexate compared with each treatment alone in patients with rheumatoid arthritis: double-blind randomised controlled trial. Lancet 2004;363(9410):675–81.
58. Clair S, van der Heijde DM, Smolen JS, et al. Combination of infliximab and methotrexate therapy for early rheumatoid arthritis: a randomized, controlled trial. Arthritis Rheum 2004;50(11):3432–43.
59. Breedveld F, Weisman M, Kavanaugh A, et al. The PREMIER study: a multicenter, randomized, double-blind clinical trial of combination therapy with adalimumab plus methotrexate versus methotrexate alone or adalimumab alone in patients with early, aggressive rheumatoid arthritis who had not had previous methotrexate treatment. Arthritis Rheum 2005;54(1):26–37.
60. Bongartz T, Sutton A, Sweeting M, et al. Anti-TNF antibody therapy in rheumatoid arthritis and the risk of serious infections and malignancies: systematic review and meta-analysis of rare harmful effects in randomized controlled trials. JAMA 2006;295(19):2275–85.
61. Flynn J, Goldstein M, Chan J, et al. Tumor necrosis factor-alpha is required in the protective immune response against *Mycobacterium tuberculosis* in mice. Immunity 1995;2(6):561–72.
62. Winthrop K. Risk and prevention of tuberculosis and other serious opportunistic infections associated with the inhibition of tumor necrosis factor. Nat Clin Pract Rheumatol 2006;2(11):602–10.
63. Singh J, Hossain A, Ghogomu T, et al. Biologic or tofacitinib monotherapy for rheumatoid arthritis in people with traditional disease-modifying anti-rheumatic drug (DMARD) failure: A Cochrane systematic review and network meta-analysis (NMA). Cochrane database Syst Rev 2016;(11):CD012437.
64. Smitten A, Simon T, Hochberg M, et al. A meta-analysis of the incidence of malignancy in adult patients with rheumatoid arthritis. Arthritis Res Ther 2008;10(2):R45.
65. Simon T, Thompson A, Gandhi K, et al. Incidence of malignancy in adult patients with rheumatoid arthritis: a meta-analysis. Arthritis Res Ther 2015;17:212.

Systemic Lupus Erythematosus for Primary Care

Ruba Kado, MD

KEYWORDS

- Systemic lupus erythematosus • Antinuclear antibody • Pleuritis • Lupus nephritis
- Pericarditis • Malar rash • Jaccoud arthropathy

KEY POINTS

- Systemic lupus erythematosus is a chronic autoimmune condition that can affect multiple organ systems, including but not limited to the skin, joints, marrow, heart, lungs, kidneys, and brain.
- Common presenting features of systemic lupus in primary care are rash, fatigue, and joint pain.
- Diagnosis can be made by assessment of clinical presentation, assessment of end-organ involvement with imaging and laboratory tests, and the presence of supportive serology.
- Early diagnosis can lead to implementation of measures to help prevent progression of disease.

Systemic lupus erythematosus (SLE) is an autoimmune condition with variable and often extensive manifestations and is characterized by autoantibodies to nuclear components and immune complex deposition. Primary care physicians often encounter the initial presentation of this systemic condition; recognition that certain presentations may be attributable to underlying SLE is of prime importance, so that appropriate testing, referrals, and treatments are implemented. The American College of Rheumatology (ACR) modified its classification criteria for SLE most recently in 1997.[1] In 2012, the Systemic Lupus International Collaborating Clinics (SLICC) proposed its own set of criteria, focusing on the importance of immunologic data by requiring at least 1 immunologic criterion for the diagnosis of SLE[2,3] (**Table 1**).

Cohort and registry analyses have revealed a prevalence of lupus at 0.07% to 0.18%; the Michigan Lupus Epidemiology and Surveillance Program and the Georgia Lupus Registry reported a lower prevalence of disease, closer to 0.07%. Studies of the

Disclosures: No funding or conflicts of interests to disclose.
Division of Rheumatology, Department of Internal Medicine, University of Michigan, Suite 7C27 North Ingalls Building, 300 North Ingalls SPC 5422, Ann Arbor, MI 48109-5422, USA
E-mail address: kador@med.umich.edu

Table 1 Diagnostic criteria for systemic lupus erythematosus	
SLICC Classification System[2]	1997 Update of the 1982 ACR Criteria for Classification of SLE[1]
Must meet 4 criteria, including 1 clinical and 1 immunologic	Must meet 4 of 11 criteria
Clinical criteria	
Acute cutaneous lupus (1 or more of the following) • Malar rash • Bullous lupus • Maculopapular rash • Photosensitive rash *Chronic cutaneous lupus* (1 or more of the following) • Classic discoid (localized vs generalized) • Hypertrophic lupus • Lupus panniculitis • Mucosal lupus • Lupus erythematous tumidus • Chilblains lupus • Discoid lupus/lichen planus overlap Oral or nasal ulcers Nonscarring alopecia *Synovitis OR tendonitis:* 2 or more joints + morning stiffness *Serositis:* pleural or pericardial Renal • Urine protein-to-creatinine ratio with more than 500 mg protein/24 h OR • Red blood cell casts *Neurologic* (1 or more of the following) • Seizures • Psychosis • Mononeuritis multiplex • Myelitis • Neuropathy • Acute confusional state *Hematologic* • Hemolytic anemia OR • Leukopenia (<4000/mm^3 at least once) OR • Lymphopenia (<1000/mm^3 at least once) OR • Thrombocytopenia (<100,000/mm^3)	Malar rash Discoid rash Photosensitivity Oral or nasal ulcers Nonerosive arthritis: 2 or more joints *Serositis:* pleural or pericardial Renal disorder • Persistent proteinuria >500 mg/24 h OR >3 + quantification OR • Cellular cast: red cell, hemoglobin, granular, tubular or mixed Neurologic disorder • Seizure OR • Psychosis Hematologic disorder • Hemolytic anemia with reticulocytosis OR • Leukopenia (<4000/mm^3 or more than 2 occasions) OR • Lymphopenia (<1500/mm^3 on more than 2 occasions) OR • Thrombocytopenia (<100,00/mm^3)
Immunologic criteria	
ANA positivity Anti-dsDNA positivity Anti-Sm positivity Antiphospholipid antibody positivity Low complement Direct Coombs (in absence of hemolytic anemia)	ANA positivity Anti-DNA, anti-Sm, OR antiphospholipid antibody positivity

Abbreviations: ACR, American College of Rheumatology; ANA, antinuclear antibody; dsDNA, double-stranded DNA; SLE, systemic lupus erythematosus; SLICC, Systemic Lupus International Collaborating Clinics.

American Indian and Alaska Native people registry, adults with Medicaid, and the lupus population in Rochester, MN, revealed a slightly higher prevalence of 0.12% to 0.18%.[4–8] Prevalence of lupus was higher in black persons than in white persons; black patients with SLE tend to present at a younger age. There is a higher prevalence of renal disease and tendency for end-organ damage in black and ethnic minority SLE populations.[4,6,8–10] A subanalysis of the Hopkins Lupus Cohort revealed that men with SLE were more likely to be diagnosed at a later age, and more likely to experience neuropsychiatric, renal, and cardiovascular manifestations of disease.[11]

Although this discussion is focused on the more common manifestations of SLE, it is important to note that this disease process can involve virtually any organ system.

UTILITY OF THE ANTINUCLEAR ANTIBODY

Although a positive antinuclear antibody (ANA) is necessary, it is a critically important point that it is not sufficient for a diagnosis of SLE by itself. In a 2013 retrospective study, fewer than 10% of patients referred to a tertiary care center for a positive ANA titer of $\geq$1:40 by indirect fluorescence were diagnosed with an ANA-associated rheumatic disease. Moreover, a cutoff ANA titer of 1:640 had positive predictive value of just more than 25%, and a subanalysis revealed that ANA was tested in some patients who had nonspecific symptoms that did not suggest SLE (including hand pain, diffuse pain, knee pain, back pain, headache, fatigue).[12] Depending on the testing method, the specificity and sensitivity of the ANA may vary.[12,13] Higher elevations in titer and certain antibody profiles are more predictive of activity and severity of disease.

Anti-Smith and anti–double-stranded DNA (anti-dsDNA) antibodies are specific for systemic lupus, and rarely found to be positive in people without SLE.[14–16] Antibody clusters in SLE may be predictive of disease manifestations; antibody clusters with anti-dsDNA tend to correlate with an increased frequency of nephrotic syndrome and clusters with clinically significant antiphospholipid antibodies (cardiolipin antibody, B2GP1, and lupus anticoagulant) correlate with an increased frequency of thrombotic disease and cardiac valvular disease.[17,18] In a 2016 study, 117 of 317 patients with SLE had what was defined as a clinically significant antiphospholipid serologic profile.[18] Lymphopenia, neutropenia, and myocarditis have been linked to the presence of anti–Sjögren syndrome–related antigen A (anti-SSA) antibodies.[19–23]

In a patient suspected to have systemic lupus, serologic testing can be useful before evaluation in rheumatology. This testing includes an anti-dsDNA, anti-Smith antibody, anti-RNP antibody, anti-SSA/SSB antibody, cardiolipin antibody, B2GP1, and dilute Russell viper venom time in addition to the ANA. Anti-Jo 1, anti–ScL 70, and anti-centromere antibodies correlate with other ANA-positive rheumatic diseases, and can be tested in primary care if myositis or scleroderma are suspected. Extractable nuclear antigen (ENA) panels are available laboratory tests to help characterize ANA subsets.

MUCOCUTANEOUS MANIFESTATIONS OF LUPUS

Cutaneous manifestations occur in most patients with SLE and often occur early in the disease course.[24,25] One meta-analysis concluded that cutaneous manifestations may be more common in early-onset SLE, with the exception of sicca symptoms.[26]

Cutaneous lupus erythematosus (CLE) can be classified under acute CLE (ACLE) (photosensitive malar and macular rash), subacute CLE (SCLE) (photosensitive papulosquamous or annular lesions), and chronic CLE (CCLE) (discoid lupus erythematosus, lupus profundus/panniculitis, chilblain lupus, and lupus tumidus).[25,27] Discoid lupus is the most common form of CCLE.[28,29] The SLICC classification system is inclusive of these subtypes.[2] Cutaneous vasculitis, urticarial vasculitis, livedo reticularis, Raynaud, periungual telangiectasias, erythema multiforme, and calcinosis can also be manifestations of lupus, but are not specific to lupus erythematosus.[25] Raynaud is most likely the most common nonspecific cutaneous manifestation in SLE, with reported occurrence in 18% to 46% of patients with SLE.[30] These nonspecific lupus erythematosus skin changes should prompt concern for other diagnoses such as antiphospholipid antibody syndrome, scleroderma, or dermatomyositis.[25]

Systemic symptoms of lupus erythematosus are most often found in patients manifesting with ACLE, and less in SCLE and CCLE.[31,32]

Ultraviolet light exposure and smoking are known triggers for CLE.[25,33] Photoprotection and cessation of smoking needs to be emphasized as part of the treatment plan for CLE.

Oral and nasal ulcers are included in the ACR and SLICC criteria for diagnosis of SLE. Oral ulcers are usually painless.[1,2] Additionally, nonscarring alopecia is a criterion for the diagnosis of SLE in the SLICC system.[2]

In the treatment of CLE, photoprotection is of prime importance, as UV light is a known trigger for disease. Treatment of active CLE can include topical or oral steroids, antimalarials, dapsone, or immunosuppression, depending on acuity and severity of disease. For long-term management in less severe CLE, Plaquenil (hydroxychloroquine) and quinacrine are often used as first-line therapies. Antimalarials are immunomodulatory and not immunosuppressive, making them attractive options for treatment.[29]

CYTOPENIA IN LUPUS

Hematological abnormalities are common in SLE.[19,20] In the ACR and SLICC criteria, leukopenia, thrombocytopenia, and autoimmune hemolytic anemia are included for the diagnosis of SLE.[1,2]

Lymphopenia is perhaps the most common hematologic manifestation in SLE. However, treatment with steroids and immunosuppressive medications can also lead to lymphopenia. The mechanisms that contribute to lymphopenia are not well understood, although anti-lymphocyte antibodies and impaired apoptosis have been described as underlying factors.[19,20] Lymphopenia has been linked to disease activity.[19] Severe lymphopenia can predispose to opportunistic infections.[19] Neutropenia in SLE is likely also multifactorial; margination, anti-neutrophil antibodies, and diminished marrow production have been described as pathologic mechanisms. Normally, neutropenia is mild and mere observation will suffice; however, severe neutropenia, which can predispose to infection, may have to be treated with glucocorticoids $\pm$ colony stimulating factor.[19]

Thrombocytopenia in SLE can result from peripheral destruction, sequestration, and decreased production. The presence of thrombocytopenia has been shown to be associated with an increased frequency of neuropsychiatric lupus, lupus nephritis, antiphospholipid antibody syndrome, and hemolytic anemia, and even in the absence of life-threatening hemorrhage, portends a poorer prognosis in SLE.[19,20,34–37] Idiopathic thrombocytopenic purpura (ITP) and thrombotic thrombocytopenic purpura (TTP) can be initial manifestations of SLE.[19,20,38] One study reported that the presence of anti-dsDNA antibodies and anti-SSA antibodies in TTP were linked to the development of an autoimmune disorder, with SLE being most frequent.[39] It is thus important that serologic testing be performed in patients with TTP or ITP to determine the risk of developing SLE. Patients with immune-mediated thrombocytopenia should be periodically monitored to assess for the emergence of symptoms that could correlate with the development of SLE.

Thrombocytopenia above a certain level (usually 50,000/mm^3), usually does not necessitate specific medical treatment, but does necessitate close observation. Glucocorticoid therapy is the first-line therapy if treatment is needed, but usually does not result in a sustained response as the dose is tapered. Steroid-sparing therapy with danazol, Plaquenil, immunosuppression, rituximab, or intravenous immunoglobulin (IVIG) can be used to achieve the desired long-term response.[19] Splenectomy for long-term treatment is controversial.

Hemolytic anemia is another hematologic manifestation of SLE, and tends to occur in younger patients.[40,41] The discovery of anemia in a patient with suspected SLE should prompt a workup for hemolysis, especially if thrombocytopenia is present. Patients with SLE who present with constitutional symptoms, dyspnea, or fatigue should be assessed not only for cardiopulmonary manifestations of disease, but also for anemia. If hemoglobin is low, haptoglobin, lactate dehydrogenase, reticulocyte count, and peripheral smear should be checked as markers of hemolysis. If there is an indication of hemolysis, antibody-mediated disease can be determined by checking the direct antiglobulin test. Steroid therapy is first line for treatment of autoimmune hemolytic anemia and most patients achieve sustained remission; for refractory disease, other therapies, such as IVIG or immunosuppressive agents, can be given.[19,41] It should be noted that pure red cell aplasia and autoimmune myelofibrosis can occur as disorders secondary to SLE.[42,43]

MUSCULOSKELETAL MANIFESTATIONS OF SYSTEMIC LUPUS ERYTHEMATOSUS

Arthralgia and arthritis are common features of SLE. Most of the time, arthritis is not deforming and nonerosive. Hand joints and knee joints are often affected.[40] Treatment of arthritis depends on the severity, but can include nonsteroidal anti-inflammatory drugs (NSAIDs), antimalarials, corticosteroids, or immunosuppressive therapy.[44,45]

A small subset of patients may develop a deforming arthropathy later in the disease course called Jaccoud arthropathy. This arthropathy was initially described in patients with rheumatic fever, and is characterized by reducible joint subluxation resulting from ligamentous laxity. Some deformities in Jaccoud arthropathy can be corrected surgically.[46] Frankly erosive and destructive arthritis mimicking rheumatoid arthritis can be seen in SLE, with an estimated prevalence of 1%.[44,47]

Avascular necrosis (AVN) can cause joint pain and needs to be considered in patients who are immunosuppressed and in patients who have been taking corticosteroids for an extended period. The risk of AVN may increase in the presence of antiphospholipid antibodies.[44] Depending on the stage of disease, treatment may include nonoperative or operative modalities.[44]

LUPUS NEPHRITIS

In an inception cohort of 1827 patients with SLE, 38.3% developed lupus nephritis (LN). LN more often occurred in the early years after diagnosis of SLE.[48] The ACR defines lupus nephritis as persistent proteinuria greater than 0.5 g per day or 3 + on dipstick, and/or red cell, hemoglobin, granular, tubular, or mixed casts on examination of urine. For practicality purposes, however, a spot urine protein-to-creatinine ratio of greater than 0.5 and an active urinary sediment with >5 red blood cells (RBCs), >5 white blood cells (WBCs) per high-power field (without infection), WBC casts, or RBC casts can serve as surrogate markers for proteinuria and casts.[49]

The optimal diagnostic tool, however, is a renal biopsy; LN is defined by the presence of immune complex–mediated glomerulonephritis. LN can be classified as Class I–VI, based on the location and extent of immune complex deposition: Class III and IV require immunosuppression. Class V LN may not be treated with immunosuppression, as long as proteinuria is in the non-nephrotic range and renal function has not declined.[49]

Initial induction immunosuppressive therapy for Class III and IV LN includes glucocorticoids and mycophenolate mofetil or cyclophosphamide; although studies with cyclophosphamide for induction outnumber those with mycophenolate mofetil for induction, the latter medication has been shown to be as effective in inducing remission. Both medications are teratogenic and pregnancy is contraindicated in a patient undergoing treatment with mycophenolate or cyclophosphamide.[49]

Considering that LN predicts a poorer prognosis, early diagnosis is key. A patient presenting to primary care with a suspicion of lupus must have renal function and sediment assessed by serum creatinine/glomerular filtration rate, urinalysis, and spot urine protein-to-creatinine ratio. Early implementation of treatment results in a better prognosis for patients with SLE complicated by LN.[50]

PLEUROPULMONARY DISEASE IN SYSTEMIC LUPUS ERYTHEMATOSUS

While the most common pulmonary manifestation in SLE is pleuritis with or without pleural effusion, other processes including acute pneumonitis, interstitial lung disease, shrinking lung syndrome, pulmonary embolism, pulmonary hypertension, and alveolar hemorrhage can occur.

A recent study demonstrated the prevalence of pleuritis to be 14% in a large lupus cohort of 1668 patients.[51] Chest pain, cough, shortness of breath, and fever may all be presenting features of pleuritis; imaging may show pleural effusions, but effusions are not always evident. When present, fluid accumulation is typically not large. As there are numerous other causes of pleural effusions, a thoracentesis is a helpful diagnostic tool. Pleural fluid in lupus pleuritis is exudative.

Interstitial lung disease (ILD) has been estimated to occur in 3% to 13% of patients with SLE. The typical pattern on high-resolution computed tomography (CT) scan is that of nonspecific interstitial pneumonitis, although other patterns, such as organizing pneumonia, are seen[52,53]. Pulmonary function tests will show a restrictive pattern with a decreased diffusion capacity (DLCO). SLE-ILD is usually not severe.[52]

Acute pneumonitis is a less common (incidence 1%–4%) but a more serious occurrence in SLE that affects the smaller lung units. As lupus pneumonitis can mimic infection or drug-induced pneumonitis, diagnosis and thus treatment may be delayed. Mortality can reach 50%.[52,54] Treatment of a critically ill patient with pneumonitis may initially include high-dose steroids and treatment of infection simultaneously, as the diagnosis is being clarified.

Diffuse alveolar hemorrhage (DAH) is another less common but life-threatening complication of SLE that can result from capillaritis. Based on a retrospective chart review, DAH tends to occur in patients with SLE with high disease activity otherwise.[55] It may be very difficult to distinguish DAH from other causes of acute lung disease on imaging, which may show nonspecific diffuse ground glass or patchy opacities on CT. An acute decrease in hemoglobin in the presence of such imaging findings should prompt concern for hemorrhage. In DAH, bronchoscopy will show increase in blood and hemosiderin-laden macrophages on serial aliquots. Critically ill or unstable patients with DAH require prompt treatment with high-dose steroids and other forms of immunosuppression (eg, cyclophosphamide or plasmapheresis). As in acute pneumonitis, it is not unusual to concomitantly treat infection.[52,54,56]

Pulmonary arterial hypertension (PAH) can be secondary in SLE and is likely related to endothelial dysfunction. Diagnosis is made by right heart catheterization, although transthoracic echocardiograms can be used to screen and follow trends in pressure. SLE-related PAH has a somewhat better prognosis than PAH related to mixed connective tissue disease or scleroderma.[52,57] Treatment consists of vasodilatory therapy; immunosuppression with cyclophosphamide may be of benefit. Chronic thromboembolic disease can exacerbate PAH.[52,57]

Shrinking lung syndrome (SLS) is an unusual complication of SLE; dyspnea, small lung volumes without ILD, and a restrictive pattern on pulmonary function tests should raise concern for this diagnosis. In one study, a history of pleural involvement was associated with SLS.[58] Diaphragmatic elevation on imaging may be seen; however, steroid myopathy and myositis are not thought to cause the diaphragmatic weakness that leads to SLS. As it is a rare manifestation, there is no standardized treatment approach; however, glucocorticoid therapy is often initiated, followed by steroid-sparing immunosuppression.[52,58]

Patients with SLE may have an increased risk of pulmonary embolism, with a higher risk of thrombosis in patients with antiphospholipid antibodies.[52]

CARDIAC MANIFESTATIONS

SLE can involve the pericardium, myocardium, valves, and coronary vessels. Pericarditis is included in the ACR and SLICC diagnostic criteria for systemic lupus.[1,2]

Pericarditis is perhaps the most common cardiac manifestation of SLE; a 2017 study reported a prevalence of 9.7%.[51] Symptomatic pericarditis most often causes pleuritic positional chest pain; accompanying symptoms can include dyspnea, fever, and tachycardia. On examination, a rub may or may not be heard. The presence of diffuse ST elevation on electrocardiogram and a pericardial effusion or pericardial thickening from acute inflammation on transthoracic echocardiography or CT scan can help solidify the diagnosis, but these findings may not be present. Progression to constrictive pericarditis or tamponade can occur, and can be prevented by early diagnosis and treatment of disease. Initial treatment normally includes NSAIDs and corticosteroids with taper; however, for more severe or recurrent disease, higher doses of steroids and steroid-sparing immunosuppression with medications such as azathioprine, mycophenolate mofetil, methotrexate, and cyclophosphamide are used.[59–62]

Lupus myocarditis is not a common clinical entity, although prevalence may be more common than thought due to subclinical disease.[60,61,63] Untreated myocarditis can result in cardiomyopathy, making early detection and treatment key. Patients can present with nonspecific dyspnea, chest pain, tachycardia, or arrhythmia. Fever or other signs of disease activity may accompany these manifestations of myocarditis. Myocarditis can be due to other causes, including infection. Echocardiography showing global hypokinesis in the absence of other causes of depressed function (eg, coronary artery disease) is suggestive of myocarditis. Delayed enhancement of the myocardium on cardiac MRI suggests myocarditis, but does not confirm lupus-related disease. Endomyocardial biopsy can be helpful, although may not be a feasible or necessary diagnostic method. If cardiomyopathy is present, other causes of disease need to be considered, included coronary artery disease, drug toxicity, microvascular disease related to lupus, and valvular disease. Due to the potential consequences of untreated myocarditis, treatment with high-dose steroids should be implemented.[64] Steroid-sparing therapy can help to maintain control of disease.[59-61]

Valvular pathology can occur in SLE. Sterile verrucous endocarditis (Libman-Sacks endocarditis) most commonly affects the mitral valve.[65] The prevalence of lupus-related sterile endocarditis decreased in the time after the advent of steroid treatment; a report of an autopsy series in 1985 demonstrated the presence of Libman-Sacks endocarditis in 59% of patients (51/86) in the "pre-steroid era" and 36% of patients in the "steroid era" (86/236).[63] Libman-Sacks endocarditis can best be detected by transesophageal echocardiogram. Murmurs may or may not be heard, depending on whether the lesion occludes the valvular opening.[59,60] If a valvular lesion is detected, infectious endocarditis must be ruled out. In clinically evident lupus sterile endocarditis, steroids may be used in the early states, as it has been shown that lesions can resolve.[66] It is not common for Libman-Sacks endocarditis to lead to embolization or valvular dysfunction, but the risk is there. Valve replacement may be indicated in situations of hemodynamic compromise.[59,60]

Although coronary vasculitis is an important entity to consider in a patient with SLE who suffers a myocardial infarction, it does not occur commonly. If present, coronary vasculitis may be difficult to distinguish from atherosclerotic pathology, and may require repeat angiography to assess the hemodynamics of the vessel. If detected, coronary vasculitis is treated with aggressive immunosuppression and possible anticoagulation.[67]

Another potential cardiac consequence of SLE is congenital heart block in the fetuses of women with lupus. Circulating maternal anti-SSA and anti-SSB antibodies can cross the placenta and cause varying degrees of fetal heart block; the incidence of complete heart block is 2% in the presence of anti-SSA antibodies, and increases to 18% with a prior affected pregnancy.[68] It is important to note that first-degree and second-degree heart block can progress to irreversible third degree, which can carry a mortality rate of 15% to 30% in utero or soon after birth; consequences of complete heart block include myocarditis, pericarditis, and cardiomyopathy.[61,69,70] A 2016 study demonstrated a higher incidence of pregnancy loss in mothers with primary Sjögren syndrome.[71] Bradycardia on fetal doppler may be an indication of the presence of SSA antibodies in asymptomatic pregnant women. It is controversial whether surveillance fetal echocardiography is warranted; disease penetrance is low and efficacy of treatment of incomplete heart block is questionable.[72] Detection of a conduction system abnormality in utero should prompt consideration of treatment of the mother with steroids, although the potential undesirable consequences of steroids should be kept in mind.[60,61] Hydroxychloroquine may reduce the risk of recurrent congenital heart block.[73]

CORONARY ARTERY DISEASE IN SYSTEMIC LUPUS ERYTHEMATOSUS

Patients with SLE are at increased risk of developing atherosclerotic coronary artery disease and myocardial infarction.[74-76] A recent study demonstrated more atherosclerotic plaque in the femoral and carotid arteries in patients with SLE when compared with controls; the risk of atherosclerosis was deemed comparable to patients with diabetes mellitus.[77] Active inflammatory states, such as in SLE, may contribute to premature atherosclerosis; however, the mechanisms for accelerated atherosclerotic disease in lupus are not fully understood, and so the traditional modifiable risk factors need to be addressed in patients with SLE. Lipid control, hypertension control, exercise, and smoking cessation are of prime importance.[61,63] Steroid use should be minimized because long-term use of systemic steroids increases the risk of developing hypertension, hyperlipidemia, and weight gain, all of which predispose to atherosclerotic coronary artery disease.[59,60,78]

NEUROPSYCHIATRIC LUPUS

Neuropsychiatric manifestations are included in the 1997 ACR and SLICC criteria for diagnosis of SLE, with seizures and psychosis being common to both sets.[1,2] Additional neurologic criteria include myelitis, cranial neuropathy, mononeuritis multiplex, peripheral neuropathy, and acute confusional state.[2,79] The frequency of neuropsychiatric SLE has been hard to define, due to variation in symptomatology, definition of disease, and difficulty determining whether the disease is directly attributable to underlying lupus.[36,80] Between 1970 and 1975, 140 patients with SLE were studied and 52 (37%) of 140 developed a neuropsychiatric event over the course of 5 years.[36] In a cohort study by Hanly and colleagues,[80] 158 (28%) of 572 patients had a neuropsychiatric incident early in the disease course, close to the time of diagnosis; the investigators recognized that only a minority of events were directly related to the systemic autoimmune condition.

Patients with a history of neuropsychiatric lupus erythematosus have been shown to have worse cognitive function and worse patient-reported outcomes when compared with patients with lupus without a history of neurologic disease.[80,81]

PLAQUENIL THERAPY

Hydroxychloroquine, a nonimmunosuppressive antimalarial drug, has become standard therapy in patients with SLE. The myriad of benefits most of the time outweighs the potential risks of use. In 1998, a study demonstrated that withdrawal of Plaquenil from patients with inactive SLE resulted in an increased risk of major flare.[82] Additional benefits may include blood glucose control, reduction of hyperlipidemia, and an antithrombotic effect,[83] although a systemic review did not find a definite beneficial effect on lipid levels.[84]

Retinal toxicity is a potential side effect that requires ophthalmologic screening; the risk increases with higher cumulative doses and thus weight-based dosing is recommended (to a maximum of 400 mg daily). Other potential risks over time include cytopenia and myopathy.

SUMMARY

SLE is a widely variable disease that can fluctuate in severity over time. Recognition of disease manifestations and monitoring of disease activity are needed to detect potentially life-threatening illness. Certain laboratory abnormalities, such as anti-dsDNA antibodies and complement levels, may be predictive of flare, although these levels do not vary in all patients with SLE. Although some clinical indicators of active SLE can be detected on physical examination, others may not be readily evident. In a young woman presenting with features common to SLE, we suggest obtaining an ANA screen, ENA 10 panel, ADNA, C3, and C4 levels. Monitoring for end-organ pathology includes routine testing for hematuria, proteinuria, impaired renal function, and cytopenia. The decision to test for other organ disease, such as serositis or cerebritis, is driven by symptomatology.

Long-term, primary care providers and rheumatologists share the responsibilities of flare recognition, coronary artery disease risk factor modification, and diabetes and osteoporosis screening in patients with SLE.

REFERENCES

1. 1997 Update of the 1982 American College of Rheumatology revised criteria for classification of systemic lupus erythematosus. Available at: http://www.rheumatology.org/Practice-Quality/Clinical-Support/Criteria/ACR-Endorsed-Criteria.
2. Petri M, Orbai A-M, Alarcon GS, et al. Derivation and validation of systemic lupus international collaborating clinics classification criteria for systemic lupus erythematosus. Arthritis Rheum 2012;64(8):2677–86.
3. Yu C, Gershwin ME, Chang C. Diagnostic criteria for systemic lupus erythematosus: a critical review. J Autoimmun 2014;48-49:10–3.
4. Somers EC, Marder W, Cagnoli P, et al. Population-based incidence and prevalence of systemic lupus erythematosus: the Michigan Lupus Epidemiology and Surveillance program. Arthritis Rheumatol 2014;66(2):369–78.
5. Uramoto KM, Michet CJ, Thumboo J, et al. Trends in the incidence and mortality of systemic lupus erythematosus, 1950-1992. Arthritis Rheum 1999;42(1):46–50.
6. Lim SS, Bayakly AR, Helmick CG, et al. The incidence and prevalence of systemic lupus erythematosus, 2002-2004: the Georgia lupus registry. Arthritis Rheumatol 2014;66(2):357–68.
7. Ferucci ED, Johnston JM, Gaddy JR, et al. Prevalence and incidence of systemic lupus erythematosus in a population-based registry of American Indian and Alaska Native people, 2007-2009. Arthritis Rheumatol 2014;66(9):2494–502.
8. Feldman CH, Hiraki LT, Liu J, et al. Epidemiology and sociodemographics of systemic lupus erythematosus and lupus nephritis among US adults with Medicaid coverage, 2002-2004. Arthritis Rheum 2013;65(3):753–63.
9. Bruce IN, O'Keeffe AG, Farewell V, et al. Factors associated with damage accrual in patients with systemic lupus erythematosus: results from the Systemic Lupus International Collaborating Clinics (SLICC) Inception Cohort. Ann Rheum Dis 2015;74(9):1706–13.
10. Alacron GS, McGwin G Jr, Petri M, et al. Baseline characteristics of a multiethnic lupus cohort: PROFILE. Lupus 2002;11(2):95–101.
11. Tan TC, Fang H, Magder LS, et al. Differences between male and female systemic lupus erythematosus in a multiethnic population. J Rheumatol 2012;39(4):759–69.
12. Abeles A, Abeles M. The clinical utility of a positive antinuclear antibody test result. Am J Med 2013;126:342–8.
13. Meroni PL, Schur PH. ANA screening: an old test with new recommendations. Ann Rheum Dis 2010;69:1420–2.
14. Arbuckle MR, McClain MT, Rubertone MV, et al. Development of autoantibodies before the clinical onset of systemic lupus erythematosus. N Engl J Med 2003;349:1526–33.
15. Pietsky DS. Anti-DNA antibodies—quintessential biomarkers of SLE. Nat Rev 2016;12:102–10.
16. Benito-Garcia E, Schur PH, Lahita R, et al. Guidelines for immunologic laboratory testing in the rheumatic diseases: anti-Sm and anti-RNP antibody tests. Arthritis Rheum 2004;51(6):1030–44.
17. To CH, Petri M. Is antibody clustering predictive of clinical subsets and damage in systemic lupus erythematosus? Arthritis Rheum 2005;52(12):4003–10.
18. Taraborelli M, Lazzaroni MG, Martinazzi N, et al. The role of clinically significant antiphospholipid antibodies in systemic lupus erythematosus. Rheumatismo 2016;68(3):137–43.

19. Fayyaz A, Igoe A, Kurien BT, et al. Haematological manifestations of lupus. Lupus Sci Med 2015;2:e000078.
20. Kao AH, Manzi S, Ramsey-Goldman R. Review of ACR hematologic criteria in systemic lupus erythematosus. Lupus 2004;13:865–8.
21. Martin M, Guffroy A, Argemi X, et al. Systemic lupus erythematosus and lympho-penia: clinical and pathophysiological features. Rev Med Interne 2017;38(9): 603–13.
22. Rivero S, Diaz-Jouanen E, Alacron-Segovia D. Lymphopenia in systemic lupus er-ythematosus. Arthritis Rheum 1978;21(3):295–305.
23. Logar D, Kveder R, Rozman B, et al. Possible association between anti-Ro anti-bodies and myocarditis or cardiac conduction defects in adults with systemic lupus erythematosus. Ann Rheum Dis 1990;49:627–9.
24. Sebastiani GD, Prevete I, Iuliano A, et al. The importance of an early diagnosis in systemic lupus erythematosus. Isr Med Assoc J 2016;18(3–4):212–5.
25. Hejazi EZ, Werth VP. Cutaneous lupus erythematosus: an update on pathogen-esis, diagnosis, and treatment. Am J Clin Dermatol 2016;17:135–46.
26. Medlin JL, Hansen KE, Fitz SR, et al. A systematic review and meta-analysis of cutaneous manifestations in late- versus early-onset systemic lupus erythemato-sus. Semin Arthritis Rheum 2016;45:691–7.
27. Stannard JN, Kahlenberg JM. Cutaneous lupus erythematosus: updates on path-ogenesis and associations with systemic lupus. Curr Opin Rheumatol 2016;28: 453–9.
28. Ribero S, Sciascia S, Borradori L, et al. The cutaneous spectrum of lupus erythe-matosus. Clinic Rev Allergy Immunol 2017;53(3):291–305.
29. Nutan F, Ortega-Loayza AG. Cutaneous lupus: a brief review of old and new med-ical therapeutic options. J Investig Dermatol Symp Proc 2017;18:S64–8.
30. Pavlov-Dolijanovic S, Damjanov NS, Stupar NZV, et al. Is there a difference in sys-temic lupus erythematosus with and without Raynaud's phenomenon? Rheumatol Int 2013;33:859–65.
31. Szczech J, Rutka M, Samotij D, et al. Clinical characteristics of cutaneous lupus erythematosus. Postepy Dermatol Allergol 2016;33(1):13–7.
32. Patskinakidis N, Gambichler T, Lahner N, et al. Cutaneous characteristics and as-sociation with antinuclear antibodies in 402 patients with different subtypes of lupus erythematosus. J Eur Acad Dermatol Venereol 2016;30:2097–104.
33. Bourre-Tessier J, Peschken CA, Bernatsky S, et al. Association of smoking with cutaneous manifestations in systemic lupus erythematosus. Arthritis Care Res 2013;6(8):1275–80.
34. Abdel Galil SM, Edrees AM, Ajeeb AK, et al. Prognostic significance of platelet count in SLE patients. Platelets 2017;28(2):203–7.
35. Miller MH, Urowitz MB, Gladman DD. The significance of thrombocytopenia in systemic lupus erythematosus. Arthritis Rheum 1983;26(10):1181–6.
36. Feinglass EJ, Arnett FC, Dorsch CA, et al. Neuropsychiatric manifestations of sys-temic lupus erythematosus: diagnosis, clinical spectrum, and relationship to other features of the disease. Medicine 1976;55(4):323–39.
37. Alger M, Alacron-Segovia D, Rivero SJ. Hemolytic anemia and thrombocytopenic purpura: two related subsets of systemic lupus erythematosus. J Rheumatol 1977;4(4):351–7.
38. Liu Y, Chen S, Sun Y, et al. Clinical characteristics of immune thrombocyto-penia associated with autoimmune disease: a retrospective study. Medicine 2016;95:50.

39. Roriz M, Landais M, Desprez J, et al. Risk factors for autoimmune diseases development after thrombocytopenic purpura. Medicine (Baltimore) 2015;94(42): e1598.

40. Gormezano NWS, Kern D, Pereira OL, et al. Autoimmune hemolytic anemia in systemic lupus erythematosus at diagnosis: differences between pediatric and adult patients. Lupus 2016;26(4):1–5.

41. Rattarittamrong E, Eiamprapai P, Tantiworawit A, et al. Clinical characteristics and long-term outcomes of warm-type autoimmune hemolytic anemia. Hematology 2016;21(6):368–74.

42. Koduri P, Parvez M, Kaza S, et al. Autoimmune myelofibrosis in systemic lupus erythematosus: report of two cases and review of the literature. Indian J Hematol Blood Transfus 2016;32(3):368–73.

43. Means RT. Pure red cell aplasia. Blood 2016;128(21):51–6.

44. Grossman JM. Lupus arthritis. Best Pract Res Clin Rheumatol 2009;23(4): 495–506.

45. Sakthiswary R, Suresh E. Methotrexate in systemic lupus erythematosus; a systemic review of its efficacy. Lupus 2014;23:225–35.

46. Santiago MB, Galvao V. Jaccoud arthropathy in systemic lupus erythematosus. Medicine 2008;87:37–44.

47. van Vugt RM, Derksen RHWM, Kater L, et al. Deforming arthropathy or lupus and rhupus hands in systemic lupus erythematosus. Ann Rheum Dis 1998;57:540–4.

48. Hanly J, O'Keeffe AG, Su L, et al. The frequency and outcome of lupus nephritis: results from an international inception cohort study. Rheumatology 2016;55: 252–62.

49. Hahn BH, McMahon M, Wilkinson A, et al. American College of Rheumatology guidelines for screening, case definition, treatment and management of lupus nephritis. Arthritis Care Res 2012;64(6):797–808.

50. Esdaile JM, Joseph L, MacKenzie T, et al. The benefit of early treatment with immunosuppressive agents in lupus nephritis. J Rheumatol 1994;21(11): 2046–51.

51. Liang Y, Leng R-X, Pan H-F, et al. The prevalence and risk factors for serositis in patients with systemic lupus erythematosus: a cross sectional study. Rheumatol Int 2017;37:305–11.

52. Mira-Avendano IC, Abril A. Pulmonary manifestations of Sjogren syndrome, systemic lupus erythematosus, and mixed connective tissue disease. Rheum Dis Clin North Am 2015;41:263–77.

53. Kumar A, Khan U, Shrestha B, et al. Interstitial lung disease as initial manifestation of systemic lupus erythematosus. J Nepal Health Res Counc 2013;11(23): 83–5.

54. Wan SA, Teh CL, Jobli AT. Lupus pneumonitis as the initial presentation of systemic lupus erythematosus: case series from a single institution. Lupus 2016; 25:1485–90.

55. Andrade C, Mendonca T, Farinha F, et al. Alveolar hemorrhage in systemic lupus erythematosus: a cohort review. Lupus 2016;25:75–80.

56. Kim D, Choi J, Cho S-K, et al. Clinical characteristics and outcomes of diffuse alveolar hemorrhage in patients with systemic lupus erythematosus. Semin Arthritis Rheum 2017;46(6):782–7.

57. Tselios K, Gladman DD, Urowitz MB. Systemic lupus erythematosus and pulmonary arterial hypertension: links, risks, and management strategies. Open Access Rheumatol 2017;9:1–9.

58. Allen D, Fischer A, Bshouty Z, et al. Evaluating systemic lupus erythematosus patients for lung involvement. Lupus 2012;21:1316–25.
59. Doria A, Iaccarino L, Sarzi-Puttini P, et al. Cardiac involvement in systemic lupus erythematosus. Lupus 2005;14:683–6.
60. Miner J, Kim A. Cardiac manifestations of systemic lupus erythematosus. Rheum Dis Clin N Am 2014;40:51–60.
61. Tincani A, Rebaioli CB, Taglietti M, et al. Heart involvement in systemic lupus erythematosus, anti-phospholipid syndrome and neonatal lupus. Rheumatology 2006;45:iv8–13.
62. Man BL, Mok CC. Serositis related to systemic lupus erythematosus: prevalence and outcome. Lupus 2005;14:822–6.
63. Doherty N, Siegel RJ. Cardiovascular manifestations of systemic lupus erythematosus. Am Heart J 1985;110(6):1257–65.
64. Chaudhari MD, Madani MM, Balbissi MK, et al. Lupus myocarditis presenting as life-threatening overt heart failure: a case report with review of cardiovascular manifestations of systemic lupus erythematosus. J La State Med Soc 2015; 167(5):220.
65. Bulkley BH, Roberts WC. The heart in systemic lupus erythematosus and the changes induced in it by corticosteroid therapy a study of 26 necropsy patients. Am J Med 1975;58:243–64.
66. Roldan CA, Shively BK, Crawford MH. An echocardiographic study of valvular heart disease associated with systemic lupus erythematosus. N Eng J Med 1996;335:1424–30.
67. Caracciolo EA, Marcu CB, Ghantous A, et al. Coronary vasculitis with acute myocardial infarction in a young woman with systemic lupus erythematosus. J Clin Rheumatol 2004;10:66–8.
68. Julkunen H, Eronen M. The rate of recurrence of isolated congenital heart block: a population-based study. Arthritis Rheum 2001;44:487–8.
69. Buyon JP, Clancy RM. Neonatal lupus: review of proposed pathogenesis and clinical data from the US-based research registry for neonatal lupus. Autoimmunity 2003;36(1):41–50.
70. Buyon JP, Hiebert R, Copel J, et al. Autoimmune-associated congenital heart block: demographics, mortality, morbidity, and recurrence rates obtained from a National Neonatal Lupus Registry. J Am Coll Cardio 1998;31:1658–66.
71. Ballester C, Grobost V, Roblot P, et al. Pregnancy and primary Sjogren's syndrome: management an outcomes in a multicenter retrospective study of 54 pregnancies. Scand J Rheumatol 2017;46(1):56–63.
72. Izmirly P, Saxena A, Buyon JP. Progress in the pathogenesis and treatment of cardiac manifestations of neonatal lupus. Curr Opin Rheumatol 2017;29(5):467–72.
73. Izmirly P, Buyon JP, Saxena A. Neonatal lupus: advances in understanding pathogenesis and identifying treatments of cardiac disease. Curr Opin Rheumatol 2012;24:466–72.
74. Manzi S, Mellahn EN, Rairie JE, et al. Age-specific incidence rates of myocardial infarction and angina in women with systemic lupus erythematosus. Am J Epidemiol 1997;145(5):408–15.
75. Avina-Zubieta JA, To F, Vostretsova K, et al. Risk of myocardial infarction and stroke in newly diagnosed systemic lupus erythematosus: a general population-based study. Arthritis Care Res (Hoboken) 2017;69(6):849–56.
76. Kaul MS, Rao SV, Shaw LK, et al. Association of systemic lupus erythematosus with angiographically defined coronary artery disease: a retrospective cohort study. Arthritis Care Res 2013;65(2):266–73.

77. Tektonidou MG, Kravvariti E, Konstantonis G, et al. Subclinical atherosclerosis in systemic lupus erythematosus: comparable with diabetes mellitus and rheumatoid arthritis. Autoimmun Rev 2017;16:308–12.
78. Petri M, Lakatta C, Magder L, et al. Effect of prednisone and hydroxychloroquine on coronary artery disease risk factors in systemic lupus erythematosus: a longitudinal data analysis. Am J Med 1994;96:254–9.
79. Jeltsch-David H, Muller S. Neuropsychiatric systemic lupus erythematosus: pathogenesis and biomarkers. Nat Rev Neurol 2014;10:579–96.
80. Hanly JG, Urowitz MB, Sanchez-Guerrero J, et al. Neuropsychiatric events at the time of diagnosis of systemic lupus erythematosus. Arthritis Rheum 2007;56(1): 265–73.
81. Gao Y, Lau EYY, Wan JHY, et al. Systemic lupus erythematosus patients with past neuropsychiatric involvement are associated with worse cognitive impairment: a longitudinal study. Lupus 2016;25:637–44.
82. Tsakonas E, Joseph L, Esdaile JM, et al. A long-term study of hydroxychloroquine withdrawal on exacerbations in systemic lupus erythematosus. Lupus 1998;7: 80–5.
83. Petri M. Use of hydroxychloroquine to prevent thrombosis in systemic lupus erythematosus and in antiphospholipid antibody-positive patients. Curr Rheumatol Rep 2011;13:77–80.
84. Ruiz-Irastorza G, Ramos-Casals M, Brito-Zeron P, et al. Clinical efficacy and side effects of antimalarials in systemic lupus erythematosus: a systematic review. Ann Rheum Dis 2010;69(1):2.

The Seronegative Spondyloarthropathies

Ayyappa S. Duba, MD, Stephanie D. Mathew, DO*

KEYWORDS

- Ankylosing spondylitis • Psoriatic arthritis • Reactive arthritis • Enteropathic arthritis
- Seronegative spondyloarthropathy

KEY POINTS

- The seronegative spondyloarthropathies are characterized by inflammatory joint disease with associated extra-articular manifestations and shared genetic markers.
- Ankylosing spondylitis is the prototypical form of SpA. Other subgroups include, psoriatic arthritis, reactive arthritis, and enteropathic arthritis.
- A detailed history and physical examination along with radiographic evaluation assist best in diagnosis of SpA. HLA-B27 testing can help predict prognosis, but is not routinely recommended for diagnosis.
- In addition to pharmacologic options (NSAIDS, DMARDS, and biologics), physical therapy plays a key role in improving function and range of motion.

INTRODUCTION

The spondyloarthropathies (SpA) are a heterogeneous group of chronic inflammatory rheumatic disorders that share characteristic clinical features including inflammatory back pain, asymmetric peripheral arthritis, enthesitis, dactylitis, and tenosynovitis; genetic predisposition (HLA-B27); and extra-articular manifestations.

CLASSIFICATION

In 1974, Moll and coworkers[1] established the concept of seronegative SpA in patients with inflammatory arthritis who were rheumatoid factor (RF) negative. Moll and coworkers described five distinct subtypes of SpA: (1) ankylosing spondylitis (AS), (2) psoriatic arthritis (PsA), (3) reactive arthritis (ReA), (4) enteropathic arthritis (EnA), and (5) undifferentiated SpA.

Disclosure: No disclosures (A.S. Duba). Pfizer grant for telehealth (S.D. Mathew) (# 26218663).
Department of Rheumatology, Dartmouth-Hitchcock Medical Center, 1 Medical Center Drive, Lebanon, NH 03756, USA
* Corresponding author.
E-mail address: Smathew7@gmail.com

PREVALENCE

Global prevalence of SpA ranges from 0.2% in South-East Asia to 1.6% in Northern Arctic communities.[2] In the United States, the overall prevalence of SpA is 1%.[3] AS is the most prevalent subtype followed by PsA.

GENETIC FACTORS

The HLA-B27 allele confers the strongest genetic risk association with SpA. Twin studies in those with AS show concordance rates of 60% to 75% for monozygotic twins and 12% for dizygotic twins. Additionally, there is a 10% to 30% increased risk of disease in first-degree relatives of those afflicted with AS.[4]

The subset of HLA-B27-positive patients with SpA are at a higher risk for involvement of the axial skeleton and tend to have a younger age of onset.[5] Of those with AS, approximately 80% to 95% of white patients and 50% to 80% of nonwhite patients are HLA-B27 positive.[5] Certain subtypes of the HLA-B27 are more commonly associated with diseases, whereas others are protective. For example, 27:02 (Mediterranean), 27:04 (Chinese), and 27:05 (white) are definitely associated with disease, whereas 27:06 and 27:09 are protective.[6]

Less than 5% of the HLA-B27-positive population develops disease. The prevalence of HLA-B27 in healthy white persons is 6% to 9%, and 3% in healthy African Americans, making routine testing for HLA-B27 less valuable.[5]

CLINICAL FEATURES

Upward of 60% of Americans are affected by an episode of low back pain in the lifetime,[3,7] and recognizing symptoms of inflammatory back pain (**Table 1**) is challenging.[3,5,8] Patients can present with isolated buttock pain and stiffness in the low back with inactivity. Over time, symptoms can progress to cause significant limitation in spinal motion.

INFLAMMATORY VERSUS MECHANICAL BACK PAIN

Peripheral arthritis involves joints outside of the spine, is usually asymmetric, and may affect large and small joints. ReA and EnA tend to prefer the joints of the lower extremities, causing a large joint oligoarthritis (<5 joints).

Enthesitis, dactylitis, and tenosynovitis are cardinal manifestations of seronegative SpA. Enthesitis is characterized by inflammation where tendons, ligaments, or articular capsule attach to bone. Common areas involved include the greater trochanters, patella, calcanei, sacroiliac joints, and ligaments around the intervertebral disks. Dactylitis is characterized by synovitis of the unidigit joints along with tenosynovitis of the flexor tendon and can result in swelling of an entire digit or "sausage digit."

Table 1
Inflammatory versus mechanical low back pain

	Inflammatory Back Pain	Mechanical Back Pain
Age of onset	<40 y old	Any age
Morning stiffness	>60 min	<30 min
Nocturnal pain	Frequent	Absent
Effect of exercise	Improvement	Exacerbation

Data from Refs.[3,5,8]

Tenosynovitis is characterized by inflammation and swelling around a tendon. The seronegative SpA commonly have extra-articular manifestations, which are summarized in **Box 1** and **Fig. 1**.

PHYSICAL EXAMINATION

The physical examination can provide several clues to assist in the diagnosis of seronegative SpA.[9] A thorough musculoskeletal (axial and peripheral) exam to assess for synovitis (swelling, redness, tenderness, limitation in range of motion), enthesitis (tenderness at the insertion sites of large tendons such as Achilles, knees and elbows) and spinal mobility is key. Several special maneuvers are helpful in the assessment of inflammatory back pain:

1. Occiput to wall testing: assesses cervical range of motion in extension. Place patient's heels and shoulders against a wall, the occiput should touch the wall in this position.

Box 1
Extra-articular manifestations

Mucocutaneous:
  Psoriasis (PsA)[a]
  Nail changes: pitting, ridging, hyperkeratosis, and onycholysis (PsA)[a] (**Fig. 1**)
  Oral ulcers (ReA, EnA)
  Keratoderma blennorrhagicum, circinate balanitis (ReA, predominantly with chlamydia)[b]
  Erythema nodosum, pyoderma gangrenosum (EnA)[a]

Ocular:
  Recurrent uveitis (mostly anterior), keratitis, conjunctivitis

Gastrointestinal:
  Ulcerative colitis, Crohn disease (EnA)[b]
  Infectious or sterile ileitis/colitis (ReA)[a]
  Microscopic colitis (AS)

Genitourinary:
  Prostatitis, infectious/sterile urethritis, cervicitis, cystitis, salpingitis, vulvovaginitis (ReA)[a]

Pulmonary: (AS)[b]
  Pulmonary fibrosis (apical lung fields)

Cardiovascular:
  Aortitis, aortic root dilation, aortic regurgitation
  Conduction abnormalities
  Myocardial dysfunction
  Pericarditis

Neurologic:
  Atlantoaxial subluxation
  Cauda equine syndrome
  Ossification of the posterior longitudinal ligament with spinal stenosis

Bone
  Osteoporosis

Renal
  IgA nephropathy
  Secondary amyloidosis
  Calcium oxalate stones (Crohn disease)

  [a] More commonly associated with.
  [b] Relatively specific for.

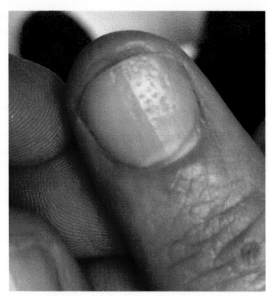

Fig. 1. Nail pitting. Nail changes, particularly nail pitting (more than 20 nail pits) and onycholysis, are associated with PsA.

2. Modified Schoeber test: detects limitation in motion of the lumbar spine. Mark a line at the dimples of Venus, and another 10 cm up from this. The patient flexes maximally forward with straight knees. The distance between the two lines should normally increase to atleast 15 cm.
3. Chest expansion: assesses rib mobility. Measure at the 4th intercostal space at maximum inhalation and exhalation. Normal is a difference of 5 cm; less than 2.5 cm is considered abnormal.
4. FABER/Patrick test: assesses for sacroiliac joint pain. With patient in the supine position, extend one leg and flex, abduct, and externally rotate the other.
5. Gaenslen maneuver: assesses sacroiliac joint pain. With the patient in the supine position, drop one leg off of the examination table and flex the opposite leg toward the chest. This elicits pain on the side of the dropped leg.

The physical examination may also reveal abnormalities in the following:

- Skin (pay attention to the scalp, extensor surfaces, gluteal cleft, skin surrounding the ears, the umbilicus, and the palms and soles) for psoriasis, keratoderma, circinate balanitis
- Nails (pitting, onycholysis)
- Ocular examination (erythema)
- Oral mucosa (ulcerations)
- Cardiac and lung examination (valvular disorders, apical lung disease)

CLASSIC RADIOGRAPHIC FINDINGS

Axial skeletal inflammation in SpA results in sacroiliitis (inflammation of the sacroiliac joints) and spondylitis. These changes are observed in any of the SpA subtypes. In AS, bilateral sacroiliitis and typical symmetric syndesmophytes are common; in ReA and PsA, asymmetric sacroiliitis and bulky asymmetric paravertebral (nonmarginal)

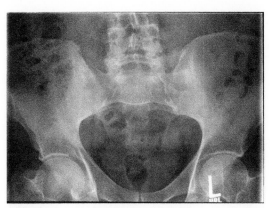

Fig. 2. Radiograph of sacroiliac joints, Ferguson view. Ankylosing spondylitis. Ankylosis of bilateral sacroiliac joints.

ossified spinal outgrowths may be observed. The axial skeletal changes of AS and EnA are often indistinguishable (**Figs. 2** and **3**).[10,11]

Peripheral joint changes in SpA are characterized by periostitis, erosions with proliferative bone changes (at the entheses), and normal bone mineralization (in contrast to rheumatoid arthritis, which typically shows erosions without associated proliferative changes and is associated with peri-articular osteopenia). These radiographic features are characteristic but may be absent early in the disease. Although x-ray imaging is the preferred initial modality, in the absence of distinctive findings, computed tomography or MRI may be considered. MRI is the most sensitive tool for detecting early axial inflammatory disease.[11]

DIAGNOSTIC CRITERIA

In 2009, the Assessment of SpondyloArthritis International Society (ASAS) Classification criteria was developed to establish the diagnosis of a seronegative SpA(**Table 2**).[12] This new criteria was developed to facilitate earlier diagnosis because the New York Criteria did not perform well in identifying pre-radiographic disease.[8]

ANKYLOSING SPONDYLITIS
Definition

AS is the prototypical disease of the seronegative SpA. It is characterized by inflammatory back pain with progressive spinal stiffness.

Epidemiology and Genetics

The disease first manifests before the age of 40, and has a male predominance of 3:1.[13] HLA-B27 and its association with AS was discovered in 1973, and is found in greater than 90% of patients with AS.[6]

Clinical Features

Nearly all patients complain of inflammatory back pain, usually affecting the sacroiliac joints and the spine. Other common sites of involvement include the hips, shoulders, costovertebral, costomanubrial, and sternoclavicular joints and 40% of patients have associated musculoskeletal chest pain.[13]

AS is divided into two groups: radiographic axial and nonradiographic axial. Radiographic sacroiliitis is considered the classic definition, but this can take 5 to 10 or more

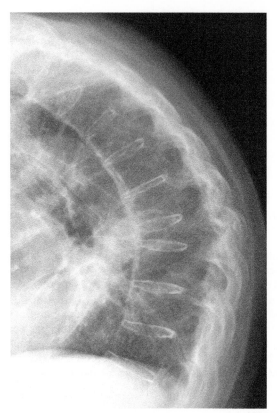

Fig. 3. Radiograph of thoracic spine, lateral. Ankylosing spondylitis. Note the vertebral body squaring and diffuse syndesmophytes and ankylosis.

years to develop. Patients without sacroiliitis on plain radiographs usually show inflammation on MRI, which is considered nonradiographic disease.[13]

Other common manifestations include enthesitis (up to 70% of patients),[13] peripheral joint involvement (up to 50% of patients; shoulders, hips, and knees are the most frequently affected),[13] and dactylitis (up to 8% of patients).[13]

Extra-articular Features

Table 1 provides a list of extra-articular features.

Differential Diagnosis

Table 3 and **Fig. 4** provide the differential diagnosis.

Diagnosis

The diagnosis is suspected in patients presenting before the age of 40 with signs and symptoms of inflammatory back pain and other classic SpA features (see **Table 2**).

Diagnostic Evaluation

Laboratory evaluation should include the following:

- Complete blood count (CBC)
- Complete metabolic panel (CMP)

Table 2
ASAS criteria for seronegative SpA

ASAS criteria:
  Only applied in patients <40 y of age with >3 mo of inflammatory back pain
  Sensitivity 82.9%, specificity 84.4%

Sacroiliitis on imaging + ≥1 spondyloarthropathy feature	OR	HLA-B27 + ≥2 spondyloarthropathy features
Spondyloarthropathy features		Sacroiliitis:
• Inflammatory back pain		• Active acute inflammation on MRI highly suggestive of sacroiliitis
• Arthritis		• Definite radiographic sacroiliitis
• Enthesitis		
• Uveitis		
• Dactylitis		
• Psoriasis		
• Crohn's/colitis		
• Good response to nonsteroidal anti-inflammatory drugs, family history of spondyloarthropathy		
• HLA-B27		
• Elevated C-reactive protein		

Data from Rudwaleit M, van der Heijde D, Landewe R, et al. The development of assessment of SpondyloArthritis international Society classification criteria for Axial Spondyloarthritis (part II): validation and final selection. Ann Rheum Dis 2009;68(6):777–83.

- Erythrocyte sedimentation rate (ESR) or C-reactive protein (CRP) (elevated in 50%–70%)[13,14]
- May consider screening with RF and anticyclic-citrullinated peptide antibodies (ACPA) (which are generally negative) in patients with peripheral arthritis
- Radiographs of the spine and sacroiliac joints

These tests help to diagnose and help to predict disease prognosis and course.

Table 3
Differential diagnosis for AS based on joint distribution

Axial Disease	Peripheral Joint Disease
Osteitis condensans ilii: radiographic finding that occurs in multiparous women Involves sclerotic bony changes found on the iliac side of the sacroiliac joint	Osteoarthritis (<30 min of morning stiffness, symptoms worse with activity)
Diffuse idiopathic skeletal hyperostosis: noninflammatory disease, more common in patients with diabetes characterized by calcification of the anterior longitudinal ligament over four consecutive vertebrae, without erosive findings (**Fig. 4**)	Rheumatoid arthritis (symmetric polyarticular, radiographic changes, lack of distal interphalangeal joint involvement)
Degenerative disk disease	Behçet syndrome (EnA) Crystalline arthropathy (gout, pseudogout)
Alternative spondyloarthropathy subtype (EnA, PsA, AS, ReA)	Sarcoidosis Infectious/postinfections Gonococcal arthritis (ReA) Poststreptococcal arthritis (ReA) Acute rheumatic fever (ReA)

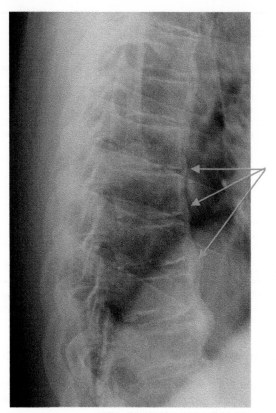

Fig. 4. Radiograph of lateral spine. Diffuse idiopathic skeletal hyperostosis (*arrows*) flowing ossification of the anterior longitudinal ligament involving the thoracic spine.

Classic Radiographic Findings

Sacroiliac joints

Changes are seen primarily in the lower two-thirds of the joint (synovial lined portion). Erosions are seen soonest on the iliac side, then the joint can look abnormally wide (pseudowidening) because of progression of the erosions, followed by bony sclerosis on both sides of the joint, and eventually fusion or ankylosis of the joint occurs (see **Fig. 2**).

Spine

The first lesion occurs where the annulus fibrosis (outer layer of the vertebral disk) inserts into the vertebral body and "shiny corners" develop, then squaring of the vertebrae occurs. Over time these outer layers become ossified and syndesmophytes form, and eventually complete fusion occurs, with "bamboo spine" (see **Fig. 3**).

Treatment

Treatment is aimed at improving function, reducing pain, and decreasing complications associated with the disease. Nonsteroidal anti-inflammatory drugs (NSAIDs) are considered first-line therapy for symptomatic axial AS and are effective in relieving pain and stiffness in 80% of patients.[13] They are also thought to be disease modifying. It is recommended to try at least two NSAIDs, for 1 to 2 weeks, before declaring a failure to respond.[14] The choice of specific nonsteroidal medication is patient dependent, but indomethacin is commonly used. NSAIDs are used on demand when side effects are less tolerable. In patients with gastrointestinal risk alone, one can consider celecoxib in conjunction with a proton pump inhibitor. In patients with high gastrointestinal and cardiovascular risk NSAIDs should be avoided.

Disease-modifying antirheumatic drugs (DMARDs) including sulfasalazine (SSZ)/methotrexate (MTX)/leflunomide (LFN) may be beneficial for peripheral arthritis, but are not as effective to treat axial disease or enthesitis.

Biologic therapies including anti–tumor necrosis factor (TNF)-α therapy are effective in reducing inflammatory component of AS; improve spinal mobility and function; reduce peripheral joint inflammation, enthesitis, and dactylitis; and can control uveitis and bowel symptoms. The 2009 ASAS guidelines recommend an anti-TNF-α inhibitor in patients with high disease activity despite a trial of two NSAIDs.[12] There are currently five anti-TNF-α agents available: adalimumab, infliximab, etanercept, certolizumab, and golimumab. The anti-TNF-α chosen depends on associated complications (eg, etanercept is not efficacious for uveitis or Crohn disease [CD]). Anti-interleukin (IL)-17A monoclonal antibody, secukinumab, recently approved for use in AS, has similar efficacy to anti-TNF-α therapy.[15]

Additional nondrug therapies are important in the management of seronegative SpA and include the following:

- Physical therapy: first-line treatment for all patients to maintain spinal range of motion and strength
- Smoking cessation
- Oral corticosteroids: limited value in AS; local injection is helpful for sacroiliitis or peripheral arthritis
- Treat and monitor for osteoporosis

Predictors of Poor Prognosis

Poor prognosis is predicted by early hip involvement[13]; ESR greater than 30, persistently high CRP, poor response to NSAIDs, and early development of syndesmophytes; and extra-articular features, such as uveitis, cardiovascular involvement, or pulmonary fibrosis, are more commonly associated with HLA-B27 positivity.

PSORIATIC ARTHRITIS
Definition

PsA is a chronic inflammatory arthritis occurring in patients with psoriasis. It occurs in up to 30% of patients with psoriasis over time. Although most (70%) patients have cutaneous disease at the time of presentation, in 10% to 15% arthritis can precede skin disease ("psoriatic arthritis sine psoriasis").[16]

Epidemiology and Genetics

The overall prevalence of PsA is estimated to be between 0.3% and 1.0%. In contrast to RA, there is no gender predilection.[17] HLA-B27 is seen in 10% to 25% of patients with PsA and is more common in patients with axial disease.[3,18] Patients with PsA or psoriasis often have a first-degree relative with the disease (40% of cases).[18]

Clinical Presentation

Patients generally present with joint pain, and stiffness (lasting >30 minutes). Both axial and peripheral joints are affected by PsA. Moll and coworkers[1] described five clinical patterns in PsA (**Table 4**). Presenting with more than one pattern or transitioning between patterns is not uncommon.

Table 4 Patterns of PsA	
Pattern of Arthritis	**Incidence**
Asymmetric oligoarticular/monoarticular arthritis	Up to 70% of cases
Symmetric polyarthritis	5%–20%, associated with a poorer prognosis
Distal interphalangeal joints joint–predominant arthritis	5%–10%
Arthritis mutilans	5%
Axial-predominant disease: spondylitis with or without sacroiliitis	Up to 50% over time when associated with peripheral disease (bilateral sacroiliitis often associated with HLA-B27 gene) 2%–4% in isolation

Data from Refs.[1,19,20]

Unlike RA, patients with PsA commonly present with asymmetric monoarticular or oligoarticular disease and distal interphalangeal joint involvement is a distinctive feature of PsA. Dactylitis occurs in 30% to 40% of patients and most commonly involves the 3rd and 4th toes.[19,20] Enthesitis and tenosynovitis occurs in up to 40% at diagnosis primarily at the Achilles insertion and plantar fascia.[19,20]

Diagnosis

Early diagnosis and treatment is critical to reducing the risk of joint damage, disability, and comorbidities.[21] Patients with psoriasis should be frequently screened for early signs of musculoskeletal disease during primary care and dermatology visits. The presence of scalp lesions, nail dystrophy, intergluteal or perianal disease, and obesity are associated with an increased risk for PsA. When PsA is suspected, early referral to a rheumatologist is valuable. Delay in diagnosis can significantly increase the risk for erosive disease and sacroiliitis.[21] The CASPAR criteria (classification criteria) are used to help facilitate the diagnosis of PsA (**Box 2**).[22]

Differential Diagnosis

Table 3 provides the differential diagnosis.

Diagnostic Evaluation

The following are recommended to help make diagnosis, predict prognosis, and assist in decision making regarding appropriate therapy:

- CBC
- CMP
- ESR and CRP: elevated in 40% and suggests a worse prognosis[23]
- RF found in less than 10% of patients with PsA[23]
- ACPA found in up to 16%[23]
- Antinuclear antibody titer $\leq$1:80 is found in 50%[23]
- HLA-B27 is generally not recommended for diagnosing PsA
- Radiographs of the affected joints

Radiographic Findings

PsA is characterized by destructive bone changes in conjunction with new bone formation. Periarticular erosions with predominant bone resorption may progress to

---

Box 2
Classification criteria for psoriatic arthritis

Established inflammatory articular disease with at least 3 points from the following features:

- Current psoriasis (2 points)

- A history of psoriasis (in the absence of current psoriasis; 1 point)

- A family history of psoriasis (in the absence of current psoriasis and history of psoriasis; 1 point)

- Dactylitis (1 point)

- Juxta-articular new-bone formation (1 point)

- RF negativity (1 point)

- Nail dystrophy (1 point)

Data from Helliwell PS, Taylor WJ. Classification and diagnostic criteria for psoriatic arthritis. Ann Rheum Dis 2005;64:ii3–8.

---

cause whittling of the bone and can lead to "pencil in cup" deformity (**Fig. 5**A). Musculoskeletal ultrasound can sometimes be useful in detecting joint inflammation, enthesitis, and tendonitis early in the disease process (**Fig. 5**B).[19] MRI can detect early bone marrow edema and soft tissue changes early on in the disease course; however, it is reserved for ambiguous axial symptoms in the setting of normal radiographs.

Treatment

Treatment strategies are generally driven by disease severity and patient's comorbidities. Conventional therapeutic strategies use NSAIDs, local steroid injections, traditional DMARDs, and biologics. Very mild disease is sometimes managed with anti-inflammatory agents alone. Patients with more severe disease and/or with evidence of joint damage require early initiation of DMARDS or biologics.

Intra-articular steroid injections are used for symptomatic relief in patients with monoarticular or enthesial disease. There are no clinical trial data supporting the

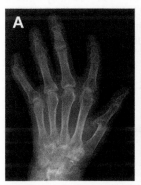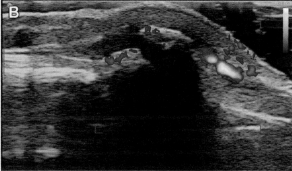

Fig. 5. (*A*) Radiograph of the hand. Destructive joint disease at distal interphalangeal joints (DIP) with "pencil in cup" deformity best seen on 5th DIP; ankylosis of interphalangeal joints (2nd, 4th) with irregular, "fuzzy" appearing proliferative bone changes around the joints; joint space narrowing at metacarpophalangeal joints and pan–carpal joint space loss. (*B*) Ultrasound DIP. Cortical irregularities with positive Doppler signal along the insertion of extensor tendon suggestive of enthesitis.

use of systemic glucocorticoids for the treatment of PsA.[24] Additionally, oral steroids are generally avoided for fear of exacerbating cutaneous psoriasis with taper (erythroderma).[25]

MTX is often a first-line agent used in patients with predominant peripheral arthritis. Other oral DMARDs, such as LFN, SSZ, and apremilast, can also be tried alone or in combination with MTX. These agents have no proven efficacy for spinal disease.[26]

Anti-TNF is recommended in patients with peripheral PsA failing traditional DMARDs and in patients with predominantly axial disease, active enthesitis, and/or dactylitis. Although anti-TNF agents are the preferred first-line biologic agents, recent data and safety profiles on newer agents (IL-12/23 inhibitor [ustekinumab] and IL-17 inhibitor [seckucunimab]) are promising and have expanded therapeutic options for PsA.[27]

Predictors of Poor Prognosis

Polyarticular disease, elevated CRP, erosive disease, and poor response to initial therapy are predictors of severe disease.[28] Patients with HLA-B27 allele tend to present at a younger age and are more likely to have severe axial disease, enthesitis, and dactylitis.[29]

ENTEROPATHIC ARTHRITIS
Definition

Inflammatory bowel diseases (IBD), specifically CD and ulcerative colitis (UC), are commonly associated with extraintestinal manifestations. Musculoskeletal complications are among the most common of these. Risk factors for the development of inflammatory arthritis in IBD patients include active bowel disease, a family history of IBD, appendectomy, cigarette smoking, and the presence of additional extraintestinal manifestations.[30]

Epidemiology and Genetics

Approximately 4 million people worldwide are diagnosed with IBD, with 1.4 million of these cases in the United States. IBD-associated arthropathy is the most common extraintestinal manifestation.[31]

Articular manifestations occur in 6% to 46% of patients with IBD.[32] Joint symptoms can precede clinically overt bowel disease. Peripheral joint involvement occurs in 5% to 14% of patients with UC, and 10% to 20% of patients with CD. Axial involvement is seen more often in patients with CD versus patients with UC and is more often associated with HLA-B27.[30]

Clinical Presentation

Table 5 provides the clinical presentation.

Extra-articular Manifestations

Box 1 lists extra-articular manifestations of IBD.

Differential Diagnosis

Table 3 provides the differential diagnosis.

Diagnosis

Although there are no set diagnostic criteria, the ASAS criteria can serve as a starting point in those patients with axial disease (see **Table 2**). In those patients without clear inflammatory back pain, diagnosis relies on history and physical examination.

Table 5			
Clinical presentation			
Type of Arthritis	Characteristics	Percentage IBD Patients	Onset
Type 1	Oligoarticular asymmetric larger joint arthritis (<5 joints), course follows that of the IBD	5%	More commonly acute in onset, and one-third occur before the bowel disease
Type 2	Polyarticular symmetric small joint arthritis, independent of IBD	3%–4%	More chronic in nature

Data from Gionchetti P, Calabrese C, Rizzello F. Inflammatory bowel disease and spondyloarthropathy. J Rheum 2015;42(suppl 93):21–2; and Arvikar SL, Fisher MC. Inflammatory bowel disease associated arthropathy. Curr Rev Musculoskelet Med 2011;4(3):123–31.

Clinicians should be alert for a family history of IBD, chronic diarrhea with rectal bleeding, abdominal pain, weight loss, chronic low back pain, peripheral joint pain and swelling, dactylitis, or enthesitis. Early referral to a gastroenterologist and/or rheumatologist is recommended for those who develop these signs and symptoms.

Diagnostic Evaluation

The following diagnostic tests are useful in identifying inflammatory arthritis and deciding on course of treatment: CBC, CMP, ESR and CRP, radiographs of affected joints, and endoscopy if appropriate.

Radiographic Findings

Radiographic findings are similar to AS.

Treatment

Treatment is similar to the other seronegative SpA and begins with NSAIDs and cyclo-oxygenase-2 inhibitors. A recent review suggests that cyclo-oxygenase-2 inhibitors are safe for most patients with IBD but close follow-up is recommended to ensure bowel disease does not worsen.[33] Disease-modifying agents to include SSZ, MTX, and AZA are effective for gastrointestinal and joint involvement.

The anti-TNF-α therapies infliximab, adalimumab, and certolizumab are Food and Drug Administration–approved to treat IBD and arthritis and are usually initiated early in the disease course if traditional DMARDs fail or the disease severity is high.[34] More recently, the IL-12/23 inhibitor, ustekinumab, was approved to treat IBD and arthritis.[34]

Surgical Options

Total colectomy of affected colon can induce remission of peripheral arthritis in UC, but not in CD. Surgery provides no benefit for axial involvement in IBD.

Prognosis

Prognosis largely depends on the severity of the underlying bowel disease. Those with well-controlled bowel disease rarely develop serious EnA.[31,32]

REACTIVE ARTHRITIS

ReA, previously called Reiter's syndrome, is an aseptic inflammatory arthritis which presents 1 to 4 weeks following an extra-articular bacterial infection. It is commonly known by the clinical triad of conjunctivitis, nongonococcal urethritis, and arthritis following gastrointestinal or urogenital infection, although only one-third of patients present with the complete triad.

Pathogenesis, Epidemiology, and Genetics

The most common organisms implicated with ReA include *Chlamydia trachomatis* (urogenital), *Yersinia*, *Salmonella*, *Shigella*, and *Campylobacter*. *Escherichia coli*, *Clostridium difficile*, and *Chlamydia pneumoniae* have also been described but are less common. No infectious agent is identified in approximately 40% of patients.[35] Accurate estimates of prevalence of ReA are limited by the lack of universally accepted diagnostic criteria and the frequency of subclinical infections.[36] However, according to population-based studies, the annual incidence of ReA is 0.6 to 27/100,000.[35,36] As in other seronegative SpA, HLA-B27 allele confers additional risk.[35,36]

Clinical Features

ReA should always be considered in young adults presenting with inflammatory arthritis. Men and women are equally affected. Symptoms usually manifest within days to weeks following a urogenital or enteric infection.

Musculoskeletal Manifestations

ReA typically presents as an asymmetric oligoarticular arthritis predominantly involving the large joints of lower extremities, although associated upper extremity involvement is seen in half of cases. Dactylitis, enthesitis, bursitis, and tenosynovitis can occur along with arthritis or in isolation. Like PsA, axial disease is less common; when present it tends to be asymmetric and is associated with HLA-B27.

Extra-articular Manifestations

Box 1 lists extra-articular manifestations.

Diagnostic Evaluation

The diagnostic evaluation should include the following:

- ESR and CRP
- CBC
- Arthrocentesis and synovial fluid analysis to exclude septic or crystalline arthritis; synovial fluid testing for gonococcal, chlamydial infections, and Lyme disease (in the appropriate clinical setting)
- Culture and/or polymerase chain reaction of synovial fluid, urine, urethra/cervix, throat, sputum
- RF and ACPA
- HLA-B27 is not routinely recommended; it can support the diagnosis when in doubt and is used to predict prognosis in those diagnosed
- Electrocardiogram (carditis or conduction block)
- Radiographs of involved joints
- Musculoskeletal ultrasound can help when patients present with subtle or ambiguous signs of enthesitis, tenosynovitis, dactylitis, or synovitis

Radiographic Findings

Radiographic findings are similar to PsA.

Treatment

A key difference between the evaluation and management of ReA and the other SpA is the assessment for active infection. Infection must be treated if present. Antibiotics should be used to treat all patients and partners with active *C trachomatis* infection. Use of combination antibiotics for *Chlamydia* shows benefit.[37] Current data do not support the use of antibiotics for treatment of other urogenital or enteric forms of ReA.

NSAIDs are often the first-line agents used to control symptoms and improve function. Indomethacin, 50 to 75 mg twice daily, is commonly used. Intra-articular corticosteroid injections are considered in the absence of a joint. Oral steroids are not particularly effective in controlling disease.

DMARDs are used, and SSZ is the drug of choice in patients with persistent disease despite adequate NSAID dosing, although others are used (MTX and LFN).[38,39] Anti-TNF-α agents have been used off-label in patients with persistent symptoms despite adequate alternative strategies.[40]

Cutaneous and ocular manifestations are often responsive to topical steroids. HLA-B27-positive patients can have recurrent or persistent uveitis and may require systemic immunosuppressive therapy.

Prognosis

Unlike other common chronic inflammatory arthritidies, more than 50% of patients with ReA are in permanent remission by 6 months. Of the remaining 50%, two-thirds can have recurrent symptoms and one-third develop a chronic disease course requiring use of immunosuppressive agents. Patients with ReA on DMARDs should be re-evaluated at frequent intervals to assess the continued need for DMARDs.[40,41]

A total of 60% of patients are HLA-B27 positive. These patients have more severe disease, are at an increased risk for extra-articular manifestations, and have a higher prevalence of sacroiliitis and a prolonged disease course.[35,41]

UNDIFFERENTIATED SPONDYLOARTHROPATHY

This diagnosis is used to describe a seronegative SpA that does not fit the criteria for a definitive diagnosis of AS or defined subtypes of SpA.

SUMMARY

The seronegative SpA are a group of diseases with a strong genetic predisposition, characterized by inflammatory back pain, peripheral arthritis, and various extra-articular features. Early recognition and referral are key to limit disability and co-management with primary care and rheumatology offers the best outcomes.

REFERENCES

1. Moll JM, Haslock I, Macrae IF, et al. Associations between ankylosing spondylitis, psoriatic arthritis, Reiter's disease, the intestinal arthropathies, and Behcet's syndrome. Medicine (Baltimore) 1974;53(5):343–64.
2. Stolwijk C, van Onna M, Boonen A, et al. Global prevalence of spondyloarthritis: a systematic review and meta-regression analysis. Arthritis Care Res 2016;68(9): 1320–31.
3. Weisman MH, Witter JP, Reveille JD. The prevalence of inflammatory back pain: population-based estimates from the US National Health and Nutrition Examination Survey, 2009–10. Ann Rheum Dis 2013;72(3):369–73.

4. Brown M, Kennedy G, Macgregor A, et al. Susceptibility to ankylosing spondylitis in twins the role of genes, HLA and the environment. Arthritis Rheum 1997;40(10): 1823–8.

5. Rudwaleit M, Haibel H, Baraliakos X, et al. The early disease stage in axial spondylarthritis: results from the German Spondyloarthritis Inception Cohort. Arthritis Rheum 2009;60(3):717–27.

6. Bowness P. HLA-B27. Annu Rev Immunol 2015;33:29–48.

7. Kinkade S. Evaluation and treatment of acute low back pain. Am Fam Physician 2004;74(8):1181–8.

8. Rudawaleit M, Metter A, Listing J, et al. Inflammatory back pain in ankylosing spondylitis: a reassessment of the clinical history for application as classification and diagnostic criteria. Arthritis Rheum 2006;54(2):569–78.

9. van der Linden S, Brown M, Kenna T, et al. Ankylosing spondylitis. In: Firestein GS, Budd RC, Gabriel SE, et al, editors. Kelley and Firestein's textbook of rheumatology. [Chapter 75]. Elsevier; 2017. p. 1256–79.

10. Kettering JM, Towers JD, Rubin DA. The seronegative spondyloarthropathies. Semin Roentgenol 1996;31(3):220–8.

11. Resnick D. Radiology of seronegative spondyloarthropathies. Clin Orthop Relat Res 1979;(143):38–45.

12. Rudwaleit M, van der Heijde D, Landewe R, et al. The development of assessment of SpondyloArthritis International Society classification criteria for axial spondyloarthritis (part II): validation and final selection. Ann Rheum Dis 2009; 68(6):777–83.

13. Taurog J, Chhabra A, Colbert R. Ankylosing spondylitis and axial spondyloarthropathies. N Engl J Med 2016;374:2563–74.

14. Braun J, Kiltz U, Sarholz M, et al. Monitoring ankylosing spondylitis: clinically useful markers and prediction of clinical outcomes. Expert Rev Clin Immunol 2015; 11(8):935–46.

15. Baeten D, Sieper J, Braun J, et al. Secukinumab, an interleukin-17A inhibitor, in ankylosing spondylitis. N Engl J Med 2015;373:2534–48.

16. Gladman DD, Shuckett R, Russell ML, et al. Psoriatic arthritis (PSA): an analysis of 220 patients. Q J Med 1987;62(238):127–41.

17. Mease PJ, Gladman DD, Papp KA, et al. Prevalence of rheumatologist-diagnosed psoriatic arthritis in patients with psoriasis in European/North American dermatology clinics. J Am Acad Dermatol 2013;69(5):729–35.

18. Gladman DD, Anhorn KA, Schachter RK, et al. HLA antigens in psoriatic arthritis. J Rheumatol 1986;13(3):586–92.

19. Torre A, Rodriguez PA, Arribas C, et al. Psoriatic arthritis (PA): a clinical, immunological and radiological study of 180 patient. Br J Rheumatol 1991;30(4):245–50.

20. Veale D, Rogers S, Fitzgerald O. Classification of clinical subsets in psoriatic arthritis. Br J Rheumatol 1994;33(2):133–8.

21. Haroon M, Kirby B, FitzGerald O. High prevalence of psoriatic arthritis in patients with severe psoriasis with suboptimal performance of screening questionnaires. Ann Rheum Dis 2013;72(5):736–40.

22. Helliwell PS, Taylor WJ. Classification and diagnostic criteria for psoriatic arthritis. Ann Rheum Dis 2005;64:ii3–8.

23. Bogliolo L, Alpini C, Caporali R, et al. Antibodies to cyclic citrullinated peptides in psoriatic arthritis. J Rheumatol 2005;32(3):511.

24. Joshi P, Dhaneshwar SS. An update on disease modifying antirheumatic drugs. Inflamm Allergy Drug Targets 2014;13(4):249–61.

25. Raychaudhuri SP, Wilken R, Sukhov AC, et al. Management of psoriatic arthritis: early diagnosis, monitoring of disease severity and cutting-edge therapies. J Autoimmun 2017 Jan;76:21–37.
26. Coates LC, Gossec L, Ramiro S, et al. New GRAPPA and EULAR recommendations for the management of psoriatic arthritis: process and challenges faced. Rheumatology (Oxford) 2017;56:1251–3.
27. Mease P. Biologic therapies for psoriatic arthritis. Rheum Dis Clin North Am 2015; 41:723–38.
28. Gladman DD, Antoni C, Mease P, et al. Psoriatic arthritis and psoriasis: classification, clinical features, pathophysiology, immunology, genetics. Psoriatic arthritis: epidemiology, clinical features, course, and outcome. Ann Rheum Dis 2005;64: ii14–7.
29. Haroon M, Winchester R, Giles JT, et al. Clinical and genetic associations of radiographic sacroiliitis and its different patterns in psoriatic arthritis. Clin Exp Rheumatol 2017;35(2):270–6.
30. Gionchetti P, Calabrese C, Rizzello F. Inflammatory bowel disease and spondyloarthropathy. J Rheumatol 2015;42(suppl 93):21–2.
31. Arvikar SL, Fisher MC. Inflammatory bowel disease associated arthropathy. Curr Rev Musculoskelet Med 2011;4(3):123–31.
32. Colia R, Corrado A, Cantore FP. Rheumatologic and extraintestinal manifestations of inflammatory bowel diseases. Ann Med 2016;48:1–10.
33. Ribaldone DG, Fagoonee S, Astegiano M, et al. Coxib safety in patients with inflammatory bowel disease: a meta-analysis. Pain Physician 2015;18:599–607.
34. DeFilippis E, Longman R, Harbus M, et al. Crohn's disease: evolution, epigenetics and the emerging role of microbiome targeted therapies. Curr Gastroenterol Rep 2016;18:13.
35. Hannu T. Reactive arthritis. Best Pract Res Clin Rheumatol 2011;25(3):347–57.
36. Söderlin MK, Börjesson O, Kautiainen H, et al. Annual incidence of inflammatory joint diseases in a population based study in Southern Sweden. Ann Rheum Dis 2002;61(10):911–5.
37. Carter JD, Espinoza LR, Inman RD, et al. Combination antibiotics as a treatment for chronic chlamydia-induced reactive arthritis: a double-blind, placebo-controlled, prospective trial. Arthritis Rheum 2010;62(5):1298–307.
38. Clegg DO, Redo DJ, Abdellatif M. Comparison of sulfasalazine and placebo for the treatment of axial and peripheral articular manifestations of the seronegative spondyloarthropaties. Arthritis Rheum 1999;42(11):2325–9.
39. Meyer A, Chatelus E, Wnedling D, et al. Safety and efficacy of anti-tumor necrosis factor alpha therapy in then patients with recent-onset refractory reactive arthritis. Arthritis Rheum 2011;63:1274–80.
40. Rihl M, Klos A, Köhler L, et al. Infection and musculoskeletal conditions: reactive arthritis. Best Pract Res Clin Rheumatol 2006;20(6):1119–37.
41. Leirisalo M, Skylv G, Kousa M, et al. Follow up study on patients with Reiter's disease and reactive arthritis, with special reference to HLA-B27. Arthritis Rheum 1982;25(3):249–59.

Common Soft Tissue Musculoskeletal Pain Disorders

Matthew J. Hubbard, DO[a],*, Bernard A. Hildebrand, MD[b],
Monica M. Battafarano, PT, DPT, CSOMT[c],
Daniel F. Battafarano, DO, MACP[d]

KEYWORDS

- Soft tissue rheumatism • Soft tissue pain • Localized pain disorders
- Musculoskeletal pain disorders

KEY POINTS

- Most soft tissue musculoskeletal pain syndromes can be diagnosed by history and physical examination.
- The overall goal for management of musculoskeletal pain is to improve comfort and restore, maximize, and preserve function.
- The mainstay of therapy for these syndromes is a combination of avoidance of the aggravating activity, education, and physical therapy.
- A formal physical therapy evaluation provides patient-centered care for each syndrome, which may manifest as unique musculoskeletal impairments.
- Analgesics and nonsteroidal anti-inflammatory drugs (NSAIDs) can be used judiciously. Corticosteroid injections and surgical therapies should be considered with failure of conservative therapy.

Disclosure Statement: The authors have nothing to disclose. The views expressed herein are those of the authors and do not reflect the official policy or position of Brooke Army Medical Center, the US Army Medical Department, the US Army Office of the Surgeon General, Department of the Air Force, Department of the Army, Department of Defense, or the US government.
[a] Rheumatology, San Antonio Uniformed Services Health Education Consortium (SAUSHEC), San Antonio Military Medical Center, 3551 Roger Brooke Drive, San Antonio, TX 78234, USA;
[b] Department of Clinical and Applied Science Education, University of the Incarnate Word School of Osteopathic Medicine, 4301 Broadway, CPO 121, San Antonio, TX 78209, USA;
[c] Sports Center Physical Therapy, 1600 West 38th Street, Suite 201, Austin, TX 78731, USA;
[d] Rheumatology Fellowship, San Antonio Uniformed Services Health Education Consortium (SAUSHEC), Uniformed Services University of the Health Sciences, San Antonio Military Medical Center, 3551 Roger Brooke Drive, San Antonio, TX 78234, USA
* Corresponding author.
E-mail address: matthew.j.hubbard14.mil@mail.mil

Prim Care Clin Office Pract 45 (2018) 289–303
https://doi.org/10.1016/j.pop.2018.02.006
0095-4543/18/Published by Elsevier Inc.

INTRODUCTION

Musculoskeletal complaints account for up to 30% of all primary care office visits.[1] Soft tissue musculoskeletal pain syndromes manifest in isolation or secondary to underlying mechanical derangements or systemic inflammatory disease. Common causes of soft tissue musculoskeletal pain include tendinitis, enthesitis, and bursitis. Tendinitis is a clinical and pathologic disorder with common features of local pain, dysfunction, tenderness, inflammation, and degeneration, often resulting from overuse and injury.[1] Enthesitis is defined as inflammation occurring at the bony insertional sites of tendons and ligaments, and bursitis is inflammation of bursae that protect soft tissues from bony prominences and friction associated with structural motion. Tendinitis, enthesitis, and bursitis may have overlapping clinical features of local tenderness, swelling, pain with motion and/or at rest, and regional loss of active motion.[1]

The purpose of this article is to give a brief overview of the most common soft tissue musculoskeletal pain syndromes that primary care providers will encounter, to be used as a reference and guide. The authors used a regional approach to organize the material, as providers will encounter these syndromes with complaints of pain referring to an anatomic location (eg, neck, shoulder, or hip pain). A comprehensive review of soft tissue pain syndrome is not possible in this article, but a list of soft tissue causes of pain by region is organized in **Table 1**.

Table 1			
List of common localized soft tissue pain disorders by anatomic region			
Head and Neck	Temporomandibular joint syndrome	Carotodynia	Stylohyoid syndrome
	Omohyoid syndrome	Muscle contraction headache	Occipital neuralgia
	Torticollis	Cervical nerve root impingement	Thoracic outlet syndrome
Chest Wall	Costochondritis	Xiphodynia	Tietze syndrome
Shoulder	Rotator cuff tendinopathy	Bicipital tendinopathy	Deltoid tendinopathy
	Subacromial bursitis	Rotator cuff tear	Adhesive capsulitis
Elbow	Olecranon bursitis	Lateral and medial epicondylitis	Cubital tunnel syndrome
Wrist	De Quervain disease	Intersection syndrome	Carpal tunnel syndrome
Hand	Stenosing tenosynovitis (trigger finger and thumb)	Dupuytren contracture	
Hip and Pelvic Girdle	Trochanteric bursitis	Ischial bursitis	Iliopectineal bursitis
	Piriformis syndrome	Meralgia paresthetica	
Knees	Prepatellar bursitis	Pes anserine bursitis	Patellofemoral syndrome
	Iliotibial band syndrome	Baker cyst	Shin splints
Ankle/Foot	Retrocalcaneal bursitis	Achilles tendinopathy	Plantar fasciitis
	Metatarsalgia	Tarsal tunnel syndrome	Morton neuroma

EPIDEMIOLOGY

Population studies reveal a high prevalence of soft tissue musculoskeletal pain syndromes. The proportion of pain caused by specific disorders in comparison with nonspecific pain is less clear. Upper limb pain is common, with a high prevalence in the shoulder (18% to 26%), elbow (8% to 12%), and wrist/hand (9% to 17%) at any point in time.[2] The myofascial pain syndrome (MPS), defined as local or regional pain with tender spots that recreate symptoms when palpated, has an estimated prevalence of 32%, with a lifetime prevalence of 85%.[3,4] Over the age of 60, hip pain is reported in more than 14% of the population,[5] and knee pain affects 25% of the adult population.[6] Finally, 10% of all adults report significant foot pain, and the prevalence increases with aging; middle-age and elderly adults have a prevalence of foot and ankle pain that is 24% and 15%, respectively.[7]

MYOFASCIAL PAIN SYNDROME

Myofascial pain syndrome (MPS) is distinct from central pain disorders such as fibromyalgia, in that there is often a focal trigger point; additionally, it does not require multiple pain generators, and it is associated with taut bands of skeletal muscle.[8] MPS may manifest as acute or chronic pain in the cervical region; upper, middle or lower back; shoulder or hip regions; pelvic floor; or chest wall (eg, an MPS in the trapezius muscle or gluteus muscle).

Conservative therapy for MPS includes education on restful sleep, cardiovascular fitness, proper body mechanics, and physical therapy. Recognition and treatment of underlying psychosocial factors may be necessary. Topical nonsteroidal anti-inflammatory drugs (NSAIDs) and lidocaine patches may effectively control MPS symptoms; however, there are inadequate data to support the efficacy of systemic NSAIDs, muscle relaxants, tramadol, benzodiazepines, selective serotonin reuptake inhibitors (SSRIs), or serotonin norepinephrine reuptake inhibitors (SNRIs).[8] Needling or trigger point injections may provide some benefit for patients with MPS when performed by clinicians with appropriate expertise and training; the greatest benefit is noted when accompanied by stretching and manual physical therapy.[9]

SHOULDER PAIN
Rotator Cuff Tendinopathy

The rotator cuff is comprised of the supraspinatus, infraspinatus, teres minor, and subscapularis tendons. Rotator cuff tendinopathy refers to injury of any of these 4 tendons, with the supraspinatus being most commonly affected. In chronic tendinopathy, the rotator cuff muscles are weakened; the deltoid is unopposed, and the humeral head becomes malaligned, leading to impingement of the supraspinatus tendon by the acromion with overhead limb movement.[10]

Symptoms vary by age and cause of injury. Younger patients usually identify a specific activity associated with an acute onset of symptoms. Older patients often report insidious onset of symptoms without a known inciting event. Pain occurs in the posterolateral shoulder and deltoid regions and is exacerbated by arm abduction greater than 90°, overhead limb movement, and lying on the affected shoulder.[11] Several provocative tests can be performed to identify rotator cuff tendinopathy (**Fig. 1**), the most sensitive provocative test being the painful arc test.[11]

If acute tendinopathy is related to a known traumatic injury, shoulder radiographs may help identify a fracture. Ultrasound and MRI have shown similar efficacy for identifying a full or partial tear of the rotator cuff,[12] and are typically reserved for refractory tendinopathy unresponsive to conservative therapy.

Treatment is classically directed toward alleviating pain by analgesic therapy and avoiding aggravating activities. Chronic rotator cuff disease or refractory symptoms may require NSAID treatment or a subacromial corticosteroid injection.[13] Once severe tendinitis pain subsides, rehabilitative physical therapy is necessary. In general, all

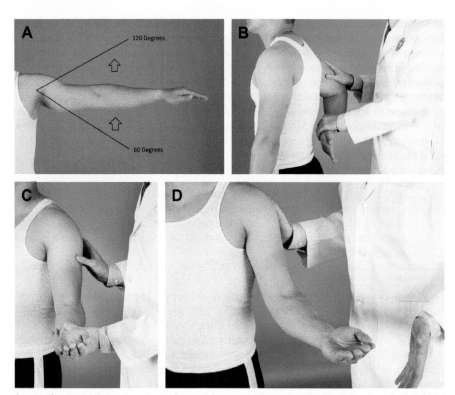

Fig. 1. The Painful Arc Test is performed by passively and actively abducting the patient's arm from 0 to 180 degrees. A positive test is elicited between 60–120 degrees of abduction with indicates the presence of a subacromial or rotator cuff disorder (*A*). The Internal Rotation Lag Test is performed by placing the hand of the affected arm behind the patient's back and pulling the hand away from the back until it is in a "lift off" position as shown. The test is positive if the patient cannot hold the "lift off" position without help and indicates a subscapularis disorder (*B*). The External Rotation Resistance Test is performed by having the patient flex the affected arm at 90 degrees, then active external rotation is resisted by the examiner. The test is positive if there is pain or weakness, indicating an infraspinatus disorder (*C*). The External Rotation Lag Test is performed by having the patient flex the elbow to 90 degrees, then it is passively rotated into full external rotation, and patient is instructed to hold that placement. It is positive if the patient is unable to maintain external rotation, which indicates a supraspinatus and infraspinatus disorder (*D*).

shoulder syndromes require physical therapy assessment for the anatomic positioning of the glenohumeral joint and the scapulothoracic joint. Manual therapy may be necessary prior to exercises to correct any movement impairment. Motor control of the rotator cuff muscles is vital to stabilize and position the humeral head in the center of the glenoid with emphasis on external rotators to counterbalance any anterior glide problems. For scapulothoracic problems, the trapezius and serratus anterior muscles should be trained to maximize the upward rotation and control during dynamic movement.[14]

Bicipital Tendinopathy

Bicipital tendon injury most commonly occurs in 18- to 35-year-old individuals who participate in overhead sports, with secondary impingement of the biceps tendon from scapular and capsule instability.[15–17] Although bicipital tendinopathy may be an independent ailment, 95% of cases occur concomitantly with other injuries.[18] Biceps tendinopathy manifests with pain of the anterior shoulder that often radiates down to the biceps muscle or toward the deltoid. The pain may be worse at night and exacerbated by pulling or lifting activities. An audible click can be noted with upper limb motion, as the bicipital tendon slips in and out of the bicipital groove.[19] Palpation of the humeral bicipital groove and directly over the biceps tendon may reproduce the pain. Provocative testing includes the Yergason and Speed tests (**Fig. 2**).[15]

Identifying concomitant rotator cuff tendinopathy is important to direct therapy. As with rotator cuff tendinopathy, treatment entails resting from overhead and aggravating activities, judicious use of analgesics or NSAIDs, and formal physical therapy. Corticosteroid injection of the bicipital tendon sheath may be considered for refractory response to therapy. Failure of conservative management may require an MRI to assess for tendon tear and referral to orthopedic surgery.[15]

Subacromial Bursitis

The subacromial bursa lies between the rotator cuff tendons and the undersurface of the acromion. Subacromial bursitis usually develops concomitantly with rotator cuff tendinopathy or shoulder impingement. Pain occurs at the insertion of the deltoid muscle, and is exacerbated by shoulder abduction.[1] Treatment is similar to that of rotator cuff tendinopathy. A meta-analysis found musculoskeletal ultrasound-guided injections resulted in better pain control and improvement in shoulder function compared to those who underwent blind injection.[20]

ELBOW PAIN
Olecranon Bursitis

The olecranon bursa is a superficial bursa posterior to the ulnar olecranon process. There are various causes of olecranon bursitis: acute trauma, chronic microtrauma,

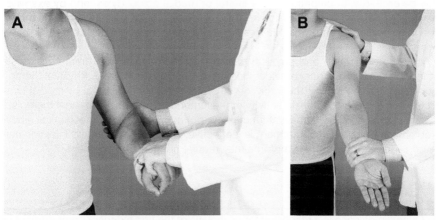

Fig. 2. Yergason's Test is performed by having the patient flex their elbow to 90 degrees in pronation, and the examiner resists supination of the forearm. A positive test elicits pain at the long head of the biceps and indicates bicipital tendinopathy (*A*). Speed's Test is performed by having the patient extend the affected arm and fully supinate, followed by flexion at the shoulder and resistance by the examiner. Pain in the anterior shoulder is a positive response and indicates bicipital tendinopathy (*B*).

gout, rheumatoid arthritis, or infection.[21] Patients often report a history suggestive of one of these etiologies and almost universally experience bursal edema, erythema, and tenderness. Elbow motion may only elicit pain with extreme flexion as the bursa is compressed. Erythema over the olecranon is common in inflammation or infection. Pain throughout full elbow range of motion, or supination/pronation of the radial head, may be more indicative of intra-articular involvement.[22]

Aspiration of the olecranon bursa fluid can exclude gout and septic bursitis. The bursal fluid should be analyzed for cell count, crystals, and microorganisms by Gram stain and culture prior to consideration of antibiotics. Radiographs of the elbow may be performed when considering fracture or bony abnormality causing the inflammation.[22]

Septic bursitis requires treatment with antibiotics with initial empiric antibiotic selection based on efficacy against *Staphylococcus* and *Streptococcus* species. Conservative antibiotic management is usually effective; however, persistent infections may require serial aspirations or incision and drainage.[22] When infection is unsuspected, olecranon bursitis can be managed conservatively with rest, compression, splinting, and avoidance of aggravating activity. A short course of NSAIDs can be effective. A corticosteroid injection may be considered in patients with severe culture negative bursitis. Chronic painful aseptic olecranon bursitis may require bursectomy.

Lateral and Medial Elbow Tendinopathy (Epicondylitis)

Lateral and medial elbow tendinopathies (epicondylitis) are considered chronic tendinosis disorders rather than tendinitis based on histologic studies.[23] The extensor carpi radialis brevis muscle (wrist extensors) originates at the distal, lateral humerus, and is most commonly affected in lateral epicondylitis or tennis elbow. The pronator teres and flexor carpi radialis tendons (wrist flexors) contribute to medial epicondylitis or golfers' elbow. Both disorders are caused by overuse activities associated with occupations, hobbies, or athletics.

Patients typically describe pain of the lateral or medial elbow just anterior to the respective epicondyle that may radiate along the affected muscles. Tenderness may be elicited with palpation of the lateral or medial epicondyles, and by examiner resistance to active wrist extension in lateral epicondylitis, or resistance to active wrist flexion in medial epicondylitis. Plain radiographs rarely identify bony abnormalities or loose bodies.

Activity modification and physical therapy are the mainstays of treatment. Acetaminophen or NSAIDs may provide short-term benefit with therapy. Physical therapy focuses on strengthening the wrist in neutral position for the lateral or medial syndrome and increasing intrinsic activity of the lumbrical muscles.[24] Physical therapists always assess shoulder and wrist function for optimal treatment of mechanical elbow problems. If conservative treatment is ineffective, a local corticosteroid injection can be considered. Refractory symptoms may require surgical management.[25]

HAND AND WRIST PAIN
De Quervain Disease

De Quervain disease is a stenosing tenosynovitis of the first extensor compartment of the wrist. Resisted gliding of the abductor pollicis longus (APL) and extensor pollicis brevis (EPB) tendons within the narrowed fibro-osseous canal causes pain (**Fig. 3**). De Quervain disease may result from repetitive microtrauma (usually occupational), inflammatory disease, and increased volume states including pregnancy, trauma, and anatomic abnormalities.[26] Women are affected more often than men.[27] Patients

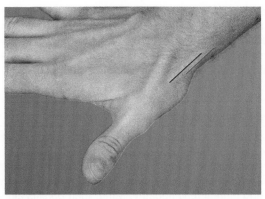

Fig. 3. De Quervain results from resisted gliding of the abductor pollicus longus (*red*) and extensor pollicus brevis (*blue*) within a narrowed fibro-osseous canal.

usually report a gradual onset of pain along the radial aspect of the wrist worsened by grasping and lifting objects.

On physical examination, pain may be elicited on palpation of the first extensor compartment over the radial styloid that radiates to the thumb or forearm. Pain may be reproduced with repetitive movement of the thumb, and extensor triggering or locking may be noted. The Finkelstein test is positive when lateral wrist pain is reproduced by passive ulnar deviation of the hand and wrist while the patient encloses his or her flexed thumb in a fist. Carpometacarpal (CMC) joint osteoarthritis may be differentiated from de Quervain disease by the presence of direct palpatory pain of the first CMC joint.[26] Chronic or recurrent disease should be assessed with imaging to identify or exclude other causes of symptoms.[26]

Conservative therapy requires avoiding aggravating activities. Analgesics and NSAIDs may be helpful for 2 to 4 weeks. A radial thumb spica splint extending to the forearm may be prescribed to immobilize the thumb and wrist. The patient may benefit from further education and rehabilitation from an occupational or physical therapist. Corticosteroid injection into the tenosynovial sheath may be effective if conservative treatments fail. When improvement is noted with an initial injection but resolution is incomplete, a repeat injection can be performed 4 to 8 weeks later. Prolonged, refractory disease may require surgery for release of the first dorsal compartment.[26,28]

Trigger Finger (Stenosing Tenosynovitis)

Trigger finger results when there is a mismatch between the size of the flexor tendon sheath and its contents.[29] The cause of trigger fingers is debated, with histologic studies identifying an underlying primary tendinopathy, and other studies revealing a paucity of inflammatory cells. This suggests that the term tenosynovitis is a misnomer, and the problem is more of a fibrocartilage abnormality.[30]

Patients with diabetes mellitus, renal disease, thyroid disease, repetitive trauma, inflammatory disease, and female gender are at greatest risk of developing trigger fingers.[29–31] A locking or clicking sensation with finger movement is reported with progression to painful triggering. Pain is localized in the palm, metacarpophalangeal joints, or the proximal interphalangeal joints.[29] Triggering may or may not be evident on physical examination.

Early or mild cases can be treated with activity avoidance[31] and splinting of the involved digit. One study found improvement in 93% of patients who were splinted for a 6- to 10-week period.[32] NSAIDs may be used, but studies are lacking to support their efficacy. Local corticosteroid injections may only be effective in 57% of patients,[33] and a recurrence rate of 56% up to 1 year after injections has been reported.[34] Conservative treatments are most effective early in the clinical course; surgical release may provide a 97% success rate if persistent.[35]

HIP PAIN
Greater Trochanteric Pain Syndrome (Tronchanteric Bursitis)

Greater trochanteric pain syndrome (GTPS) manifests with pain at and around the greater trochanter that may radiate to the lateral thigh and is exacerbated by physical activity or lying on the affected side. The term trochanteric bursitis has been replaced by GTPS, as advanced imaging of the lateral hip more consistently reveals peritrochanteric edema and gluteal tendinopathy, rather than bursitis alone.[36] Physical examination reveals tenderness on palpation of the greater trochanter. A single-legged stance test and resisted external rotation test can differentiate the pain from a gluteal tendinopathy (**Table 2**).[37]

Avoidance of provocative activities, stretching, and physical therapy are the mainstays of therapy. Illiotibial band stretching, gluteal strengthening, straight leg raises, and assisted squats enabled 34% of patients to return to normal activity within 6 months.[38] Local corticosteroid injections may be effective.[39] Surgery is reserved for refractory symptoms despite conservative treatments.[40]

KNEE PAIN
Knee Bursitis

The prepatellar bursa (**Fig. 4**) is anterior to the knee between the patella and subcutaneous tissues. The differential diagnosis for prepatellar bursitis is similar to olecranon bursitis: acute trauma, chronic microtrauma, gout, rheumatoid arthritis, or infection. People in specific occupations requiring repetitive kneeling are most often diagnosed with prepatellar bursitis, particularly fishermen, roofers, carpet layers, house cleaners, and coal miners.[41]

Prepatellar bursitis is painful mostly on flexion of the knee because of compression of the bursa, but the knee joint is not painful. There is erythema over the patellar surface. The bursal fluid should be analyzed for cell count, crystals, and microorganisms by Gram stain and culture. Septic bursitis requires conventional antibiotic therapy for *Staphylococcus* and *Streptococcus* species. Broad-spectrum antibiotics are necessary with a penetrating injury. Conservative antibiotic

Table 2			
Provocative tests to assess for gluteal causes of greater trochanteric pain syndrome			
Test	**How to Perform**	**Positive Test**	**Sensitivity and Specificity for Gluteal Tendinopathy**
Single leg stance test[37]	Patient stands on the affected leg for 30 s	Pain in affected lateral hip	100%, 97.3%
Resisted external rotation[37]	Patient lies supine, hip and knee flexed to 90°, then the hip is externally rotated. The examiner resists patient effort to internally rotate	Pain in affected lateral hip	88%, 97.3%

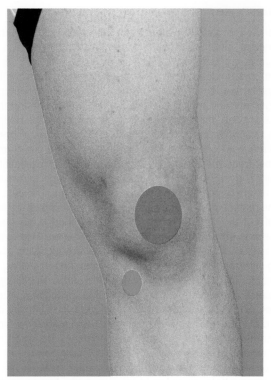

Fig. 4. The anterior knee with markers identifying the location of the prepatellar bursa (*red*) and pes anserine bursa (*blue*).

management is usually effective, but sometimes serial aspirations or incision and drainage may be indicated.[22] When infection is unsuspected, olecranon bursitis can be managed conservatively with rest, compression, and avoidance of aggravating activity. A short course of NSAIDs can be considered if safely prescribed. A corticosteroid injection may be considered in patients with severe, culture-negative prepatellar bursitis.

Pes Anserine Bursitis

The pes anserine bursa (see **Fig. 4**) overlies the medial tibia metaphysis just inferior to the tibial plateau, and just deep to the tendons of the sartorius, gracilis, and semitendinosus muscles. It is believed to result from overuse friction to the bursa caused by excessive valgus or rotatory stresses to the knee or by direct contusion.[42] The pain mimics medial knee joint pain by history; however, the pain is located distal to the joint line. Obese patients with underlying knee osteoarthritis or rheumatoid arthritis are at highest risk. The most commonly affected athletes are middle-aged, female long-distance runners.[43]

On physical examination, pain occurs with direct palpation of the affected bursa, and mild swelling and warmth may be present. Any inciting activities should be avoided, and analgesics may be helpful. Physical therapy should assess the hip and ankle joint function to be most effective for the treatment of pes anserine bursitis, mechanical knee problems, or associated osteoarthritis. Corticosteroid injections can be helpful to treat severe pes anserine bursitis. Bursectomy is rarely necessary for recurrent bursitis.[43]

Popliteal Cysts (Baker Cysts)

Popliteal cysts, or Baker cysts, develop when the gastrocnemio-semimembranosus bursa of the medial popliteal fossa distends with fluid. The gastrocnemio-semimembranosus bursa communicates with the knee joint via a 1-way valvelike mechanism that allows unidirectional flow of synovial fluid from the knee joint to the cyst. Popliteal cysts commonly develop in the setting of concomitant knee joint pathology or derangement and may become inflamed. Differentiating the popliteal cyst from other causes of posterior knee mass is important, because deep venous thrombosis, aneurysms, ganglion or meniscal cysts, and tumors may present similarly.[44] Further, the popliteal cyst can compress various anatomic structures, the popliteal vein being the most frequent target, and thrombophlebitis may develop.[45]

Often, the popliteal cyst will develop insidiously over time and may be secondary to chronic inflammatory or noninflammatory knee pathology. The cyst may be increasingly notable to the patient as the fluid mass expands, causing posterior knee swelling, stiffness, discomfort, and limited range of motion. Once large enough, it can be observed with the patient standing and/or on examination. However, patients may also present with acute popliteal cyst rupture manifesting with acute calf muscle pain and swelling with resolution of previous posterior knee swelling.

Treatment of the popliteal cyst is conservative and supportive as resolution may be spontaneous. In some cases, specific treatment of an associated intra-articular knee disorder is required to facilitate popliteal cyst resolution. In patients with knee osteoarthritis complicated by popliteal cysts, aspiration of the popliteal cyst followed by intra-articular corticosteroid injection may facilitate significant reduction of pain and cyst size.[46] Use of ultrasound to guide cyst aspiration is recommended to avoid complications. A comparison study of osteoarthritis patients with popliteal cysts who underwent intra-articular or intracystic corticosteroid injections identified beneficial effect from both procedures, with intracystic injections resulting in greater reduction of cyst size.[47] Refractory popliteal cysts may be effectively treated with surgical cyst excision.

ANKLE/FOOT PAIN
Plantar Fasciitis

Plantar fasciitis is a chronic degenerative process involving the dense, fibrous, collagenous connective tissue (aponeurosis) of the foot that originates at the medial tubercle of the calcaneus and fans distally toward its insertion at the base of each proximal phalanx.[48] The thick proximal origin of the plantar fascia is the segment most likely to be affected in plantar fasciitis, and histopathologic studies have shown degenerative features with an absence of inflammatory cells suggesting *plantar fasciosis* better reflects an accurate diagnostic term.[49] The classic presentation of plantar fasciitis involves medial heal pain with greatest severity in the morning with initial steps. Sharp, intense pain occurs at the heel and plantar arch with improvement upon resting. Pes planus, pes cavus, overpronation of the foot and leg-length discrepancies may predispose to the development of plantar fasciitis, and exercise training errors may lead to symptoms in athletes.[49]

On physical examination, pain is reproduced with palpation of the plantar medial aspect of the heel and with passive dorsiflexion of the ankle and toes (windlass test). Pain at a location other than the plantar fascia origin suggests an alternative diagnosis.[48,49]

Treatment should be individualized and may include stretching (**Figs. 5** and **6**), weight loss in obese patients, rest and training correction in athletes, arch supports, heel cups, and NSAIDs for pain control. Ultrasonography, iontophoresis,

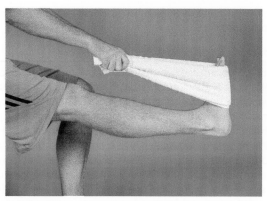

Fig. 5. Calf and foot arch stretch using a towel. The knee is maintained in extension while the patient gently stretches the plantar fascia before weight bearing.

extracorporeal shockwave therapy, custom orthoses, and night splints may be prescribed when patient stretching is suboptimal. Corticosteroid, platelet-rich plasma, and botulinum toxin injections have limited data supporting their use in the management of plantar fasciitis.[49] Prolonged conservative management for over 6 months

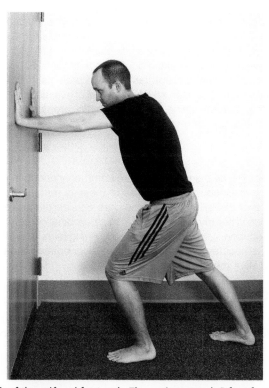

Fig. 6. Wall stretch of the calf and foot arch. The patient stands 3 feet from a wall, places his or her hands against the wall, and steps forward with one foot. With the feet pointed toward the wall and the rear heel on the floor, the calf muscles are stretched with the knee in partial flexion and extension.

results in complete pain relief in 85% to 90% of patients.[49] Surgical plantar fascia release is rarely indicated.

Achilles Tendinopathy

Several different predisposing factors may contribute to the development of Achilles tendinopathy. High-intensity running, previous trauma, sedentary lifestyle, high-healed shoes, anatomic variance, reactive arthritis, rheumatoid arthritis, and the use of fluoroquinolones or systemic corticosteroids have been associated with Achilles tendinopathy. Symptoms of Achilles tendinopathy include pain, diffuse or localized Achilles regional swelling, or decline in various activities. An acute rupture of the Achilles tendon is perceived as sudden-onset posterior calcaneal pain during a high-impact activity, whereas chronic tendinopathy develops insidiously and may be unprovoked in sedentary or elderly individuals.[50] The midportion of the Achilles tendon is affected in 55% to 65% of all injuries, and insertional Achilles tendinopathy (enthesopathy) occurs in 20% to 25% of cases.[51] Palpation of the full length of the Achilles tendon may localize pain in the area of 2 cm to 6 cm proximal to the insertion into the posterior calcaneus. The examiner should assess for tendon fullness, irregularity, and gapping or tenderness; additionally, active and passive range of motion should be assessed with strength and gait testing.[50] Chronic Achilles tendon ruptures may be more difficult to identify by physical examination than acute ruptures, as scarring may bridge any gaps in the torn tendon fibers.[51]

Conservative management of Achilles tendinopathy is the mainstay in the majority of cases and includes rest, icing, analgesics, bracing, ankle-foot orthoses, and activity modification. Physical therapy should be initiated soon after diagnosing Achilles tendinopathy to improve ankle dorsiflexion, recruitment of anterior tibialis, and intrinsic foot muscles with gradual progression of ankle plantarflexor strengthening.[24,50] Acute Achilles tendon rupture requires walking boot immobilization. Surgical reconstruction is often essential for acute tendon ruptures in active patients.[50] Chronic Achilles tendinopathy is typically treated conservatively. The use of injections with corticosteroids, platelet-rich plasma, normal saline, and anesthetic preparations is controversial without evidence to support long-term benefit.

SUMMARY

Soft tissue musculoskeletal pain disorders are commonly encountered in the primary care setting. Early recognition and diagnosis of these common syndromes will minimize patient pain and disability. These disorders can be diagnosed by history and physical examination. Therapy typically requires a combination of avoiding the aggravating activity, education, and physical therapy. Analgesics and NSAIDs should be used judiciously. Corticosteroid injections and surgical options should be considered only when conservative therapy is ineffective.

ACKNOWLEDGMENTS

Special thanks go to Grace Balfour (SAMMC photography) for her assistance with instructional photos in this article. Thanks also go to Jose Ruiz for modeling the physical maneuvers.

REFERENCES

1. Sheon RP, Moskowitz RW, Goldberg VM. Soft tissue rheumatic pain: recognition, management, and prevention. 3rd edition. Baltimore (MD): Williams & Wilkins; 1996.

2. Walker-Bone KE, Palmer KT, Reading I, et al. Soft-tissue rheumatic disorders of the neck and upper limb: prevalence and risk factors. Semin Arthritis Rheum 2003;33(3):185–203.
3. Gerwin RD. Myofascial trigger point pain syndromes. Semin Neurol 2016;36(5): 469–73.
4. Rivers WE, Garrigues D, Graciosa J, et al. Signs and symptoms of myofascial pain: an international survey of pain management providers and proposed preliminary set of diagnostic criteria. Pain Med 2015;16(9):1794–805.
5. Christmas C, Crespo CJ, Franckowiak SC, et al. How common is hip pain among older adults? Results from the Third National Health and Nutrition Examination Survey. J Fam Pract 2002;51(4):345–8.
6. Nguyen US, Zhang Y, Zhu Y, et al. Increasing prevalence of knee pain and symptomatic knee osteoarthritis: survey and cohort data. Ann Intern Med 2011; 155(11):725–32.
7. Thomas MJ, Roddy E, Zhang W, et al. The population prevalence of foot and ankle pain in middle and old age: a systematic review. Pain 2011;152(12):2870–80.
8. Borg-Stein J, Iaccarino MA. Myofascial pain syndrome treatments. Phys Med Rehabil Clin N Am 2014;25(2):357–74.
9. Edwards J, Knowles N. Superficial dry needling and active stretching in the treatment of myofascial pain–a randomised controlled trial. Acupunct Med 2003; 21(3):80–6.
10. Frontera WR, Silver JK, Rizzo TD. Essentials of physical medicine and rehabilitation: musculoskeletal disorders, pain, and rehabilitation. 3rd edition. Philadelphia: Elsevier/Saunders; 2015.
11. Hermans J, Luime JJ, Meuffels DE, et al. Does this patient with shoulder pain have rotator cuff disease?: The Rational Clinical Examination systematic review. JAMA 2013;310(8):837–47.
12. Lenza M, Buchbinder R, Takwoingi Y, et al. Magnetic resonance imaging, magnetic resonance arthrography and ultrasonography for assessing rotator cuff tears in people with shoulder pain for whom surgery is being considered. Cochrane Database Syst Rev 2013;(9):CD009020.
13. Boudreault J, Desmeules F, Roy JS, et al. The efficacy of oral non-steroidal anti-inflammatory drugs for rotator cuff tendinopathy: a systematic review and meta-analysis. J Rehabil Med 2014;46(4):294–306.
14. Sahrmann S. Diagnosis and treatment of movement impairment syndromes. St Louis: Mosby; 2002.
15. Churgay CA. Diagnosis and treatment of biceps tendinitis and tendinosis. Am Fam Physician 2009;80(5):470–6.
16. Kibler WB. Scapular involvement in impingement: signs and symptoms. Instr Course Lect 2006;55:35–43.
17. Abrams JS. Special shoulder problems in the throwing athlete: pathology, diagnosis, and nonoperative management. Clin Sports Med 1991;10(4):839–61.
18. Patton WC, McCluskey GM 3rd. Biceps tendinitis and subluxation. Clin Sports Med 2001;20(3):505–29.
19. McFarland EG, Borade A. Examination of the biceps tendon. Clin Sports Med 2016;35(1):29–45.
20. Wu T, Song HX, Dong Y, et al. Ultrasound-guided versus blind subacromial-subdeltoid bursa injection in adults with shoulder pain: a systematic review and meta-analysis. Semin Arthritis Rheum 2015;45(3):374–8.
21. Larson RL, Osternig LR. Traumatic bursitis and artificial turf. J Sports Med 1974; 2(4):183–8.

22. Reilly D, Kamineni S. Olecranon bursitis. J Shoulder Elbow Surg 2016;25(1): 158–67.

23. Doran A, Gresham GA, Rushton N, et al. Tennis elbow. A clinicopathologic study of 22 cases followed for 2 years. Acta Orthop Scand 1990;61(6):535–8.

24. Sahrmann S. Movement system impairment syndromes of the extremities, cervical and thoracic spines. St Louis (MO): Elsevier/Mosby; 2011.

25. Vaquero-Picado A, Barco R, Antuna SA. Lateral epicondylitis of the elbow. EFORT Open Rev 2016;1(11):391–7.

26. Ilyas AM, Ast M, Schaffer AA, et al. De quervain tenosynovitis of the wrist. J Am Acad Orthop Surg 2007;15(12):757–64.

27. Wolf JM, Sturdivant RX, Owens BD. Incidence of de Quervain's tenosynovitis in a young, active population. J Hand Surg Am 2009;34(1):112–5.

28. Huisstede BM, Coert JH, Friden J, et al. Consensus on a multidisciplinary treatment guideline for de Quervain disease: results from the European HANDGUIDE study. Phys Ther 2014;94(8):1095–110.

29. Ryzewicz M, Wolf JM. Trigger digits: principles, management, and complications. J Hand Surg Am 2006;31(1):135–46.

30. Sampson SP, Badalamente MA, Hurst LC, et al. Pathobiology of the human A1 pulley in trigger finger. J Hand Surg Am 1991;16(4):714–21.

31. Giugale JM, Fowler JR. Trigger finger: adult and pediatric treatment strategies. Orthop Clin North Am 2015;46(4):561–9.

32. Colbourn J, Heath N, Manary S, et al. Effectiveness of splinting for the treatment of trigger finger. J Hand Ther 2008;21(4):336–43.

33. Fleisch SB, Spindler KP, Lee DH. Corticosteroid injections in the treatment of trigger finger: a level I and II systematic review. J Am Acad Orthop Surg 2007; 15(3):166–71.

34. Rozental TD, Zurakowski D, Blazar PE. Trigger finger: prognostic indicators of recurrence following corticosteroid injection. J Bone Joint Surg Am 2008;90(8):1665–72.

35. Turowski GA, Zdankiewicz PD, Thomson JG. The results of surgical treatment of trigger finger. J Hand Surg Am 1997;22(1):145–9.

36. Klontzas ME, Karantanas AH. Greater trochanter pain syndrome: a descriptive MR imaging study. Eur J Radiol 2014;83(10):1850–5.

37. Lequesne M, Mathieu P, Vuillemin-Bodaghi V, et al. Gluteal tendinopathy in refractory greater trochanter pain syndrome: diagnostic value of two clinical tests. Arthritis Rheum 2008;59(2):241–6.

38. Rompe JD, Segal NA, Cacchio A, et al. Home training, local corticosteroid injection, or radial shock wave therapy for greater trochanter pain syndrome. Am J Sports Med 2009;37(10):1981–90.

39. Furia JP, Rompe JD, Maffulli N. Low-energy extracorporeal shock wave therapy as a treatment for greater trochanteric pain syndrome. Am J Sports Med 2009; 37(9):1806–13.

40. Redmond JM, Chen AW, Domb BG. Greater trochanteric pain syndrome. J Am Acad Orthop Surg 2016;24(4):231–40.

41. Reid CR, Bush PM, Cummings NH, et al. A review of occupational knee disorders. J Occup Rehabil 2010;20(4):489–501.

42. Rennie WJ, Saifuddin A. Pes anserine bursitis: incidence in symptomatic knees and clinical presentation. Skeletal Radiol 2005;34(7):395–8.

43. Hong E, Kraft MC. Evaluating anterior knee pain. Med Clin North Am 2014;98(4): 697–717, xi.

44. Herman AM, Marzo JM. Popliteal cysts: a current review. Orthopedics 2014; 37(8):e678–84.

45. Fritschy D, Fasel J, Imbert JC, et al. The popliteal cyst. Knee Surg Sports Traumatol Arthrosc 2006;14(7):623–8.
46. Acebes JC, Sanchez-Pernaute O, Diaz-Oca A, et al. Ultrasonographic assessment of Baker's cysts after intra-articular corticosteroid injection in knee osteoarthritis. J Clin Ultrasound 2006;34(3):113–7.
47. Bandinelli F, Fedi R, Generini S, et al. Longitudinal ultrasound and clinical follow-up of Baker's cysts injection with steroids in knee osteoarthritis. Clin Rheumatol 2012;31(4):727–31.
48. Thompson JV, Saini SS, Reb CW, et al. Diagnosis and management of plantar fasciitis. J Am Osteopath Assoc 2014;114(12):900–6.
49. Young C. In the clinic. Plantar fasciitis. Ann Intern Med 2012;156(1 Pt 1):ITC1-1. ITC1-2, ITC1-3, ITC1-4, ITC1-5, ITC1-6, ITC1-7, ITC1-8, ITC1-9, ITC1-10, ITC11-11, ITC11-12, ITC11-13, ITC11-14, ITC11-15; [quiz: ITC11-16].
50. Saini SS, Reb CW, Chapter M, et al. Achilles tendon disorders. J Am Osteopath Assoc 2015;115(11):670–6.
51. Maffulli N, Via AG, Oliva F. Chronic achilles tendon disorders: tendinopathy and chronic rupture. Clin Sports Med 2015;34(4):607–24.

Primary Care Vasculitis
Polymyalgia Rheumatica and Giant Cell Arteritis

Mathilde H. Pioro, MDCM, MSc, FRCPC[a,b],*

KEYWORDS

- Polymyalgia rheumatica • Giant cell arteritis • Temporal artery biopsy
- Corticosteroids • Tocilizumab

KEY POINTS

- Polymyalgia rheumatica (PMR) and giant cell arteritis (GCA) are related inflammatory diseases of adults aged 50 years or older.
- PMR presents with pain and stiffness of proximal shoulders with or without hip involvement, elevated inflammatory markers (occasionally normal), and a characteristic dramatic response to corticosteroids.
- GCA presents with cranial vessel ischemia, causing headache, jaw claudication, and visual disturbances. Not all clinical features may be present; hence, a high index of suspicion must be maintained.
- If GCA is suspected, corticosteroids must be promptly initiated to avert irreversible vision loss. Treatment should be initiated before temporal artery biopsy if clinical suspicion is high.
- GCA may also present with predominantly constitutional symptoms, including fever of unknown origin. Treatment includes corticosteroids, aspirin, and tocilizumab.

INTRODUCTION

Polymyalgia rheumatica (PMR) is an inflammatory syndrome of older adults characterized by aching pain and morning stiffness of the shoulder and pelvic girdles associated with increased acute phase reactants and rapid response to steroids. It can be associated with giant cell arteritis (GCA), and the 2 conditions may constitute different manifestations of a disease spectrum.

Disclosure Statement: No disclosure.
[a] Department of Rheumatology, Orthopedic and Rheumatologic Institute, Cleveland Clinic, 9500 Euclid Avenue A50, Cleveland, OH 44195, USA; [b] Cleveland Clinic Lerner College of Medicine of Case Western Reserve University, 9500 Euclid Avenue A50, Cleveland, OH 44195, USA
* Orthopedic and Rheumatologic Institute, Cleveland Clinic, 9500 Euclid Avenue A50, Cleveland, OH 44195.
E-mail address: piorom@ccf.org

Prim Care Clin Office Pract 45 (2018) 305–323
https://doi.org/10.1016/j.pop.2018.02.007
0095-4543/18/© 2018 Elsevier Inc. All rights reserved.

EPIDEMIOLOGY

PMR is the second most common inflammatory autoimmune syndrome after rheumatoid arthritis with a lifetime risk in the United States of 2.4% in women and 1.1% in men,[1] based on a primarily white population of mainly Scandinavian descent. The incidence is more poorly defined but much less common in other ethnic groups. PMR is very rare at less than 50 years of age, with mean age of onset approximately 70 years old, and increasing prevalence with older age.[2] Consideration of PMR in a patient less than 50 years of age should prompt careful review of other diagnostic entities (see later discussion of differential diagnosis).

PATHOGENESIS

Systemic inflammation is the hallmark of PMR, manifesting as constitutional symptoms in many patients. The cause of PMR is unknown. The higher prevalence of PMR in white populations suggests a genetic predisposition, and PMR is associated with specific alleles of the human leukocyte antigen, including HLA-DR4.[3,4] Onset of disease late in life suggests that environmental factors influence disease expression; however, there is no known association with any infectious agent or toxin. As with other chronic autoimmune diseases, there appears to be an imbalance between the immunosuppressive T-regulatory lymphocytes and the pro-inflammatory T-helper 17 lymphocytes.[5] Evidence of subclinical inflammation (increased expression of proinflammatory cytokines, including interleukin-6 [IL-6])[6] has been demonstrated in the temporal arteries of PMR patients without clinical evidence of GCA. Some studies have suggested relative adrenal insufficiency with inadequate cortisol production in response to inflammation.[7,8]

HISTORY

Patients with PMR present with the classic inflammatory symptoms of morning stiffness and night pain, involving primarily the posterior neck and shoulders and frequently the pelvic girdle. Onset of PMR may be abrupt over days, at times overnight, or insidious over weeks to months. Shoulder pain is frequently referred to the upper arms. Pelvic girdle pain can include the hips (groin) and lateral and posterior thighs, but is not required for diagnosis. The pain is deep and aching and can be so severe that simply rolling in bed from one side to the other becomes difficult and may wake the patient from sleep. Pain may be unilateral at onset but generally becomes bilateral and symmetric, which helps to differentiate it from focal musculoskeletal syndromes, such as rotator cuff tendinitis.

MORNING STIFFNESS AND FUNCTIONAL LIMITATIONS

The characteristic proximal aching and stiffness of PMR is thought to result from referred pain from inflamed joints and periarticular tissues of the shoulders and hips. Morning stiffness typically lasts well beyond 45 minutes, often persisting into the afternoon or all day, and worsens or recurs with immobility (eg, car ride, movie). A marked decline in functional status from baseline is characteristic, with patients reporting decreased ability to perform activities of daily living, especially in the morning, sometimes to the point of requiring assistance. Decrease in overall mobility is also prominent. Patients frequently complain of severe proximal weakness, with difficulty lifting arms overhead to dress and groom, and difficulty arising from chairs and climbing stairs. The weakness is often described as painful or aching, unlike primary myopathies, which are painless.

CONSTITUTIONAL SYMPTOMS

Constitutional symptoms may include malaise, fatigue, depression, low-grade fever, and sometimes striking weight loss. Before attributing fever and weight loss to PMR, other causes, such as infection, malignancy, and vasculitis, should be considered.

PHYSICAL EXAMINATION

Findings on physical examination are often considerably milder than would be expected from the intensity of symptoms. Tenderness to palpation of the neck and shoulders may be present. Severely decreased shoulder abduction is a particularly prominent feature. Decreased range of motion (ROM) and pain with active ROM more than passive ROM are present in the cervical spine, shoulders, and hips. With longer duration of illness, capsular contraction may occur, limiting passive ROM.

Mild distal joint inflammation can be present in approximately one-half of patients,[9] with upper greater than lower extremity involvement, typically at the wrists and metacarpophalangeal (MCP) joints, rarely at the knees with associated effusions. Wrist involvement may result in carpal tunnel syndrome. Joint tenderness to palpation exacerbated by passive ROM suggests underlying joint inflammation. Ankle and metatarsophalangeal (MTP) synovitis are very rare and should trigger consideration of other diagnoses. Although patients frequently complain of weakness, careful neurologic examination with prompting and encouragement reveals normal strength limited by pain. Strength can be tested by asking the patient to provide bursts of maximal strength for a few seconds as tolerated (eg, shoulder abduction, hip flexion), advising the patient that this may provide brief discomfort but will aid in diagnosis. Longstanding symptoms may result in disuse atrophy with resultant weakness.

REMITTING SERONEGATIVE SYMMETRIC SYNOVITIS WITH PITTING EDEMA

Remitting seronegative symmetric synovitis with pitting edema (RS3PE) is an uncommon PMR variant in approximately 10% of patients.[9,10] RS3PE presents with severe, sometimes dramatic, swelling and edema of the hands and fingers, resulting in inability to make a fist. The swelling and edema (usually pitting) can result in disappearance of bony landmarks and a "boxing glove" appearance reminiscent of acute gout without erythema or warmth, and not as painful. Proximal inflammation and pain in the shoulders are usually present but subtle. Ultrasound and MRI demonstrate extensor tenosynovitis and synovitis of the forearms and wrists, and to a lesser degree in the MCPs and proximal interphalangeal joints.[11,12]

LABORATORY TESTS: ERYTHROCYTE SEDIMENTATION RATE AND C-REACTIVE PROTEIN

The most characteristic laboratory finding in PMR is an elevated erythrocyte sedimentation rate (ESR). Twenty percent of patients in one study had ESR greater than 104 mm/h (and C-reactive protein [CRP] >8.8 mg/dL).[13] A normal sedimentation rate does not rule out PMR. ESR less than 40 mm/h has been reported in 6% to 22% of patients.[13-17] It is important to remember that ESR increases with age. A simple adjustment to the ESR can be easily calculated (Box 1).[18]

CRP, which is a more specific marker for inflammation than ESR, may also be considered. Studies have shown tight concordance of elevated ESR and CRP in patients with PMR.[13,14] In addition, PMR patients with normal ESR have been found to have a modestly elevated CRP (median 1.4 mg/dL).[13] Having both normal ESR and normal CRP in PMR is extremely rare, occurring in 1.2% of cases in a prospective study.[19] Similar to ESR, CRP increases with age (see Box 1).[20] ESR declines

---

Box 1
Correction of acute phase reactants for age

Sedimentation rate[18]
　　Adjusted upper limit of normal ESR for age
　　Age/2 for men, ([age+10]/2) for women
　　Units: mm/h

C-reactive protein[20]
　　Adjusted upper limit of normal CRP for age
　　Mexican-Americans & non-Hispanic whites:
　　Age/50 for men, ([age/50]+0.6) for women
　　Non-Hispanic blacks:
　　Age/30 for men, ([age/50]+1.0) for women
　　Units: mg/dL

---

much more slowly than CRP after inflammation subsides (half-life ESR 7 days, CRP 18 hours).[21]

OTHER LABORATORY TESTS

In keeping with systemic inflammation, common findings include normochromic normocytic anemia and thrombocytosis. Liver function test abnormalities may be seen in up to one-third of patients.[19] Tests for rheumatoid factor, cyclic citrullinated peptide antibodies, and antinuclear antibodies are negative. Creatine kinase is normal. Synovial fluid when obtained is inflammatory with negative crystal examination and culture. Although the term PMR appears to imply muscle abnormality, muscle biopsies either are normal or show nonspecific changes without evidence of inflammation.[22]

IMAGING

Imaging is not routinely used to support a diagnosis of PMR. Radiographs are unremarkable. Multiple studies have confirmed inflammation of shoulder and hip joints, bursae, and tendons in PMR by ultrasound, MRI, and PET scanning, with subdeltoid/subacromial bursitis detected in more than two-thirds of patients.[23–25] The use of shoulder ultrasound marginally improves the sensitivity and specificity of PMR diagnostic criteria.[26] PET scan has revealed subclinical inflammation of the subclavian arteries in a subset of PMR patients.[27] Although this finding is consistent with the known association between PMR and GCA, the clinical and prognostic significance of this is not clear. The current standard of care does not support obtaining advanced vascular imaging in PMR patients without clinical features of GCA.

DIFFERENTIAL DIAGNOSIS

Conditions to consider in the differential diagnosis are presented in **Table 1**. If the diagnosis of PMR is considered, the clinician must always consider the possibility of associated GCA.

ESTABLISHING THE DIAGNOSIS OF POLYMYALGIA RHEUMATICA

Classification criteria for PMR have been defined for use in research.[16,28] In practice, however, the diagnosis of PMR is a clinical one, based on the following features:

- Age older than 50 years
- Proximal bilateral aching and morning stiffness lasting at least 30 to 45 minutes

Table 1
Differential diagnosis of polymyalgia rheumatica

Diagnosis	Characteristic Features (Not All May Be Present)
Shoulder osteoarthritis, rotator cuff syndrome, subacromial bursitis, frozen shoulder	Limited morning stiffness; no constitutional symptoms; more likely unilateral; normal ESR/CRP; abnormal radiographs
Fibromyalgia	Longstanding symptoms, often years; no constitutional symptoms; tender myofascial points; normal ESR, CRP, and hemoglobin
Bone metabolism abnormalities: hyperparathyroidism, osteomalacia	Underlying history of renal/GI disease; hypercalcemia and elevated parathyroid hormone; vitamin D; abnormal radiographs (chondrocalcinosis, pseudofractures)
Malignancy (especially lymphoma, myeloma)	Past history of malignancy; fever; adenopathy; leukopenia; thrombocytopenia; elevated total protein/decreased albumin in serum; abnormal protein electrophoresis in serum/urine; abnormal bone scan
Infection (tuberculosis, HIV, endocarditis)	Fever, murmur; abnormal cultures and serologies
Statin-induced myalgias and myopathy	Statin use; no morning stiffness; preserved range of motion of proximal joints; increased CK if myopathy
Inflammatory myopathy	Painless; elevated CK; abnormal EMG and muscle biopsy
Spondyloarthropathy	Low back pain; inflammatory GI symptoms; psoriasis; dactylitis, enthesitis; uveitis; abnormal spine and sacroiliac joint radiographs; HLAB27
Hypothyroidism	Delayed tendon reflexes; elevated thyroid stimulating hormone; decreased T4; normal ESR/CRP
Parkinson disease	Tremor; rigidity; decreased blink; shuffling gait
Crowned dens syndrome (calcium hydroxyapatite or pyrophosphate deposition in periodontoid soft tissue)	Past history of intermittent inflammatory joint symptoms; may have radiographic chondrocalcinosis of joints (wrists, shoulders, knees); abnormal CT scan at C1-2
Depression	No morning stiffness; normal joint ROM; normal laboratory tests
Vasculitis	Fever; bruits; decreased pulses; palpable purpura; pulmonary renal syndrome; mononeuritis multiplex; active urinary sediment
Rheumatoid arthritis	Distal greater than proximal joint involvement; synovitis of wrists, MCPs, ankles, MTPs; recurrent joint pain and swelling on low doses of prednisone; positive RF and CCP; joint space narrowing and erosions on radiograph

- Involvement of the neck, shoulders or proximal arms, hips or proximal thighs (generally 2 of the 3 areas, shoulders being most common)
- ESR ≥40 mm/h and/or elevated CRP
- Rapid, usually dramatic, response to steroids; absence of the characteristic response to steroids should prompt reevaluation of the diagnosis

In addition to eliciting the classic symptoms of aching pain and stiffness of the upper and lower extremities, the clinician must enquire about symptoms suggestive of GCA (new headache, scalp tenderness, jaw claudication, visual change, arm claudication). Review of systems should be directed to evaluation of possible mimics as outlined in **Table 1**. Physical examination should include vascular examination (temporal artery pulses, bruits, asymmetric blood pressure) and musculoskeletal examination of proximal and distal joints for ROM and synovitis. Basic laboratory testing includes complete blood count, ESR, CRP, renal and hepatic function tests, and glucose. Other testing may include RF, CCP, calcium, creatine kinase (CK), urinalysis, and other tests as guided by the clinical picture and differential diagnosis. Glucose, hemoglobin A1c, and lipid profile may be obtained in anticipation of prolonged steroid treatment.

ATYPICAL CLINICAL PRESENTATIONS

In general, if 1 or 2 clinical features are atypical (eg, asymmetric presentation, normal acute phase reactants), clinical diagnosis relies on the remainder of the presentation (history, physical examination, laboratory tests, response to steroids) to be as classical as possible. The more atypical the clinical presentation, the greater the concern for another underlying condition.

In the setting of normal ESR, the diagnosis of PMR can be made if there is a textbook history and physical examination, unequivocal dramatic response to steroids, and mimics have been considered and determined to be unlikely. Following CRP when ESR is normal would be reasonable. If both ESR and CRP are normal, the diagnosis is uncertain. Continued follow-up is warranted with close attention to development of new symptoms, especially as steroids are tapered down. PMR patients generally respond to 15 to 20 mg daily of prednisone and normalize their ESR within 30 days and CRP within 1 week (see later discussion). A substantial subset of patients however responds in an incomplete or delayed fashion. In one prospective study of 129 patients with newly diagnosed PMR, 26% still reported proximal myalgias 3 weeks after starting steroids, and 29% still had more than 30 minutes of morning stiffness after 3 weeks of treatment.[29] In another prospective study of 125 patients, 71% of patients met the definition for a complete response to steroids at 4 weeks.[28] Fever, failure to respond to steroids, and/or continued elevation of acute phase reactants suggest an alternative diagnosis, in particular, GCA or malignancy such as lymphoma.

TREATMENT OF POLYMYALGIA RHEUMATICA

Glucocorticoids are the mainstay of treatment of PMR, and rapid, often dramatic response to steroids is the norm, with many patients reporting their effect as a "miracle." There have been no controlled trials comparing steroids to other medications; however, decades of use have confirmed their efficacy. There is no consensus on initial steroid dosing, maintenance therapy, or tapering schedule.

INITIAL TREATMENT

Published guidelines recommend a starting dose in the range of 12.5 to 25 mg of daily prednisone equivalent.[30] A benefit of 50% to 70% improvement in pain and stiffness has been reported within 1 to 3 days even with longstanding symptoms. Although some patients respond within 1 to 2 doses, up to 25% will take several days (1–2 weeks or more) to reach effectiveness.[31] Fifteen milligrams once daily of prednisone equivalent is an appropriate starting dose for most patients, with modifications as needed for comorbidities, such as diabetes, congestive heart failure, or severe hypertension. An increased dose (20 mg, at times even 30 mg daily prednisone equivalent) may be considered after approximately 1 week if only a partial effect is reported and clinical suspicion remains high. Continued failure to respond should prompt reevaluation of the diagnosis. Systematic reviews have reported lower cumulative doses and fewer glucocorticoid-related adverse effects in patients treated with prednisone 15 mg daily or less.[31] Patients reporting a wearing off effect of the prednisone toward the end of the day may benefit from splitting the dose twice daily, with subsequent consolidation to daily dosage after a few weeks. One study has reported a comparable efficacy of oral glucocorticoids and intramuscular methylprednisolone with lower cumulative GC doses and less weight gain in the methylprednisolone group (intramuscular methylprednisolone 120 mg every 4 weeks reduced by 20 mg every 3 months if symptoms and ESR/CRP remain normal).[32] In the authors' experience, empirical use of oral methylprednisolone may sometimes be effective if prednisone fails to produce a dramatic improvement in a patient with high clinical suspicion for PMR.

MAINTENANCE AND TAPER

Glucocorticoid taper is based on the patient's clinical response, with monitoring of PMR symptoms and ESR/CRP. ESR is most commonly followed. In occasional patients, CRP may be a more useful monitoring parameter. The initial dose is generally maintained for 2 to 4 weeks after acute phase reactants normalize and symptoms have fully resolved.[31] Prednisone is then decreased by 2.5 mg every 2 to 4 weeks until a dose of 10 mg daily is attained (**Box 2**). Subsequent tapering should be very slow by 1 mg every 1 to 2 months.[31] Patients often reach a threshold dose below which symptoms recur, whereupon an increase in dose by 1 to 2 mg generally results in rapid relief. Repeat slower taper may be attempted after approximately 1 month. In the author's experience, stepwise alternate day decrease by 1 mg over 2 to 4 weeks may help facilitate the taper when at very low doses. Slight adjustments in the total dose by 1 to 2 mg for long stretches of cold weather may also be helpful.

DISEASE MONITORING DURING TREATMENT

Patients should be monitored for recurrence of their original PMR symptoms as well as symptoms suggestive of GCA. Unmasking of pain from unrelated entities (eg, rotator cuff tendinitis, osteoarthritis) is common during glucocorticoid taper and should be assessed as outlined in **Table 1**. Distal rather than proximal articular symptoms, such as recurrent pain and stiffness in the wrists and MCPs, with attempted steroid taper should suggest evolution to rheumatoid arthritis and a need for careful examination of the joints. In general, PMR patients should respond to 15 to 20 mg daily of prednisone and normalize their ESR within 30 days and CRP within 1 week.

Box 2
Sample steroid tapering schedule for polymyalgia rheumatica

Prednisone 15 mg daily until disease is controlled and ESR/CRP are normal approximately (2–4 weeks)

Less than 15 mg daily taper by 2.5 mg every 2 to 4 weeks

Less than 10 mg daily taper by 1 mg every 1 to 2 months

Consider alternate day tapering at very low doses

Inability to discontinue or taper steroids to low doses (approximately 5 mg daily or less of prednisone equivalent) should prompt reevaluation of the diagnosis.

Comprehensive management of patients with PMR includes prophylaxis and monitoring of steroid side effects, including hypertension, glucose intolerance, and osteoporosis. In a population-based incidence cohort of 232 elderly patients with PMR with mean prednisone dosage of 9.6 mg daily, the risk of diabetes and fragility fractures (vertebrae, hip) was 2 to 5 times greater than in age- and sex-matched control patients.[33] In another retrospective study of PMR patients with a mean prednisone dose of 3.4 mg daily, steroid side effects were common (24.7% hypertension, 5.0% diabetes, 4.1% myocardial infarction).[34]

FREQUENCY OF ERYTHROCYTE SEDIMENTATION RATE/C-REACTIVE PROTEIN MONITORING

ESR/CRP should be measured at baseline and then approximately 1 to 2 months later after initiation of treatment to confirm normalization (**Box 3**). Subsequent testing can be done less frequently (approximately every 3–4 months) than every 4 to 6 months in asymptomatic patients on low-steroid doses. Patients off steroids do not need testing unless a change in clinical status prompts reevaluation. An increase in ESR/CRP during steroid taper in an asymptomatic patient should not justify an increase in prednisone, but rather a search for the cause of the increased acute phase reactant.

RELAPSE DURING TREATMENT

Too rapid steroid tapering may result in relapse. If relapse occurs and is quickly identified, disease control is often achieved by a small increase in dosage to just above that at which symptoms occurred. If severe relapse occurs, the initial dosage required to achieve disease control should be resumed. A prolonged period of dose stability (at least 3–6 months, sometimes longer) should be maintained before attempting steroid taper again.

CLINICAL COURSE OF POLYMYALGIA RHEUMATICA

Most patients (60%–75%) have a monophasic illness with gradual discontinuation of glucocorticoids after 1 to 2 years.[2] Others may require very low-dose prednisone (prednisone 5 mg daily or less) for many years, more than 4 years in 40% of patients in one study,[35] up to 6 years in another study.[36] Patients with prolonged duration of treatment are more likely to have polyphasic illness with partial relapses and requirement for temporary increase in glucocorticoids. Relapses are common, occurring in approximately 50% of patients,[14,37] and may occur months or even years after

---

Box 3
Sample erythrocyte sedimentation rate/C-reactive protein monitoring schedule for polymyalgia rheumatica

At diagnosis	Baseline ESR/CRP[a]
1–2 mo after diagnosis	To confirm normalization of ESR/CRP
Every 3–4 mo after normalization	To monitor patients being tapered
Every 4–6 mo	Asymptomatic patients on low-dose steroids
No monitoring necessary[b]	Patients off steroids

[a] Both ESR and CRP do not need to be monitored; one or the other is sufficient.
[b] Unless change in clinical status prompts reevaluation.

discontinuation of steroids.[38] Approximately 5% of patients evolve into rheumatoid arthritis.[39] The RS3PE variant of PMR has been reported to represent a possible paraneoplastic phenomenon in some patients. Although this association is not definitive, it is prudent to pursue an age-appropriate malignancy workup in patients presenting with this condition.[40–43]

STEROID-SPARING THERAPY

Unlike its role in rheumatoid arthritis, methotrexate (MTX) has a limited effect on PMR. The only randomized controlled study of MTX in PMR (using a low dose of 10 mg orally weekly) showed a higher proportion of patients discontinuing glucocorticoids after 18 months and fewer flares. The mean reduction in prednisone dose however was very modest (1 mg per day compared with the control group).[44] MTX may be considered in rare instances of refractory disease or in patients at high risk for glucocorticoid side effects.[23] There are no data on its use at higher doses, similar to those used in RA. There are insufficient data to support the use of other adjunctive medications, such as tumor necrosis factor (TNF) inhibitors in the treatment of PMR.

GIANT CELL ARTERITIS
Introduction

GCA is a vasculitis of large- and medium-sized arteries often associated with PMR.

GCA should be considered in any patient older than the age of 50 years with new headache, jaw claudication, abrupt change in vision (especially transient monocular loss of vision), unexplained fever, unexplained elevated ESR/CRP, or history of PMR.

Epidemiology

GCA is the most common vasculitis, and the most likely to be encountered and recognized by primary care providers. Similar to PMR, GCA is a condition of older adults, primarily older than 50 years, with a peak incidence after 70 years of age.[45–47] Women are affected 2- to 3-fold more than men, and the disease is most common in Caucasians.[48]

Pathophysiology

The pathologic hallmark of vasculitis is inflammatory infiltration and disruption of the vessel wall, with the degree of disruption correlating with the severity of the clinical presentation. In GCA, dendritic cells within the vessel wall appear to trigger the inflammatory cascade and recruit T cells and macrophages to form granulomatous infiltrates. Proinflammatory cytokines, including IL-1, IL-6, and interferon gamma (the latter not found in PMR), and other inflammatory mediators, such as nitric oxide, result in arterial injury. The vessel wall destruction is coupled with a repair mechanism from activated endothelial cells, vascular smooth muscle cells, and fibroblasts, resulting in intimal proliferation and wall remodeling obstructing the vessel lumen.[48]

Relationship Between Polymyalgia Rheumatica and Giant Cell Arteritis

Almost half of patients with GCA have symptoms of PMR.[49] Conversely, 10% to 20% of patients with PMR develop GCA.[50,51]

History

GCA can have a variety of presentations, ranging from classic cranial ischemic findings, to large vessel inflammation, to constitutional symptoms alone (**Box 4**). Similar to PMR, symptoms may be acute or subacute in onset.[19]

> **Box 4**
> **Clinical presentations of giant cell arteritis**
>
> Systemic
> - Fever, night sweats
> - Weight loss
>
> Myalgic
> - Polymyalgia rheumatica
> - Proximal symmetric muscle pain and stiffness
>
> Arteritic
> - Localized pain, swelling, and tenderness
> - Partial occlusion with claudication
> - Complete occlusion with ischemia and distal necrosis

Cranial Symptoms

The most characteristic symptoms of GCA arise from inflammation of small muscular arteries from cranial branches of the aortic arch. Symptoms include superficial temporal headache, scalp tenderness (eg, while combing hair, resting head on pillow), jaw and tongue claudication, and transient visual loss (amaurosis fugax). In a prospective study of 31 patients with GCA, symptoms at diagnosis included headache (85%), fever (43%), fatigue (41%), weight loss (41%), jaw claudication (28%), night sweats (26%), and visual impairment (18%).[19] Jaw claudication is the most specific symptom for GCA and may be described by the patient as fatigue or tiredness of the jaw when chewing continuously (eg, on a piece of bread). Jaw pain at rest is more likely to be from nonischemic causes such as bruxism. Other presentations include nonspecific aching facial pain mimicking sinusitis or ear pain, unusual pain in the face, throat, or tongue. A new headache in an older patient should always prompt consideration of GCA. Although the classic headache is constant and bitemporal, it can occur in any distribution and chronologic pattern. In patients with chronic preexisting headache, a change in headache from baseline should be enquired about.

Visual Symptoms

The most dreaded presentation of GCA, visual loss, occurs in 15% of patients.[52,53] The blindness is sudden and painless and results from inflammatory occlusion of optic nerve arterial supply. Blindness may be preceded by premonitory symptoms, including blurring of vision, scotomata, visual field cut (eg, lowered blind effect), and diplopia.[54] In a retrospective study, two-thirds of patients reported premonitory visual symptoms lasting an average of 9 days before vision loss. The remaining one-third had no preceding visual symptoms.[53] New-onset diplopia in an elderly patient is a red flag for GCA. Transient monocular visual loss (confirmed by covering one eye) is of particular concern and mandates urgent evaluation.[52]

Large Vessel Inflammation

In approximately 20%[38] of patients, symptomatic inflammation of large vessels can result in arm and leg claudication (subclavian and iliac arteries), hypertension (renal), angina (coronary), dizziness (vertebral, basilar), or abdominal pain (mesenteric).[38] Stroke is very rare in GCA. Asymptomatic large vessel involvement has been demonstrated by PET scan in 50% to 80% of patients.[55] Large vessel inflammation can result in stenosis, dissection, and aneurysms of the affected arteries. Aortic aneurysm and dilatation should be considered in any GCA patient with unexplained new abdominal pain or back pain.

Systemic Manifestations

GCA may present solely with nonspecific constitutional symptoms, including fever, night sweats, weight loss (5–20 kg),[38] and fatigue. Fever occurs in almost one-half of GCA patients and is generally low grade (1–2° above baseline), but has been reported up to a median of 102.4 F/39.1 C.[38,56] GCA accounts for fever of unknown origin in 17% of elderly patients.[57]

Physical Examination

Examination should include blood pressure in both arms. Temporal artery pulses, tenderness, swelling, and nodularity should be assessed. A newly tender, ropelike temporal artery with beading is rare but characteristic and may be unilateral or bilateral. The carotid and subclavian vessels should be examined for bruits and tenderness (carotidynia). Tender small pea-sized nodules from underlying arterial inflammation may develop anywhere on the scalp, reflecting the scalp's extensive arterial circulation (as evidenced by abundant bleeding with scalp laceration).[38] Arterial bruits and diminished or absent pulses, although common in the elderly, lend support to the diagnosis of GCA in the appropriate clinical setting but are often challenging to differentiate from underlying atherosclerosis. In practice, it is difficult even for experienced clinicians to differentiate between diminished and absent pulses without use of Doppler. An aortic insufficiency murmur may occur.

Laboratory Tests

Elevated ESR and CRP are characteristic, with mean values of 93 mm/h and 9.4 mg/dL, respectively.[56,58] A normal ESR has been reported in 5% of cases[59]; therefore, normal acute phase reactants do not rule out the diagnosis. Other nonspecific findings include anemia, leukocytosis, thrombocytosis, hypoalbuminemia, and elevated alkaline phosphatase. Antinuclear antibody, rheumatoid factor, and anti-CCP are negative.

Diagnostic Considerations

Temporal artery biopsy

In cases of predominantly cranial involvement, definitive diagnosis is made by biopsy of the temporal artery. Temporal arteries are biopsied because they are the most easily accessible arteries. Pathology of affected arteries in GCA classically reveals a transmural granulomatous inflammatory reaction with intimal thickening, smooth muscle hyperplasia, and luminal occlusion. Not all biopsy specimens are diagnostic, however, in part because the inflammatory process is patchy and may not involve the segments being examined.

Biopsy should be performed on the most symptomatic side, as identified by the patient. Overall, temporal artery biopsy is diagnostic in approximately 85% of patients. In patients with negative biopsy and high clinical suspicion, biopsy of the contralateral temporal artery may be considered, although the additional yield is only 5%.[60] Patients with primarily posterior headaches may have posterior occipital arterial involvement. An important clinical point is that the decision to obtain a biopsy should not delay starting steroids when clinical suspicion is high. Inflammation on biopsy can still be detected 2 weeks after starting high-dose steroids and diminishes after 4 weeks.[61–63] Appropriate referral for biopsy should be made as soon as possible after initiation of steroids to expedite the process.

Imaging

In cases with predominantly extracranial large vessel involvement, temporal biopsy yield is considerably lower (~60%),[64] and imaging with computed tomographic (CT) angiography or magnetic resonance angiography is necessary to demonstrate inflammation.[60,65] Imaging should be performed early in the course of treatment because, unlike pathology findings, imaging evidence of inflammation decreases markedly after 4 days of high-dose steroids.[66] Ultrasonography of the inflamed temporal artery can demonstrate a "halo" corresponding to edema of the arterial intima. In experienced hands, sensitivity and specificity are comparable to temporal artery biopsy; however, in practice, this test should be limited to centers with expertise in performing and interpreting this study.[67] PET scanning provides excellent images but is limited by clinical and financial considerations, including intravenous (IV) contrast use and radiation exposure.[68]

Differential Diagnosis

Differential diagnosis of GCA includes infection (especially endocarditis), medium vessel vasculitides involving the temporal artery, infiltrative diseases such as amyloidosis, and malignancy (particularly lymphoma). Note that amyloidosis has been reported to cause jaw claudication.[69] Although most vision loss in GCA is due to anterior ischemic optic neuropathy (AION), most AIONs in clinical practice are related to atherosclerosis.[54] Unlike GCA-related AION, atherosclerosis-related AION is often reversible.

Treatment

Glucocorticoids

Dosage regimen depends on whether vision loss is present or suspected. Response to steroids is dramatic and rapid within days, usually 1 week.[59]

Vision loss at diagnosis

If there is concern for possible vision loss (eg, amaurosis fugax, diplopia), treatment should be initiated with IV methylprednisolone 1 g daily for 3 days followed by oral prednisone equivalent of 1 mg/kg/d for at least 2 weeks, usually 4 weeks, followed by slow taper (**Box 5**). Treatment goal is primarily to protect the unaffected eye. The secondary goal is to try stabilizing or reversing vision loss in the affected eye.

No vision loss at diagnosis

Treatment is initiated at 1 mg/kg/d oral prednisone equivalent, usually 60 mg daily for 2 weeks and then slowly tapered (see **Box 5**). Tapering too rapidly results in increased risk of flare.

Aspirin

Daily low-dose acetylsalicylic acid (ASA; 81–100 mg daily) has been shown in several studies to reduce ischemic events in GCA, including cardiovascular events and blindness[70,71]; however, data from randomized studies are not available.[72] If clinically appropriate, cytoprotection should be used in conjunction with aspirin.

Statins

There are no data supporting the use of statins in the management of GCA. In a retrospective analysis, statin use did not appear to modify the clinical presentation or disease course of patients with GCA.[73]

Steroid-sparing medications

The long-term use of steroids in GCA patients has prompted extensive search for adjunctive immunosuppressants. MTX overall had a modest effect.[74,75] TNF inhibitors

---

Box 5
Suggested treatments

Suggested treatment, GCA with visual symptoms
  Intravenous methylprednisolone 1 g daily × 3 days, then
  Prednisone 1 mg/kg/d (usually prednisone 60 mg daily) × 4 weeks, then
  Decrease prednisone by 10 mg daily every 2 weeks until prednisone 20 mg daily, then
  Decrease prednisone by 2.5 mg daily every 2 weeks until prednisone 10 mg daily, then
  Decrease prednisone by 1 mg daily every 4 weeks as tolerated
  Close clinical monitoring (history, physical examination)
  Close laboratory monitoring (ESR CRP every month, then every 2-3 months off medications)
  ASA 81 mg daily
  Consider adjuvant treatment for steroid sparing

Suggested treatment, GCA without visual symptoms
  Prednisone 1 mg/kg/d (usually prednisone 60 mg daily) × 2 weeks, then
  Decrease prednisone by 10 mg daily every 2 weeks until prednisone 20 mg daily, then
  Decrease prednisone by 2.5 mg daily every 2 weeks until prednisone 10 mg daily, then
  Decrease prednisone by 1 mg daily every 4 weeks as tolerated
  Close clinical monitoring (history, physical examination)
  Close laboratory monitoring (ESR CRP every month, then every 2–3 months off medications)
  ASA 81 mg daily
  Consider adjuvant treatment for steroid sparing

(infliximab, etanercept, adalimumab) were unsuccessful.[76–78] Most recently, tocilizumab, an IL-6 inhibitor used for treatment of rheumatoid arthritis, was found in a randomized placebo controlled trial to successfully enable steroid tapering in GCA patients while successfully inducing and maintaining disease control.[79] Based on these data, tocilizumab (administered subcutaneously every 2 weeks) has been approved by the US Food and Drug Administration for treatment of GCA. Potential adverse effects of tocilizumab include liver function test elevations, cytopenias, hyperlipidemia, and gastrointestinal (GI) perforation. Tocilizumab is contraindicated in the setting of diverticulitis. Importantly, because of the inhibitory effect of tocilizumab on IL-6, one of the main proinflammatory cytokines, use of tocilizumab results in normalization of ESR and CRP, which can no longer be used as monitoring parameters.

General Measures

Routine preventive measures should be instituted to limit glucocorticoid-related toxicity, including diabetes mellitus, hypertension, hyperlipidemia, osteoporosis, infection, steroid myopathy, and cataracts. In a retrospective review of a population-based incidence cohort of 120 patients with GCA, 86% developed steroid-related adverse effects after a median treatment duration of 6.5 months to reach a prednisone dose of 7.5 mg daily. Adverse effects included cataract (41%), fragility fracture (38%), infection (31%), hypertension (22%), diabetes (9%), and GI bleeding (4%).[80]

Vaccinations against influenza and streptococcus should be administered. In patients not on tocilizumab and taking less than 20 mg of prednisone daily, immunization against varicella zoster virus should be considered. In patients receiving prednisone 20 mg or more daily, prophylaxis against *Pneumocystis jirovecii* pneumonia should be considered.[81]

Clinical Course: Visual Symptoms

Even after aggressive treatment with IV steroids, it takes approximately 1 week for steroids to stop the disease process in the arterial wall. In a prospective study of GCA patients with vision loss, approximately one-quarter of patients experienced continued visual deterioration in the first 6 days despite treatment with 3 days of IV pulse steroids followed by high-dose oral steroids.[82] In addition, 9% of patients lost vision in the unaffected eye. Other reports have confirmed that less than 5% of patients with visual symptoms at diagnosis achieve significant visual recovery despite treatment.[82,83] Early initiation of steroids is effective for prevention of future visual loss. If vision is intact after initiation of treatment with high-dose steroids, the probability of future vision loss at 5 years is reduced to 1%.[84]

LONG-TERM FOLLOW-UP
Disease Flares

Disease flares are common, occurring in 50% of patients over a period of 2 to 5 years.[85] Close follow-up with a rheumatologist is essential.

Aortic Aneurysms and Dissection

Cohort studies have reported a 2- to 17-fold increase in abdominal and thoracic aortic aneurysms, respectively, in GCA patients,[86–88] with an estimated incidence of dissection and rupture between 2% and 6%.[87] Although there are no specific recommendations for aneurysm screening, clinical judgment suggests that patients with risk factors, such as smoking and hypertension, may benefit from screening. The choice of screening modality, whether chest radiograph, echocardiogram, or CT abdomen, is not clear, and the frequency of serial monitoring, if any, is controversial.

Other Monitoring

Patients should be monitored for signs and symptoms of progressive aortic insufficiency. Development of refractory hypertension should prompt consideration of renal artery stenosis. Follow-up and monitoring of GCA patients require multidisciplinary management by primary care providers and other specialists, including rheumatologists.

SUMMARY

PMR and GCA are related inflammatory conditions affecting individuals aged 50 years and older. Careful attention to history and physical examination is critical to diagnosis, because laboratory abnormalities may occasionally be absent. Mimics should be considered and excluded. Timely diagnosis is essential if visual impairment from GCA is suspected, followed by rapid initiation of corticosteroids. Active management and close follow-up of patients are essential to prevent and minimize complications of corticosteroid use and monitor for relapse or disease evolution.

REFERENCES

1. Crowson CS, Matteson EL, Myasoedova E, et al. The lifetime risk of adult-onset rheumatoid arthritis and other inflammatory autoimmune rheumatic diseases. Arthritis Rheum 2011;63(3):633–9.
2. Chuang TY, Hunder GG, Ilstrup DM, et al. Polymyalgia rheumatica: a 10-year epidemiologic and clinical study. Ann Intern Med 1982;97(5):672–80.
3. Weyand CM, Hunder NN, Hicok KC, et al. HLA-DRB1 alleles in polymyalgia rheumatica, giant cell arteritis, and rheumatoid arthritis. Arthritis Rheum 1994;37(4):514–20.

4. Gonzalez-Gay MA, Amoli MM, Garcia-Porrua C, et al. Genetic markers of disease susceptibility and severity in giant cell arteritis and polymyalgia rheumatica. Semin Arthritis Rheum 2003;33(1):38–48.

5. Samson M, Audia S, Fraszczak J, et al. Th1 and Th17 lymphocytes expressing CD161 are implicated in giant cell arteritis and polymyalgia rheumatica pathogenesis. Arthritis Rheum 2012;64(11):3788–98.

6. Weyand CM, Hicok KC, Hunder GG, et al. Tissue cytokine patterns in patients with polymyalgia rheumatica and giant cell arteritis. Ann Intern Med 1994; 121(7):484–91.

7. Cutolo M, Montecucco CM, Cavagna L, et al. Serum cytokines and steroidal hormones in polymyalgia rheumatica and elderly-onset rheumatoid arthritis. Ann Rheum Dis 2006;65(11):1438–43.

8. Demir H, Tanriverdi F, Ozogul N, et al. Evaluation of the hypothalamic-pituitary-adrenal axis in untreated patients with polymyalgia rheumatica and healthy controls. Scand J Rheumatol 2006;35(3):217–23.

9. Salvarani C, Cantini F, Macchioni P, et al. Distal musculoskeletal manifestations in polymyalgia rheumatica: a prospective followup study. Arthritis Rheum 1998; 41(7):1221–6.

10. Salvarani C, Gabriel S, Hunder GG. Distal extremity swelling with pitting edema in polymyalgia rheumatica. Report on nineteen cases. Arthritis Rheum 1996;39(1): 73–80.

11. Klauser A, Frauscher F, Halpern EJ, et al. Remitting seronegative symmetrical synovitis with pitting edema of the hands: ultrasound, color Doppler ultrasound, and magnetic resonance imaging findings. Arthritis Rheum 2005;53(2):226–33.

12. Agarwal V, Dabra AK, Kaur R, et al. Remitting seronegative symmetrical synovitis with pitting edema (RS3PE) syndrome: ultrasonography as a diagnostic tool. Clin Rheumatol 2005;24(5):476–9.

13. Cantini F, Salvarani C, Olivieri I, et al. Erythrocyte sedimentation rate and C-reactive protein in the evaluation of disease activity and severity in polymyalgia rheumatica: a prospective follow-up study. Semin Arthritis Rheum 2000;30(1):17–24.

14. Salvarani C, Cantini F, Niccoli L, et al. Acute-phase reactants and the risk of relapse/recurrence in polymyalgia rheumatica: a prospective followup study. Arthritis Rheum 2005;53(1):33–8.

15. Helfgott SM, Kieval RI. Polymyalgia rheumatica in patients with a normal erythrocyte sedimentation rate. Arthritis Rheum 1996;39(2):304–7.

16. Gonzalez-Gay MA, Rodriguez-Valverde V, Blanco R, et al. Polymyalgia rheumatica without significantly increased erythrocyte sedimentation rate. A more benign syndrome. Arch Intern Med 1997;157(3):317–20.

17. Proven A, Gabriel SE, O'Fallon WM, et al. Polymyalgia rheumatica with low erythrocyte sedimentation rate at diagnosis. J Rheumatol 1999;26(6):1333–7.

18. Miller A, Green M, Robinson D. Simple rule for calculating normal erythrocyte sedimentation rate. Br Med J (Clin Res Ed) 1983;286(6361):266.

19. Myklebust G, Gran JT. A prospective study of 287 patients with polymyalgia rheumatica and temporal arteritis: clinical and laboratory manifestations at onset of disease and at the time of diagnosis. Br J Rheumatol 1996;35(11):1161–8.

20. Wener MH, Daum PR, McQuillan GM. The influence of age, sex, and race on the upper reference limit of serum C-reactive protein concentration. J Rheumatol 2000;27(10):2351–9.

21. Gabay C, Kushner I. Acute-phase proteins and other systemic responses to inflammation. N Engl J Med 1999;340(6):448–54.

22. Gordon I, Rennie AM, Branwood AW. Polymyalgia rheumatica: biopsy studies. Ann Rheum Dis 1964;23(6):447.
23. Buttgereit F, Dejaco C, Matteson EL, et al. Polymyalgia rheumatica and giant cell arteritis: a systematic review. JAMA 2016;315(22):2442–58.
24. Cantini F, Salvarani C, Olivieri I, et al. Shoulder ultrasonography in the diagnosis of polymyalgia rheumatica: a case-control study. J Rheumatol 2001;28(5): 1049–55.
25. Cantini F, Niccoli L, Nannini C, et al. Inflammatory changes of hip synovial structures in polymyalgia rheumatica. Clin Exp Rheumatol 2005;23(4):462–8.
26. Weigand S, Ehrenstein B, Fleck M, et al. Joint involvement in patients with early polymyalgia rheumatica using high-resolution ultrasound and its contribution to the EULAR/ACR 2012 classification criteria for polymyalgia rheumatica. J Rheumatol 2014;41(4):730–4.
27. Blockmans D, De Ceuninck L, Vanderschueren S, et al. Repetitive 18-fluorodeoxyglucose positron emission tomography in isolated polymyalgia rheumatica: a prospective study in 35 patients. Rheumatology (Oxford) 2007;46(4):672–7.
28. Dasgupta B, Cimmino MA, Kremers HM, et al. 2012 provisional classification criteria for polymyalgia rheumatica: a European League against Rheumatism/ American College of Rheumatology collaborative initiative. Arthritis Rheum 2012;64(4):943–54.
29. Hutchings A, Hollywood J, Lamping DL, et al. Clinical outcomes, quality of life, and diagnostic uncertainty in the first year of polymyalgia rheumatica. Arthritis Rheum 2007;57(5):803–9.
30. Dejaco C, Singh YP, Perel P, et al. 2015 recommendations for the management of polymyalgia rheumatica: a European League Against Rheumatism/American College of Rheumatology collaborative initiative. Arthritis Rheumatol 2015;67(10): 2569–80.
31. Hernandez-Rodriguez J, Cid MC, Lopez-Soto A, et al. Treatment of polymyalgia rheumatica: a systematic review. Arch Intern Med 2009;169(20):1839–50.
32. Dasgupta B, Dolan AL, Panayi GS, et al. An initially double-blind controlled 96 week trial of depot methylprednisolone against oral prednisolone in the treatment of polymyalgia rheumatica. Br J Rheumatol 1998;37(2):189–95.
33. Gabriel SE, Sunku J, Salvarani C, et al. Adverse outcomes of antiinflammatory therapy among patients with polymyalgia rheumatica. Arthritis Rheum 1997; 40(10):1873–8.
34. Mazzantini M, Torre C, Miccoli M, et al. Adverse events during longterm low-dose glucocorticoid treatment of polymyalgia rheumatica: a retrospective study. J Rheumatol 2012;39(3):552–7.
35. Ayoub WT, Franklin CM, Torretti D. Polymyalgia rheumatica. Duration of therapy and long-term outcome. Am J Med 1985;79(3):309–15.
36. Cimmino MA, Salvarani C, Macchioni P, et al. Long-term follow-up of polymyalgia rheumatica patients treated with methotrexate and steroids. Clin Exp Rheumatol 2008;26(3):395–400.
37. Kremers HM, Reinalda MS, Crowson CS, et al. Relapse in a population based cohort of patients with polymyalgia rheumatica. J Rheumatol 2005;32(1):65–73.
38. Jones JG. Clinical features of giant cell arteritis. Baillieres Clin Rheumatol 1991; 5(3):413–30.
39. Gran JT, Myklebust G. The incidence and clinical characteristics of peripheral arthritis in polymyalgia rheumatica and temporal arteritis: a prospective study of 231 cases. Rheumatology (Oxford) 2000;39(3):283–7.

40. Sibilia J, Friess S, Schaeverbeke T, et al. Remitting seronegative symmetrical synovitis with pitting edema (RS3PE): a form of paraneoplastic polyarthritis? J Rheumatol 1999;26(1):115–20.
41. Kimura M, Tokuda Y, Oshiawa H, et al. Clinical characteristics of patients with remitting seronegative symmetrical synovitis with pitting edema compared to patients with pure polymyalgia rheumatica. J Rheumatol 2012;39(1):148–53.
42. Yao Q, Su X, Altman RD. Is remitting seronegative symmetrical synovitis with pitting edema (RS3PE) a subset of rheumatoid arthritis? Semin Arthritis Rheum 2010;40(1):89–94.
43. Karmacharya P, Donato AA, Aryal MR, et al. RS3PE revisited: a systematic review and meta-analysis of 331 cases. Clin Exp Rheumatol 2016;34(3):404–15.
44. Caporali R, Cimmino MA, Ferraccioli G, et al. Prednisone plus methotrexate for polymyalgia rheumatica: a randomized, double-blind, placebo-controlled trial. Ann Intern Med 2004;141(7):493–500.
45. Gonzalez-Gay MA, Miranda-Filloy JA, Lopez-Diaz MJ, et al. Giant cell arteritis in northwestern Spain: a 25-year epidemiologic study. Medicine (Baltimore) 2007; 86(2):61–8.
46. Salvarani C, Crowson CS, O'Fallon WM, et al. Reappraisal of the epidemiology of giant cell arteritis in Olmsted County, Minnesota, over a fifty-year period. Arthritis Rheum 2004;51(2):264–8.
47. Kermani TA, Schafer VS, Crowson CS, et al. Increase in age at onset of giant cell arteritis: a population-based study. Ann Rheum Dis 2010;69(4):780–1.
48. Gonzalez-Gay MA, Vazquez-Rodriguez TR, Lopez-Diaz MJ, et al. Epidemiology of giant cell arteritis and polymyalgia rheumatica. Arthritis Rheum 2009;61(10): 1454–61.
49. Gonzalez-Gay MA, Barros S, Lopez-Diaz MJ, et al. Giant cell arteritis: disease patterns of clinical presentation in a series of 240 patients. Medicine (Baltimore) 2005;84(5):269–76.
50. Salvarani C, Gabriel SE, O'Fallon WM, et al. Epidemiology of polymyalgia rheumatica in Olmsted County, Minnesota, 1970-1991. Arthritis Rheum 1995;38(3): 369–73.
51. Gonzalez-Gay MA, Garcia-Porrua C, Vazquez-Caruncho M, et al. The spectrum of polymyalgia rheumatica in northwestern Spain: incidence and analysis of variables associated with relapse in a 10-year study. J Rheumatol 1999;26(6): 1326–32.
52. Gonzalez-Gay MA, Garcia-Porrua C, Llorca J, et al. Visual manifestations of giant cell arteritis. Trends and clinical spectrum in 161 patients. Medicine (Baltimore) 2000;79(5):283–92.
53. Font C, Cid MC, Coll-Vinent B, et al. Clinical features in patients with permanent visual loss due to biopsy-proven giant cell arteritis. Br J Rheumatol 1997;36(2): 251–4.
54. Hayreh SS, Podhajsky PA, Zimmerman B. Ocular manifestations of giant cell arteritis. Am J Ophthalmol 1998;125(4):509–20.
55. Blockmans D, de Ceuninck L, Vanderschueren S, et al. Repetitive 18F-fluorodeoxyglucose positron emission tomography in giant cell arteritis: a prospective study of 35 patients. Arthritis Rheum 2006;55(1):131–7.
56. Calamia KT, Hunder GG. Giant cell arteritis (temporal arteritis) presenting as fever of undetermined origin. Arthritis Rheum 1981;24(11):1414–8.
57. Knockaert DC, Vanneste LJ, Bobbaers HJ. Fever of unknown origin in elderly patients. J Am Geriatr Soc 1993;41(11):1187–92.

58. Gonzalez-Gay MA, Lopez-Diaz MJ, Barros S, et al. Giant cell arteritis: laboratory tests at the time of diagnosis in a series of 240 patients. Medicine (Baltimore) 2005;84(5):277–90.

59. Salvarani C, Hunder GG. Giant cell arteritis with low erythrocyte sedimentation rate: frequency of occurrence in a population-based study. Arthritis Rheum 2001;45(2):140–5.

60. Niederkohr RD, Levin LA. Management of the patient with suspected temporal arteritis a decision-analytic approach. Ophthalmology 2005;112(5):744–56.

61. Achkar AA, Lie JT, Hunder GG, et al. How does previous corticosteroid treatment affect the biopsy findings in giant cell (temporal) arteritis? Ann Intern Med 1994; 120(12):987–92.

62. Jakobsson K, Jacobsson L, Mohammad AJ, et al. The effect of clinical features and glucocorticoids on biopsy findings in giant cell arteritis. BMC Musculoskelet Disord 2016;17(1):363.

63. Narvaez J, Bernad B, Roig-Vilaseca D, et al. Influence of previous corticosteroid therapy on temporal artery biopsy yield in giant cell arteritis. Semin Arthritis Rheum 2007;37(1):13–9.

64. Brack A, Martinez-Taboada V, Stanson A, et al. Disease pattern in cranial and large-vessel giant cell arteritis. Arthritis Rheum 1999;42(2):311–7.

65. Prieto-Gonzalez S, Arguis P, Garcia-Martinez A, et al. Large vessel involvement in biopsy-proven giant cell arteritis: prospective study in 40 newly diagnosed patients using CT angiography. Ann Rheum Dis 2012;71(7):1170–6.

66. Hauenstein C, Reinhard M, Geiger J, et al. Effects of early corticosteroid treatment on magnetic resonance imaging and ultrasonography findings in giant cell arteritis. Rheumatology (Oxford) 2012;51(11):1999–2003.

67. Karassa FB, Matsagas MI, Schmidt WA, et al. Meta-analysis: test performance of ultrasonography for giant-cell arteritis. Ann Intern Med 2005;142(5):359–69.

68. Prieto-Gonzalez S, Depetris M, Garcia-Martinez A, et al. Positron emission tomography assessment of large vessel inflammation in patients with newly diagnosed, biopsy-proven giant cell arteritis: a prospective, case-control study. Ann Rheum Dis 2014;73(7):1388–92.

69. Audemard A, Boutemy J, Galateau-Salle F, et al. AL amyloidosis with temporal artery involvement simulates giant-cell arteritis. Joint Bone Spine 2012;79(2):195–7.

70. Nesher G, Berkun Y, Mates M, et al. Low-dose aspirin and prevention of cranial ischemic complications in giant cell arteritis. Arthritis Rheum 2004;50(4):1332–7.

71. Lee MS, Smith SD, Galor A, et al. Antiplatelet and anticoagulant therapy in patients with giant cell arteritis. Arthritis Rheum 2006;54(10):3306–9.

72. Weyand CM, Goronzy JJ. Clinical practice. Giant-cell arteritis and polymyalgia rheumatica. N Engl J Med 2014;371(1):50–7.

73. Schmidt J, Kermani TA, Muratore F, et al. Statin use in giant cell arteritis: a retrospective study. J Rheumatol 2013;40(6):910–5.

74. Hoffman GS, Cid MC, Hellmann DB, et al. A multicenter, randomized, double-blind, placebo-controlled trial of adjuvant methotrexate treatment for giant cell arteritis. Arthritis Rheum 2002;46(5):1309–18.

75. Spiera RF, Mitnick HJ, Kupersmith M, et al. A prospective, double-blind, randomized, placebo controlled trial of methotrexate in the treatment of giant cell arteritis (GCA). Clin Exp Rheumatol 2001;19(5):495–501.

76. Hoffman GS, Cid MC, Rendt-Zagar KE, et al. Infliximab for maintenance of glucocorticosteroid-induced remission of giant cell arteritis: a randomized trial. Ann Intern Med 2007;146(9):621–30.

77. Martinez-Taboada VM, Rodriguez-Valverde V, Carreno L, et al. A double-blind placebo controlled trial of etanercept in patients with giant cell arteritis and corticosteroid side effects. Ann Rheum Dis 2008;67(5):625–30.

78. Seror R, Baron G, Hachulla E, et al. Adalimumab for steroid sparing in patients with giant-cell arteritis: results of a multicentre randomised controlled trial. Ann Rheum Dis 2014;73(12):2074–81.

79. Villiger PM, Adler S, Kuchen S, et al. Tocilizumab for induction and maintenance of remission in giant cell arteritis: a phase 2, randomised, double-blind, placebo-controlled trial. Lancet 2016;387(10031):1921–7.

80. Proven A, Gabriel SE, Orces C, et al. Glucocorticoid therapy in giant cell arteritis: duration and adverse outcomes. Arthritis Rheum 2003;49(5):703–8.

81. Kermani TA, Ytterberg SR, Warrington KJ. Pneumocystis jiroveci pneumonia in giant cell arteritis: a case series. Arthritis Care Res (Hoboken) 2011;63(5):761–5.

82. Danesh-Meyer H, Savino PJ, Gamble GG. Poor prognosis of visual outcome after visual loss from giant cell arteritis. Ophthalmology 2005;112(6):1098–103.

83. Hayreh SS, Zimmerman B, Kardon RH. Visual improvement with corticosteroid therapy in giant cell arteritis. Report of a large study and review of literature. Acta Ophthalmol Scand 2002;80(4):355–67.

84. Aiello PD, Trautmann JC, McPhee TJ, et al. Visual prognosis in giant cell arteritis. Ophthalmology 1993;100(4):550–5.

85. Kermani TA, Warrington KJ, Cuthbertson D, et al. Disease relapses among patients with giant cell arteritis: a prospective, longitudinal cohort study. J Rheumatol 2015;42(7):1213–7.

86. Evans JM, O'Fallon WM, Hunder GG. Increased incidence of aortic aneurysm and dissection in giant cell (temporal) arteritis. A population-based study. Ann Intern Med 1995;122(7):502–7.

87. Mackie SL, Hensor EM, Morgan AW, et al. Should I send my patient with previous giant cell arteritis for imaging of the thoracic aorta? A systematic literature review and meta-analysis. Ann Rheum Dis 2014;73(1):143–8.

88. Robson JC, Kiran A, Maskell J, et al. The relative risk of aortic aneurysm in patients with giant cell arteritis compared with the general population of the UK. Ann Rheum Dis 2015;74(1):129–35.

Fibromyalgia in Primary Care

Jay B. Higgs, MD

KEYWORDS

- Fibromyalgia • Pain • Sleep wake disorders • Cognitive behavioral therapy (CBT)
- Exercise • Serotonin and noradrenaline reuptake inhibitors (SNRI) • Antiepileptics
- Antidepressive agents

KEY POINTS

- Fibromyalgia is a common disorder with substantial morbidity.
- Clinical diagnosis is aided by published criteria.
- The diagnosis of fibromyalgia does not rule out comorbid conditions; history, physical examination, and limited laboratory screening are used to direct additional testing or specialty referral if indicated.
- Nonpharmacologic treatments, including cognitive behavioral therapy, sleep hygiene, and regular aerobic exercise, form the cornerstone of management; results from pharmacotherapy are variable.
- The primary care provider can use the tool kit to prepare an organized approach to management of this challenging condition.

INTRODUCTION

Fibromyalgia (FM) is a common disorder that is frustrating to patients and poses unique challenges to the primary care provider (PCP).[1,2] About one of every 20 patients in primary care suffers from FM,[3] with an average annual cost to the health care system of more than $9000 per patient.[4] The impact on quality of life is greater than rheumatoid arthritis or chronic obstructive pulmonary disease.[4] Patients with FM are facing long-term widespread pain among a myriad of other symptoms with no clear cause, no definitive diagnostic tests, and a modest response to interventions.[5] The diagnosis is delayed an average of 2 years. Patients often describe their symptoms in catastrophic terms. Many in the community, including some medical

Disclosures: The author has no financial disclosures.
The views expressed herein are those of the author and do not reflect the official policy or position of Brooke Army Medical Center, the US Army Medical Department, the US Army Office of the Surgeon General, the Department of the Army, the Department of the Air Force, and Department of Defense, or the US Government.
Brooke Army Medical Center, MCHE-ZDM-MDR, Brooke Army Medical Center, 3551 Roger Brooke Drive, JBSA Fort Sam Houston, TX 78234-4504, USA
E-mail address: jay.b.higgs.civ@mail.mil

providers, suspect them of making a conscious choice to assume the sick role.[6,7] Chronic pain and social pressures may exacerbate comorbid affective disorders.

Even now after years of research, the PCP treating FM is dealing with a "bitterly controversial condition," with numerous entities having a stake in the diagnosis and treatment.[8] The PCP is often challenged with an unhappy patient who is desperate to have a long list of often catastrophic symptoms addressed and may have 2 or more years of prior testing, alternate diagnoses, failed treatment trials, and comorbidities to review. Feeling unable to meet these challenges, some PCPs routinely refer FM patients for subspecialist care, but others overcome these challenges to manage FM independently and report achievement of an acceptable quality of life in 28% to 60% of cases.[1] The goal of this article is to offer the PCP practical tools to enhance the likelihood of successful management of FM. Off-label prescribing is recommended in this article and identified as such. Unreferenced recommendations represent current practice of the author and may not be validated by research data.

THE HISTORY OF FIBROMYALGIA

A brief review of the history of FM serves to show that this condition is not a phenomenon of modern culture.[9] In 410 BC, Hippocrates was surprisingly close to the concept of central hypersensitivity when he described the "Rheuma" (flow) theory: the brain sends liquid to the legs: the more liquid, the more pain. In 300 AD, Theophrastus described "lassitude" as widespread pain, a "soul disorder" with the brain being the center of pain.[10] In 1815, Balfour ascribed the symptoms to nociceptive (peripheral) pain from "fibrosistitis," an inflammatory disorder of fibrous tissue. In 1904, Gowers used the term fibrositis, which persisted for years among numerous other labels, including psychogenic rheumatism and pseudorheumatism. In 1976, P.K. Hench first coined "fibromyalgia," the term most widely used now. The first widely accepted research classification for FM was adopted by the American College of Rheumatology (ACR) in 1990. Although intended only for research classification, the 1990 ACR criteria were used for diagnosis despite problems with standardization of the tender point examination and the lack of inclusion of comorbidities. In 2010, the ACR endorsed preliminary diagnostic criteria that were more practical for the PCP.[11] In 2011, Wolfe and colleagues[12] modified the criteria for epidemiologic research using questionnaire format, and in 2016, proposed unification of the 2010 and 2011 criteria as described below.[13]

FIBROMYALGIA PATHOGENESIS

Although the cause or causes of FM remain unknown, the PCP should be aware of the complexity of this discussion and what is currently known about the pathogenesis of FM. Discussing with patients generally what is understood as well as acknowledging the uncertainties is part of the patient educational process vital to FM management.

One recent review of pathogenesis FM cited more than 600 references, only to conclude that the cause remains unknown.[7] The pain processing system is highly complex, and disorders of it should come as no surprise. **Table 1** lists the chief levels of pain processing that have been targets of investigation. The possibility of more than one level contributing to FM further complicates the issue. It is quite possible that clinical FM represents a range of disorders that converge in a final common pathway.

Starting at the periphery (nociceptive pain), inflammation of fibrous tissue was postulated but never convincingly documented. Searches for systemic inflammation, infection, nutrition, and endocrine disorders likewise resulted in subtle findings at best.[4,7] There is evidence that some with FM may have a small fiber neuropathy,[2,7] but this

Table 1
Potential sources of fibromyalgia pain

Source of Pain Studied	Methods of Study	Primary Findings	Conclusions
Fibrous tissue at tender points[7]	Biopsy	No inflammation	Not the source
Muscle[14,15]	Biopsy, metabolic	No inflammation; no conclusive findings for ischemia, metabolic defect	Unlikely contributor
Small nerve fibers[2]	Skin biopsy	Decreased nerve fiber density	Possible small-fiber neuropathy; controversial
Endocrine[4]	Blood testing: baseline and stress testing	Adrenal pituitary axis intact	No conclusive evidence for endocrine mechanism
Immune system[7]	Serologic testing	Normal and false positive tests are common	Not an autoimmune disorder
Infection[7]	Serologies, cultures	No infection implicated	Infection unlikely
Defective sleep[2,4,24–26]	Sleep studies	Increased sleep fragmentation; poor quality sleep independent of sleep duration; increased sleep apnea, especially in men	May be bidirectional with FM
Prior trauma[27]	Self-report historical features	Associations with posttraumatic stress disorder, adult or childhood sexual abuse. Not associated with physical trauma	Prior emotional trauma associated, but causation not established
Spinal cord[7]	Cerebrospinal fluid analysis	Increased substance P	Possible central sensitization
Autonomic nervous system[17]	Heart rate, tilt table testing	Subtle abnormalities	May contribute to orthostatic symptoms in FM
Limbic system[19,20]	Functional testing, MRI, SPEC testing	Smaller gray matter at amygdala and anterior cingulate gyrus with increased activity; defective pain inhibition pathways; abnormal hippocampus	Possible central amplification
Cerebral cortex[2,21,22]	Neuropsychological testing	Decreased attention and executive function "Type D" personality	Anxiety and depression associated but not the cause of FM; fibrofog may be from diversion of resources to pain processing

Abbreviation: SPEC, single photon emission computed tomography.

concept remains controversial. Likewise, disorders of muscle metabolism, blood flow, and inflammation have been investigated, with no conclusive findings.[7,14,15] Myofascial trigger points (distinct from the tender points of the ACR criteria) are not the cause of FM, but such nociceptive input may serve to augment centralized pain.[7,16]

Peripheral sympathetic hyperactivity at rest with adrenergic hypoactivity in response to stimulation has also been investigated. Abnormal tilt table testing in young patients with FM has been touted as an example of this.[7,17] Autonomic instability may be the reason some FM patients complain of orthostatic symptoms.

Central sensitization, pain arising from the spinal cord level after prolonged stimulation at the nociceptive level, is better documented. However, central sensitization tends to be more of a focal phenomenon and cannot alone account for the widespread pain and other symptoms of FM.[7,18]

Central amplification, pain arising from pain processing in the brain, is of most recent interest. Although many findings have not been replicated, several themes persist. The amygdala and anterior circulate gyrus are 2 limbic areas of the brain that are involved in pain processing. Anatomic studies of the gray matter of these areas demonstrate that they are smaller in FM populations than healthy controls, but functional studies indicate that these same areas are hyperactive. None of these changes, however, create a specific signature for FM.[19] Most recent imaging techniques make it possible to study "connectivity" between various regions of pain processing, which appears abnormal in FM.[7] In addition to excessive pain amplification, defective descending pain inhibitory mechanisms have been demonstrated in FM.[4,7,19] Brain neurochemistry suggests abnormal function of the hippocampus may play a key role in defective pain processing.[7,20]

Finally, the cortical brain is the level most apparent to the clinician. This area is where lower-level inputs result in thoughts and actions apparent at the bedside. In addition to somatic symptoms, up to 70% of patients will report "fibrofog," the variable feelings of reduced concentration, poor memory, and confusion.[21] Formal investigation of mentation of FM patients suggests subtle disorders of attention and executive function.[19,22] Some suggest that diversion of cognitive resources to pain processing may be responsible for this, as reviewed by Borchers and colleagues.[7] Anxiety and depression have a prevalence of 13% to 48% in FM, but it is not clear that these rates are higher than healthy controls. Whether FM and affective disorders belong to the same spectrum of central nervous system disorders is controversial.[7] A high percentage of FM patients are reported to have negative affect with social inhibition, termed the Type D personality.[2]

Also at the cortical level, some have suggested that FM represents a conscious choice to complain about common symptoms.[6] Although secondary gain may be a conscious choice in some cases, the author rejects this hypothesis for the majority. This assumption that FM is a conscious choice ("all in my head") is what FM patients fear most from their health care providers.[23]

The highest likelihood is that the generalized hypervigilance of FM arises from more than one level, and the contributions from each level may vary between patients. The more encompassing term "central amplification" has been advocated to reflect the totality of processes involved.[7,18]

Poor-quality sleep has long been associated with FM and has been thought important in both pathogenesis and treatment.[4] Sleep instability, measured by the cyclic alternating pattern, is increased in FM.[24] Sleep in FM is unrefreshing, regardless of duration.[2] Poor sleep and FM are bidirectional; both contribute to the severity to each other.[7] Restless legs syndrome and obstructive sleep apnea are more common in FM patients.[25,26]

Patients may ascribe their own case to an etiologic event in their life. A self-reported history of sexual abuse has been associated with FM.[27] Chronic stress and emotional trauma are commonly cited by FM patients.[7] Inflammatory, infectious, and physical trauma have been cited as causes of FM, with very little supportive data[7] but also no way to certainly refute these theses.

EPIDEMIOLOGY

The prevalence of FM in the United States using the 1990 ACR criteria is about 2%.[7] The disease is more common in women, but the average 3:1 ratio may have been exaggerated in the past because the 1990 ACR criteria required tender points, which are more prominent among women.[3,7] Prevalence rates using the 2010 ACR criteria may be higher than with the 1990 criteria.

FIBROMYALGIA SYMPTOMS AND CRITERIA

FM is a clinical syndrome that results in a spectrum of symptoms, including widespread pain, nonrestorative sleep, restless legs, fatigue, and numerous associated symptoms including but not limited to altered mentation ("fibrofog"), headaches, temporomandibular disorders, irritable bowel, interstitial cystitis, anxiety, and depression. Among all of these symptoms, the FM sufferers report that fatigue is the worst.[7] Given the lack of objective characteristics, The ACR has established clinical criteria. The first ACR criteria were established in 1990 for research classification.[28] The greatest weakness of the 1990 criteria was standardization of the tender point examination.[4,7] Skill is required to locate the tender points and gradually press to the maximum target pressure of 4 kg per square meter. Women have greater tender point pressure sensitivity, which may have exaggerated the female predominance of FM.[3] Finally, associated symptoms were relatively neglected in the 1990 criteria.

In 2010, in recognition of the need for a more practical tool for clinicians, the ACR published preliminary diagnostic criteria that eliminated the tender point examination, quantified widespread pain, and gave more recognition to associated symptoms.[11] There are 2 component scores, one for "widespread pain" and one for "symptom severity." The combination of scores is used to meet criteria, and the total score is advocated as a measure of "fibromyalgianess." A medical evaluation is required, and conditions that could cause the symptoms must be ruled out. The old concept of primary versus secondary FM has been abandoned.[7] To facilitate epidemiologic studies, the same group in 2011 modified the criteria so that a single questionnaire could be used for research in large populations.[12]

Finally, in 2016, Wolfe and colleagues[13] proposed further modification of the criteria to combine the 2010 and 2011 criteria and better define widespread pain. The 2010 requirement to rule out other causes for FM symptoms was eliminated, while at the same time acknowledging that the diagnosis of FM does not rule out other conditions. At this time, only the 2010 criteria are formally endorsed by the ACR and even then as "preliminary."

FIBROMYALGIA EVALUATION AND DIAGNOSIS

With lack of a standard diagnostic algorithm, 46% of PCP report uncertainty when diagnosing FM.[1] Perhaps the greatest confusion over the evaluation of FM is how to do the "complete evaluation" and what other health care screening should be done. The list of conditions that may mimic or be comorbid with FM is considerably long and to "rule out everything" is an untenable suggestion. One important principle is that FM is not a diagnosis of exclusion, requiring "rule out everything" before diagnosis.[3] Likewise, a diagnosis of FM does not rule out other comorbid conditions. For example, rheumatoid arthritis and FM may occur in the same patient, just the same as hypertension and heart disease may be comorbid.

The ACR 2010 and the 2016 criteria are useful to establish initial diagnostic criteria for FM. The author uses a questionnaire to focus the interview and cover all of the points in the criteria. The criteria are readily available and are part of the suggested tool kit discussed later. The author starts with a standard history and physical examination, including the complete review of systems by questionnaire. Clues to other underlying associated conditions are sought, understanding that the FM patient suffering from central hypersensitivity may be prone to catastrophizing,[7] requiring the practitioner to assist the patient in prioritizing symptoms. The physical examination is generally complete but focused on the most symptomatic areas. A formal tender point examination is no longer necessary, but it is valuable to be aware of the tender point locations to avoid confusion with local musculoskeletal syndromes. For example, the FM patient will commonly have bilateral greater trochanter tender points, which can appear similar to trochanteric bursitis/tendinitis. There are no standard laboratory tests required, but the author uses as a minimum those listed in **Table 2**. Some add an erythrocyte sedimentation rate (ESR) or C-reactive protein (CRP) to this list,[29] but the results are age and body weight dependent as well as nonspecific.

Note there are no serologic tests in this list; they all perform poorly as screening tools for systemic rheumatic disease.[3,30] In particular, the positive predictive value of the antinuclear antibody (ANA) as a screening test is very poor because of the low specificity and high population prevalence of this test. For example, if all patients with FM are screened for ANA with the goal of selecting those needing more testing or specialty referral, 12% to 30% will be positive.[31] Assuming a 2% FM prevalence and even the lower rate of 12% positive ANA, 780,000 persons in the United States would require further evaluation of this test alone.

Table 3 lists a partial differential diagnosis of FM, clues that might arise during the primary evaluation, and the author's suggested next step for each. Age-appropriate cancer screening should be up-to-date. For patients suspected of comorbid sleep apnea, a formal sleep study should be considered. Whatever tests are used, the ordering provider must anticipate responses to the results and explain the relevance to the patient.

FIBROMYALGIA MANAGEMENT

Optimal management of FM requires a multifaceted approach, including education, cognitive behavioral therapy (CBT), exercise, sleep hygiene, pharmacotherapeutics,

Table 2 Basic laboratory testing for fibromyalgia	
Test	Rationale
Chemistries: Creatinine, calcium, AST, ALT	Screen for renal insufficiency, hyperparathyroidism, hepatitis; renal and liver function important in medication prescribing
Sensitive thyrotropin (TSH)	Hypothyroidism may be difficult to detect by history and physical
Complete blood count	Abnormalities may be a clue to other chronic disease
Urinalysis	Systemic disorders may be manifest by renal disease not detected clinically

Table 3
Partial differential diagnosis of fibromyalgia

Condition	Clues in FM Patient That Merit Further Evaluation	Next Step in Evaluation
Hypothyroidism[4,46]	Elevated TSH	Repeat TSH, then treat or refer to specialty care if questions
Hyperparathyroidism[4,46]	Elevated serum calcium, low phosphate, history of recurrent renal stones, osteoporosis	PTH panel, then refer to specialty care if abnormal
Statin-induced myalgia[46]	Statin therapy of any duration	Consider 3 mo trial off statin; specialty referral if high cardiovascular risk
Inflammatory myositis[4]	Muscle weakness > pain	ESR, creatine kinase, specialty referral
Polymyalgia rheumatica[4,46]	Older age onset, prominent morning stiffness and gel phenomenon, extremity edema	ESR, CRP, trial of low-dose corticosteroids or rheumatology referral
Other autoimmune disease,[4,46] for example, RA, SLE	Symptoms plus objective findings, for example, skin rash, joint swelling, abnormal CBC, proteinuria, hematuria	Rheumatology and/or nephrology referral
Chronic hepatitis C	All adults born between 1945 and 1965; potential exposure history; elevated transaminases	Check serologies
Chronic hepatitis B	Potential exposure history; elevated transaminases; lived in endemic area	Check serologies

and management of comorbidities.[2,5,7] The PCP should be generally aware of the spectrum of current investigations for new therapies as well as complementary and alternative medicine approaches patients may consider. In some cases referral for specialty care may be needed. The primary care medical home model provides an opportunity for an organized team approach to this management challenge.[3] A complete medical home practice, however, requires adequate staffing that is mostly available in larger practices. The most recent clinical practice guideline on the management of FM was published by the European League Against Rheumatism (EULAR) in 2016 and is part of the recommended tool kit.[5]

Education

Education of the FM patient begins at the time of diagnosis, with the first challenge being gaining the patient's confidence. Acknowledgment that the provider understands the symptoms are not "imagined" is very important to gain the confidence of the patient, who likely has been challenged by other providers, friends, or family members as to the veracity of their pain. Reassurance that other treatable causes of the symptoms will be considered is also important. On the other hand, patients must be cautioned not to pursue excessive testing or harmful interventions. Patient responses to such counseling will vary, depending on their prior experiences. Some will be relieved that they are finally believed, and others may be anxious or angry, having been told by others that FM is "not a real diagnosis," or that their FM symptoms are from another condition, such as lupus or chronic infection. The latter group may be highly suspicious that their providers have been ignoring their symptoms and missing a diagnosis that would respond to other treatment. FM patients should be cautioned about the Internet, which contains a wide variety of misinformation about FM, including promises of rapid cure by unproven methods. Part of the initial discussion should include that FM management is a long-term multidisciplinary effort, with gradual responses to therapy. With proper diagnosis and initial education, most FM patients have improved satisfaction and decreased health care utilization.[3] The provider tool kit provides references to available education resources.

Cognitive Behavioral Therapy

CBT by a therapist who understands FM can be very helpful. CBT in a group setting has been used, with the advantage of efficiency and group support at the same time. The goals of CBT are education and improvement of the adaptive response to FM symptoms. A series of sessions spread over time allows the patient to practice adaptive techniques, report responses, and pose new questions along the way, although intensive single sessions have been used. Family member participation may allay misconceptions about FM and improve domestic support.

Exercise

Exercise has remained a mainstay of management of FM since even before the first criteria were published, and it is the only therapy to receive a "strong" recommendation from EULAR.[5] FM patients may react to exercise with excessive pain or fatigue, especially the day following their effort. Therefore, whatever exercise is chosen should be implemented at a very low level and gradually increased over time. Aerobic exercise is generally recommended over weight-based resistive exercise, but moderate resistance exercise may be beneficial as well.[4,32] Aquatic exercise has similar benefit.[4] Gradually increasing to 30 to 60 minutes of exercise 2 to 3 times per week is a reasonable goal.[3] One form of exercise that research has been shown beneficial for both FM and osteoarthritis is tai chi.[33]

Sleep Hygiene

Another cornerstone of therapy is adequate sleep. For selected patients, a sleep study may be in order to rule out underlying sleep apnea. Sleep hygiene training may be a part of CBT, the office visit, or printed material. When used, pharmacologic therapy as discussed later should be considered an adjunct and not a replacement for sleep hygiene.

Pharmacotherapeutics

Writing a prescription for FM may seem the fastest disposition in the busy clinic environment but, especially if used without other management techniques, is often doomed to failure. More than 50% of FM prescriptions are abandoned by the patient because of inefficacy or side effects. Repeatedly switching medications and polypharmacy are common, in part because of unrealistic treatment expectations.[3] Of the 3 US Food and Drug Administration (FDA) -approved medications for FM, none have yet gained such approval in Europe.[7] Understanding these caveats, pharmacologic therapy may still play a significant role in the management of FM. This discussion centers on practical aspects of pharmacologic intervention. Medication mechanisms of action and other details may be found in **Table 4**.

Table 4
Common medications for fibromyalgia

Drug	Mechanism of Action	Initial Dose	Maximum Dose	FDA Status (in US)
Amitriptyline[4,5]	Norepinephrine serotonin reuptake inhibition	10 mg qhs	75 mg 1–2 hours before bed	Off label
Cyclobenzaprine[4,5]	Similar to amitriptyline	5 mg 1–2 hours before bed	40 mg 1–2 hours before bed or divided daily	Off label
Duloxetine[4,5]	SNRI	30 mg every morning for 1 wk, then increase to 60 mg	60 mg every morning	Approved
Milnacipran[4,5]	SNRI	12.5 mg/d increasing gradually to 50 mg bid in 1 wk (See FDA label schedule)	100 mg bid	Approved
Pregabalin[4,5]	Binding to alpha2 subunit of voltage gated calcium ion channels in CNS	75 mg bid increasing to 150 mg bid in 1 wk as tolerated	225 mg po bid; consider dosing at night for sleep	Approved
Gabapentin[39]	Same as pregabalin	100 mg qhs	Gradual increase to 2400 mg/d divided tid	Off label
Tramadol (may be combined with acetaminophen)[5]	Weak opioid with mild SNRI activity	37.5–50 mg daily	Same dose up to 4 times daily	Off label

It is useful to consider what has been tried but does not work for FM. Nonsteroidal anti-inflammatory drugs do not work for FM[5] unless there is a comorbid nociceptive pain input, such as osteoarthritis, that is feeding the pain pathway with additional input. Opioids are ineffective[3,7] and may make the problem worse. Selective serotonin reuptake inhibitor (SSRI) antidepressants may treat comorbid depression but probably do not hold much benefit for FM.[2,4,5,34] Of the antileptics, topiramate has not performed well in FM. Corticosteroids have no role in FM treatment.[5]

An important part of the history of each FM case is prior treatments, including drugs tried, dose, response, and adverse reactions. Comorbidities and other medications may limit the options as well. For each medication prescribed, attention must be given to potential drug-drug and drug-comorbidity interactions. For example, antidepressants may unmask the manic side of bipolar disorder[35]; hence, pharmacologic therapy for this population should be coordinated with a psychiatrist. The same goes for any patient with a history of suicidal ideation or who is already under current treatment by a psychiatrist. Beyond the tables and clinical practice guidelines, prescribers should have a thorough knowledge of each medication used, and patients should be both counseled on principal side effects and given written information in more detail. Suicidal ideation is a risk with all of the FDA-approved FM medications, requiring discussion with patients about this complication. In addition, FM itself, especially with comorbidities, poses an increased risk of suicide.[36]

Some of the first-line and time-tested options for FM management remain off label. In fact, one meta-analysis concluded that tricyclic agents were better for FM pain than any of the FDA-approved drugs discussed below.[37] Amitriptyline[2,5] and cyclobenzaprine[5] are the most common tricyclic agents used for FM. The goal of these medications is to use the lowest possible dose to achieve higher-quality sleep and pain modification. The author advises patients that their sleep quality may improve before pain. FM patients tend to be highly sensitive to medication side effects, especially sedation the day after dosing. Hence, very low doses of tricyclic agents or CBP are advised at drug initiation, and the medications should be taken about 1–2 or more hours before bed. Standard medication sedation precautions should be discussed. The first dose should not be given the day before any critical activities, such as driving or operating dangerous machinery, are required, in case of excessive sedation. Mild sedation will likely improve with continued dosing, but severe sedation with even low doses will require a change in therapy. Dose increments may be made at variable intervals; the author's practice is to allow about 3 to 6 weeks at each dose, the shorter duration reserved for more severe symptoms with no side effects at initial doses.

Three drugs have been approved by the FDA for FM, all having similar efficacy and tolerability.[38] The dual-action serotonin and norepinephrine reuptake inhibitor (SNRI) antidepressants duloxetine and milnacipran have each achieved FDA approval for use in FM, although systematic reviews conclude that the improvement in pain is minor, and changes in fatigue, quality of life, and sleep are not significant.[4,5] As with all other medications, the principle of management is to start at the lowest dose and increase as tolerated and needed. In studies, duloxetine was not beneficial until a dose of 60 mg was achieved, and higher doses yielded no further benefit.[5] Hence, the package insert instructs to start at duloxetine 30 mg for 1 week and then increase to 60 mg. However, if there are any questions about side effects or some initial benefit at 30 mg is suspected, the author will persist at the starting dose longer than 1 week.

Pregabalin is the antileptic approved by the FDA for FM. The mechanism of action is different from the antidepressants, making pregabalin use possible either as monotherapy or in combination with antidepressants. Dose escalation is described in the package labeling. Gabapentin has also been found beneficial in FM, but is off label and less studied.[39] Patients should be cautioned not to suddenly stop an antileptic after regular use without a taper schedule, because of the risk of precipitating a seizure, even if one had never been experienced before.

Tramadol is the only pain medication that has found use in FM. The author prefers to use it as an adjunct when standard therapy fails. It is contraindicated in patients with a history of seizure disorder, because it may lower the seizure threshold. The lowest effective dose should be sought, and tramadol should be abandoned if not clearly effective.

Patience and persistence may be necessary to achieve the best therapeutic regimen for each patient. Trials of an average of 3 drug/dose modifications before at least some improvement in FM were reported by PCP.[1] It is important to recognize that there is a low compliance rate with FM medications, probably because of inadequate clinical response.[2] Education of the patient for realistic expectations of treatment goals is important.[3] A brief discussion at the time of first prescription about the role of antidepressants in FM management will avoid the issue of the patient researching the drug, finding it is psychotropic, and concluding that the provider really does think it is "all in my head."

In FM patients refractory to monotherapy, combinations of the above may be of benefit,[40] using one drug from each class. Providers not experienced with such therapy should refer the patient for specialty input.

THERAPIES UNDER CURRENT INVESTIGATION

Patients doing their own research will encounter a host of FM treatments under recent investigation.[41] Some Internet authors caution patients that their medical providers are not adequately educated about current medications for FM. Testimonials or uncontrolled studies may entice patients to request a trial of the "latest" therapies. Patients may come to their appointments armed with their own Internet reading and with unrealistic expectations about the PCP's time to keep abreast of FM clinical trials around the world. The PCP who completely avoids this discussion only feeds into the above notion of "uninformed" providers. The PCP can meet this challenge by being generally aware of the large spectrum of research treatments (**Table 5**), emphasizing to patients that recognized therapies are best to try first, and referring patients for clinical trials or specialty care when needed. Discussion with patients about the value of double-blind placebo-controlled trials can be a useful part of CBT education.

OTHER COMPLEMENTARY AND ALTERNATIVE THERAPIES

Faced with a condition with no definitive diagnostic test, no cure, and no certain promise of relief with current therapies, patients with FM understandably seek numerous complementary and alternative medical treatments for their condition (**Table 6**). Some may do so without knowledge of their traditional medical provider, but others will ask the provider's opinion. Providers can support patients by being aware of

Table 5
Selected investigational therapies fibromyalgia

Intervention	Data on Efficacy	Comment
Anodal transcranial direct current brain stimulation[47]	Improved attention, but not alertness; increased temperature pain threshold by 1.5–2°	May modulate central nervous system function; very investigational
Repetitive transcranial magnetic stimulation	Meta-analysis concluded benefit for FM separate from depression at 1 mo of therapy[48]	FDA approved for depression but not FM, further data needed
Quetiapine (antipsychotic)[49]	Limited data; better than placebo but not better than amitriptyline	
Cannabanoids (nabilone)[4,41,50]	*Cochrane Review;* no evidence for efficacy	
Sodium oxybate[41]	Effective for sleep fatigue, pain, overall function[4]	Not FDA approved for FM due to abuse potential; FDA approved for narcolepsy
S-adenosyl methionine (SAMe)	Small trials with improvement in pain and fatigue; EULAR recommendation "weak against"[5]	Side effects mild and infrequent
Low-dose opioid antagonists (naltrexone)[41]	Early studies suggest effective for pain and fatigue, but dose may have been too low to act as opioid antagonist	Theory is presumed endogenous opioid overactivity is causing opioid-induced hyperalgesia
Modafinil, armodafinil[41]	Variable results in small studies	FDA approved for narcolepsy

the modalities patients may try and the evidence for and against each. Most importantly, the PCP can steer patients away from the least beneficial and more risky options.

WHEN TO REFER FOR SUBSPECIALTY CARE

Some of the most common indications for referral to specialty care are listed in **Table 7**. This table is not comprehensive; the PCP will undoubtedly have additional valid questions and reasons for referral. Referral for specialty evaluation is more likely to answer these questions than broad spectrum testing in the absence of clinical indications just to reassure that "everything has been done." Referral also is valuable for refractory cases or when there are comorbid psychiatric disorders requiring medication.

PROGNOSIS

Patients with FM may lead satisfactory lives with this condition. FM, however, rarely remits completely. Improvement is often very gradual. Periodic exacerbations are common.[7] Comorbidities such as bipolar disorder lead to a worse prognosis. Patients treated at the primary care level have a better prognosis than that reported from tertiary care centers, probably because of patient selection.[42]

PEDIATRIC FIBROMYALGIA

Much of the research in FM has been for the adult population, but FM may occur in the pediatric age range as well.[43] The criteria for diagnosis in adults is largely applicable in children,[44] although some of the associated symptoms may differ in prevalence. The management also involves similar principles, with some important differences. The nonpharmacologic measures listed above are even more important in children and are preferable to medications. Hypermobility is more common in this age group, providing a potential target for physical therapy. The FDA-approved medications for FM are not approved for pediatric use; hence, all FM pharmacologic therapy in this age group is off label. Suicidal ideation may be more severe in adolescents taking

Table 6 Selected complementary and alternative therapies	
Intervention	**Evidence for Efficacy**
Acupuncture[2,4]	Variable reports; poor for widespread pain, possible focal benefit; not better than sham acupuncture
Electroacupuncture[2]	Poor for widespread pain, possible focal benefit
Moxibustion[2]	Poor for widespread pain, possible focal benefit
Chiropractic[2]	Poor for widespread pain, possible focal benefit; EULAR recommendation "strong against"[5]
Laser therapy, taping[51]	Improvement from baseline, but similar to placebo
Music therapy[2]	Pain relief 1–14 d
Hyperbaric oxygen[52]	Unblinded crossover study Short Form-36 quality of life score improved from a baseline of 3.15 increasing to 3.48
Massage therapy[4]	Improved pain, anxiety, depression; myofascial release techniques most beneficial; EULAR recommendation "weak against"[5]

Table 7
Selected indications for specialty referral of the fibromyalgia patient

Indication for Referral	Suggested Specialty
Patient or provider concerned about systemic rheumatic disease	Rheumatology consult more effective than broad serologic testing
Suspected bipolar disorder suicidal ideation, or psychiatric condition other than anxiety and depression	Psychiatry referral before medical therapy
Ongoing psychiatric care	Coordinate all medication therapy with psychiatrist
Narcotic-dependent pain	Pain specialist
Suspected statin myalgia in patient with known cardiovascular disease	Consultation with the specialty treating vascular problem to consider drug holiday or alternate therapy
Prominent neurologic symptoms or suspicion of primary muscle disorder	Neurology referral
Administrative disability claim	Referral to physician with training in disability evaluations
Inability to do even limited exercise	Physiatry and/or physical therapy
Provider or patient concern about chronic infection	Referral to Infectious Diseases

antidepressant or antileptic medications for FM. The prognosis for FM in younger patients may be better than in adults.

TROUBLESHOOTING PROVIDER ISSUES WITH FIBROMYALGIA MANAGEMENT

Although the challenge of living with FM takes an emotional toll on the patients, the effect on the PCP team caring for this population should be considered as well.[23,45] Common problems that may leave providers without easy answers are listed in **Table 8**, along with responses per the author's practice pattern. Recognizing the effect of FM on patient emotions may help providers accept patient behavior that would otherwise be highly frustrating. Attention to even small improvements in patient function can change the conversation to a positive light and improve the provider/patient relationship. Some FM training of the entire medical home team will improve the patient experience.

THE PRIMARY CARE PROVIDER TOOL KIT

Table 9 is the author's recommended tool kit to assist the PCP in formulating an organized approach to FM. The ACR provides the 2010 diagnostic tool, and the 2016 revision is proposed but not yet endorsed by the ACR. The PCP can choose the ACR-endorsed 2010 versus the revised 2016 criteria, which the author favors. EULAR provides the most recent treatment guideline. Patient education is available from the ACR and the Arthritis Foundation. The University of Michigan Fibroguide is a useful interactive program for patients, but requires some computer skills to navigate. Steps to an organized implementation of the tool kit include the following:

- Decide whether to use the 2010 ACR Preliminary versus the 2016 revised criteria in your practice and then create corresponding forms compatible with your electronic medical record

Table 8
Troubleshooting strategies for the primary care provider

Problematic Issue	Possible Solutions
Patient certain that another disease, not FM is causing their symptoms	Do reasonable screening for other problems Avoid serologies with poor predictive value Avoid total body scans without clinical indications Explain rationale to patient Specialty referral if above unsatisfactory
FM patient is already on chronic narcotic medication, "can't live without it"	Initiate proper FM management first and then attempt to wean from narcotics; pain specialist referral if this does not suffice
Patient resistant to trying any exercise at all	Start with CBT, encourage very low exercise to start; physical therapy or physiatry consult if problem persists
Patient is angry, leaving provider feeling helpless	Acknowledge that this feeling is common, caused by the frustration of patient and provider over lack of easy treatment options; refer patient for CBT, psychological counseling, or specialty consultation as necessary; avoid promising that consultants will have "the" answer

- Use the tool kit resources to establish a hard copy and electronic library of resources for FM patient education
- Consider demonstrating the Fibroguide program to patients in your office or as a part of CBT education to facilitate access
- Establish a referral relationship with local resources for CBT specific for FM, neurology, psychiatry, physiatry, physical therapy, rheumatology, and sleep medicine
- Establish a prescribing pattern of medications appropriate to your practice, using the EULAR clinical practice guideline, information in this article, and package insert prescribing information
- Provide education on the principles of FM to all members of your primary care team

Table 9
Primary care provider tool kit for fibromyalgia management

Resource	How to Access
American College of Rheumatology 2010 Preliminary Guidelines for Diagnosis of FM and Patient education materials (on line)	www.rheumatology.org Or see Ref.[11]
2016 Revision to 2010/2011 diagnostic criteria	See Ref.[13]
EULAR guidelines for the management of FM	http://ard.bmj.com/content/76/2/318 See also Ref.[5]
University of Michigan FibroGuide	https://fibroguide.med.umich.edu/ • Requires some computer skills • Browser must have Adobe Flash Player active • Follow navigation instructions carefully
Arthritis Foundation patient information	http://www.arthritis.org/about-arthritis/types/fibromyalgia/

SUMMARY

FM is a common disorder facing the PCP and has substantial impact on patient quality of life. The cause remains unknown, but current evidence points to multifactorial involvement of pain processing by the nervous system. Clinical diagnosis is aided by evidence-based diagnostic criteria. There is no cure for FM at this time, but management may lead to a satisfactory lifestyle. Nonpharmacologic treatment is the most important long-term modality. CBT, sleep hygiene, and regular aerobic exercise are central to management. Pharmacologic interventions are an important adjunct, but benefit is variable and side effects are common. Comorbidities and medication interactions are important to consider when tailoring therapy to the individual patient. Nontraditional therapies are frequently sought by patients desperate for relief, and the PCP must be prepared to counsel patients about the issues surrounding unproven remedies. The challenges of management can be discouraging to the patient and PCP alike, but persistence and patience can be highly rewarding. Organizing FM care within the structure of the PCP practice environment will improve chances of success.

REFERENCES

1. Hadker N, Suchita G, Chandran AB, et al. Primary care physicians' perceptions of the challenges and barriers in the timely diagnosis, treatment and management of fibromyalgia. Pain Res Manag 2011;16(6):440–4.
2. Bazzichi L, Giacomelli C, Consensi A, et al. One year in review 2016: fibromyalgia. Clin Exp Rheumatol 2016;34(2 Suppl 96):S145–9.
3. Arnold LM, Gebke KB, Choy EH. Fibromyalgia: management strategies for primary care providers. Int J Clin Pract 2016;70(2):99–112.
4. Chinn S, Caldwell W, Gritsenko K. Fibromyalgia pathogenesis and treatment options update. Curr Pain Headache Rep 2016;20(4):25.
5. Macfarlane GJ, Kronisch C, Dean LE, et al. EULAR revised recommendations for the management of fibromyalgia. Ann Rheum Dis 2017;76(2):318–28.
6. Hadler NM. Fibromyalgia" and the medicalization of misery. J Rheumatol 2003; 30(8):1668–70.
7. Borchers AT, Gershwin ME. Fibromyalgia: a critical and comprehensive review. Clin Rev Allergy Immunol 2015;49(2):100–51.
8. Wolfe F. Fibromyalgia wars. J Rheumatol 2009;36(4):671–8.
9. Inanici F, Yunus MB. History of fibromyalgia: past to present. Curr Pain Headache Rep 2004;8(5):369–78.
10. Perrot S. If fibromyalgia did not exist, we should have invented it. A short history of a controversial syndrome. Reumatismo 2012;64(4):186–93.
11. Wolfe F, Clauw DJ, Fitzcharles MA, et al. The American College of Rheumatology preliminary diagnostic criteria for fibromyalgia and measurement of symptom severity. Arthritis Care Res (Hoboken) 2010;62(5):600–10.
12. Wolfe F, Clauw DJ, Fitzcharles MA, et al. Fibromyalgia criteria and severity scales for clinical and epidemiological studies: a modification of the ACR Preliminary Diagnostic Criteria for Fibromyalgia. J Rheumatol 2011;38(6):1113–22.
13. Wolfe F, Clauw DJ, Fitzcharles MA, et al. 2016 Revisions to the 2010/2011 fibromyalgia diagnostic criteria. Semin Arthritis Rheum 2016;46(3):319–29.
14. Bandak E, Amris K, Bliddal H, et al. Muscle fatigue in fibromyalgia is in the brain, not in the muscles: a case-control study of perceived versus objective muscle fatigue. Ann Rheum Dis 2013;72(6):963–6.

15. Simms RW, Roy SH, Hrovat M, et al. Lack of association between fibromyalgia syndrome and abnormalities in muscle energy metabolism. Arthritis Rheum 1994;37(6):794–800.
16. Ge HY, Wang Y, Fernandez-de-las-Penas C, et al. Reproduction of overall spontaneous pain pattern by manual stimulation of active myofascial trigger points in fibromyalgia patients. Arthritis Res Ther 2011;13(2):R48.
17. Furlan R, Colombo S, Perego F, et al. Abnormalities of cardiovascular neural control and reduced orthostatic tolerance in patients with primary fibromyalgia. J Rheumatol 2005;32(9):1787–93.
18. Clauw DJ, Arnold LM, McCarberg BH, FibroCollaborative. The science of fibromyalgia. Mayo Clin Proc 2011;86(9):907–11.
19. Walitt B, Ceko M, Gracely JL, et al. Neuroimaging of central sensitivity syndromes: key insights from the scientific literature. Curr Rheumatol Rev 2016; 12(1):55–87.
20. Fayed N, Andres E, Rojas G, et al. Brain dysfunction in fibromyalgia and somatization disorder using proton magnetic resonance spectroscopy: a controlled study. Acta Psychiatr Scand 2012;126(2):115–25.
21. Katz RS, Heard AR, Mills M, et al. The prevalence and clinical impact of reported cognitive difficulties (fibrofog) in patients with rheumatic disease with and without fibromyalgia. J Clin Rheumatol 2004;10(2):53–8.
22. Torta RG, Tesio V, Ieraci V, et al. Fibro-fog. Clin Exp Rheumatol 2016;34(2 Suppl 96):S6–8.
23. Bernstein J, Hadler NM, Clauw DJ, et al. Not the last word: fibromyalgia is real. Clin Orthop Relat Res 2016;474(2):304–9.
24. Rizzi M, Sarzi-Puttini P, Atzeni F, et al. Cyclic alternating pattern: a new marker of sleep alteration in patients with fibromyalgia? J Rheumatol 2004;31(6):1193–9.
25. Viola-Saltzman M, Watson NF, Bogart A, et al. High prevalence of restless legs syndrome among patients with fibromyalgia: a controlled cross-sectional study. J Clin Sleep Med 2010;6(5):423–7.
26. Roizenblatt S, Neto NS, Tufik S. Sleep disorders and fibromyalgia. Curr Pain Headache Rep 2011;15(5):347–57.
27. Hauser W, Kosseva M, Uceyler N, et al. Emotional, physical, and sexual abuse in fibromyalgia syndrome: a systematic review with meta-analysis. Arthritis Care Res (Hoboken) 2011;63(6):808–20.
28. Wolfe F, Smythe HA, Yunus MB, et al. The American College of Rheumatology 1990 criteria for the classification of fibromyalgia. Report of the multicenter criteria committee. Arthritis Rheum 1990;33(2):160–72.
29. Goldenberg DL. Clinical manifestations and diagnosis of fibromyalgia in adults. In: Schur PH, editor. UpToDate®. Available at: https://www.uptodate.com/contents/clinical-manifestations-and-diagnosis-of-fibromyalgia-in-adults. Accessed November 22, 2017.
30. Clauw DJ. Fibromyalgia: a clinical review. JAMA 2014;311(15):1547–55.
31. Solomon DH, Kavanaugh AJ, Schur PH, American College of Rheumatology Ad Hoc Committee on Immunologic Testing Guidelines. Evidence-based guidelines for the use of immunologic tests: antinuclear antibody testing. Arthritis Rheum 2002;47(4):434–44.
32. Jones KD. Recommendations for resistance training in patients with fibromyalgia. Arthritis Res Ther 2015;17:258.
33. Wang C, Schmid CH, Rones R, et al. A randomized trial of tai chi for fibromyalgia. N Engl J Med 2010;363(8):743–54.

34. Walitt B, Urrutia G, Nishishinya MB, et al. Selective serotonin reuptake inhibitors for fibromyalgia syndrome. Cochrane Database Syst Rev 2015;(6):CD011735.

35. Bortolato B, Berk M, Maes M, et al. Fibromyalgia and bipolar disorder: emerging epidemiological associations and shared pathophysiology. Curr Mol Med 2016; 16(2):119–36.

36. Lan CC, Tseng CH, Chen JH, et al. Increased risk of a suicide event in patients with primary fibromyalgia and in fibromyalgia patients with concomitant comorbidities: a nationwide population-based cohort study. Medicine (Baltimore) 2016;95(44):e5187.

37. Papadopoulou D, Fassoulaki A, Tsoulas C, et al. A meta-analysis to determine the effect of pharmacological and non-pharmacological treatments on fibromyalgia symptoms comprising OMERACT-10 response criteria. Clin Rheumatol 2016; 35(3):573–86.

38. Lee YH, Song GG. Comparative efficacy and tolerability of duloxetine, pregabalin, and milnacipran for the treatment of fibromyalgia: a Bayesian network meta-analysis of randomized controlled trials. Rheumatol Int 2016;36(5):663–72.

39. Arnold LM, Goldenberg DL, Stanford SB, et al. Gabapentin in the treatment of fibromyalgia: a randomized, double-blind, placebo-controlled, multicenter trial. Arthritis Rheum 2007;56(4):1336–44.

40. Gilron I, Chaparro LE, Tu D, et al. Combination of pregabalin with duloxetine for fibromyalgia: a randomized controlled trial. Pain 2016;157(7):1532–40.

41. Ablin JN, Hauser W. Fibromyalgia syndrome: novel therapeutic targets. Pain Manag 2016;6(4):371–81.

42. Fitzcharles MA, Da Costa D, Poyhia R. A study of standard care in fibromyalgia syndrome: a favorable outcome. J Rheumatol 2003;30(1):154–9.

43. Kashikar-Zuck S, King C, Ting TV, et al. Juvenile fibromyalgia: different from the adult chronic pain syndrome? Curr Rheumatol Rep 2016;18(4):19.

44. Ting TV, Barnett K, Lynch-Jordan A, et al. 2010 American College of Rheumatology adult fibromyalgia criteria for use in an adolescent female population with juvenile fibromyalgia. J Pediatr 2016;169:181–7.e1.

45. Homma M, Ishikawa H, Kiuchi T. Association of physicians' illness perception of fibromyalgia with frustration and resistance to accepting patients: a cross-sectional study. Clin Rheumatol 2016;35(4):1019–27.

46. Goldenberg DL. Differential diagnosis of fibromyalgia. In: Schur PH, editor. UpToDate®. Available at: https://www.uptodate.com/contents/differential-diagnosis-of-fibromyalgia. Accessed June 8, 2017.

47. Silva AF, Zortea M, Carvalho S, et al. Anodal transcranial direct current stimulation over the left dorsolateral prefrontal cortex modulates attention and pain in fibromyalgia: randomized clinical trial. Sci Rep 2017;7(1):135.

48. Knijnik LM, Dussan-Sarria JA, Rozisky JR, et al. Repetitive transcranial magnetic stimulation for fibromyalgia: systematic review and meta-analysis. Pain Pract 2016;16(3):294–304.

49. Walitt B, Klose P, Uceyler N, et al. Antipsychotics for fibromyalgia in adults. Cochrane Database Syst Rev 2016;(6):CD011804.

50. Walitt B, Klose P, Fitzcharles MA, et al. Cannabinoids for fibromyalgia. Cochrane Database Syst Rev 2016;(7):CD011694.

51. Vayvay ES, Tok D, Turgut E, et al. The effect of laser and taping on pain, functional status and quality of life in patients with fibromyalgia syndrome: a placebo-randomized controlled clinical trial. J Back Musculoskelet Rehabil 2016;29(1):77–83.

52. Efrati S, Golan H, Bechor Y, et al. Hyperbaric oxygen therapy can diminish fibromyalgia syndrome–prospective clinical trial. PLoS One 2015;10(5):e0127012.

Autoimmunity Mimics
Infection and Malignancy

Jeffrey C. Eickhoff, MD[a],*, Angelique N. Collamer, MD[b]

KEYWORDS

- Mimics • Musculoskeletal • Rheumatic • Autoimmune • Infection • Cancer
- Malignancy • Paraneoplastic

KEY POINTS

- Septic joint should be considered for any acute-onset monoarticular inflammatory arthritis, prompting urgent arthrocentesis and synovial fluid analysis (level C).
- Controlled trials show no benefit of prolonged antibiotic treatment over placebo in treatment of post-Lyme disease syndrome (level A).
- Many viral infections can cause both acute and chronic arthritis as well as other extraarticular rheumatic manifestations (level B).
- Fungal and tuberculous arthritis often present as chronic monoarthritis of the knee (level B).
- Malignancy may present as isolated musculoskeletal or rheumatic features, and should be considered when features of rheumatic disease are atypical or response to therapy is limited (level C).

INTRODUCTION

Musculoskeletal syndromes are commonly encountered in the primary care setting and a broad differential is required to avoid missing potentially life-threatening diagnoses. A plethora of infectious agents can produce osteoarticular and soft tissue

Disclosure Statement: The authors declare no commercial or financial conflicts of interest. The views expressed in this article are those of the authors and do not necessarily reflect the official policy or position of the Department of the Navy, Department of the Army, Department of the Air Force, the Uniformed Services University, the Department of Defense, or the U.S. Government. We are military service members. This work was prepared as part of our official duties. Title 17 U.S.C. 105 provides that "Copyright protection under this title is not available for any work of the United States Government." Title 17 U.S.C. 101 defines a United States Government work as a work prepared by a military service member or employee of the United States Government as part of that person's official duties.

[a] Rheumatology Service, U.S. Navy, Medical Corps, Naval Medical Center Portsmouth, 620 John Paul Jones Circle, Portsmouth, VA 23708, USA; [b] Rheumatology Service, U.S. Air Force, Medical Corps, Walter Reed National Military Medical Center, Uniformed Services University, 4301 Jones Bridge Road, Bethesda, MD 20814-4799, USA
* Corresponding author.
E-mail address: Jeffrey.c.eickhoff.mil@mail.mil

manifestations. Likewise, malignancies may manifest as rheumatic symptoms via direct tumor invasion or paraneoplastic effects. Herein we focus on the recognition, diagnosis, and evaluation of infectious and malignant mimics of rheumatic disease.

BACTERIAL INFECTIONS OF THE BONE, JOINT, AND SOFT TISSUE

Bacterial infections of the bone and joint are true emergencies. Permanent disability and death may result if prompt effective treatments are not instituted.[1]

Nongonococcal Bacterial Arthritis

The incidence of native joint infections ranges from 2 to 10 cases per 100,000 annually.[2] Prosthetic joint infections occur in approximately 1% to 2% of cases. Hematogenous spread is the most common route of entry into the joint, although infection may occur via contiguous spread or through direct inoculation.[3,4] **Table 1** presents the common types of infections and their clinical features, host risk factors and example empiric treatment options.[2–6]

Clinical features

Bacterial septic arthritis usually presents as a monoarticular acutely painful and inflamed joint. Constitutional symptoms are common.[3] Large joints such as the knee, hip, shoulder, elbow, and ankle are most often involved, and both active and passive ranges of motion are limited. Prosthetic joint infections may have a more indolent presentation.[4] Sternoclavicular and sacroiliac involvement may be seen in intravenous (IV) drug users.

Diagnosis

The differential diagnosis for acute septic arthritis includes:

- Crystalline arthropathy (gout, pseudogout);
- Systemic rheumatic disease;
- Primary and metastatic malignancy; and
- Numerous rare conditions.[3]

Inflammatory markers such as the erythrocyte sedimentation rate, C-reactive protein, and white blood cell counts lack both sensitivity and specificity and blood cultures are positive in only 50% of patients. Synovial fluid analysis is essential for the diagnosis. Synovial fluid should be sent for a white blood cell count with differential, Gram stain, culture, and crystal analysis. White blood cell counts of greater than 50,000/mm^3 and polymorphonuclear cell counts of greater than 90% are suggestive.[3]

In nongonococcal bacterial arthritis, the synovial fluid gram stain is positive in 50% or more of cases, with positive cultures in more than 90%.[7] Prosthetic joint infections may present in a more indolent fashion and diagnostic imaging modalities may be more helpful in these cases.[4] See **Table 2** for comparative features of various causes of septic arthritis.[1,3,8,9]

Treatment

Treatment is targeted to the causative organism. In developed countries, *Staphylococcus aureus* is the most common cause of septic arthritis, with methicillin-resistant *S aureus* playing an increasingly important role (see **Table 1**).[2] Repeated joint aspirations and serial synovial fluid analysis or surgical drainage are often required. Treatment for prosthetic joint infections is complex and usually requires the removal of hardware with prolonged antibiotic administration. See reference[10] for Infectious Diseases Society of America guidelines for diagnosis and management of prosthetic joint infections. **Fig. 1** demonstrates an infected prosthetic knee joint.

Table 1
Nongonococcal bacterial infections of the bone, joint, and periarticular soft tissues

Common Organisms	Risk Factors	Clinical Features	Empiric Treatment Options[a]
Type of infection	**Septic joint**		
Neonates	• Drug abuse	Native joint	Based on Gram stain result (preferred):
• *Staphylococcus aureus*	• Malignancies	• Pain; erythema; usually monoarticular; fever (60%)	• GPC: Vancomycin
• GBS	• Diabetes mellitus	• Synovial fluid WBC/mm^3 usually >50,000, >75% PMNs	• GNC: Ceftriaxone
• Enterobacteriaceae	• Alcoholism/cirrhosis		• GNR: Ceftazidime, cefepime
Children:	• IV drug abuse	Prosthetic joint	• Negative Gram stain: vancomycin plus ceftazidime or cefepime
• *S aureus*	• Hemoglobinopathies	• Synovial fluid WBC/mm^3 often much lower	
• *Streptococcus pneumoniae*	• Rheumatoid arthritis	• Early: <3 mo; joint pain, erythema, warmth, fever, chills, effusion	
• GAS	• SLE	• Delayed: 3–24 mo; indolent pain	
• *Haemophilus influenza*	• Dog/cat bites	• Late: >24 mo; acute onset pain; with or without fever/leukocytosis	
• *Kingella kingae*	• Hemochromatosis		
Adults			
• *S aureus*			
• *S pneumoniae*			
• β-Hemolytic streptococcus			
• *Neisseria gonorrhoeae*			
• *Salmonella*			
• Enterobacteriaceae			

(continued on next page)

Table 1
(continued)

Type of infection	Common Organisms	Risk Factors	Clinical Features	Empiric Treatment Options[a]
Osteomyelitis	Most common • S aureus • Coagulase-negative staphylococci Less common • Streptococcus pyogenes • S pneumoniae • H influenza • Anaerobes (eg, Peptostreptococcus) • E coli • Pseudomonas	• Diabetes mellitus • Decubitus ulcers • Surgery • Trauma • IV drug use	Acute: • Children > adults • Osteonecrosis absent • Constitutional symptoms common • Progressive (days) Chronic: • Adults > children • Osteonecrosis present • Via open wound/fracture • Insidious (months)	• IV antibiotics targeted to blood or bone culture susceptibility × 4–12 wk duration • Drainage and debridement • Oral antibiotics in some cases after an IV course
Bursitis	S aureus (>80%)	• Trauma • Alcoholism • Diabetes mellitus • Preexisting bursal disease	• Olecranon bursa most common • Painful, warm, swollen, erythema • Possible overlying cutaneous injury • Joint function not typically impaired • Aspirate; WBC usually moderately elevated	• Coverage for methicillin-resistant Staphylococcus aureus • Initial IV antibiotics recommended for more severe cases • Duration 2–3 wk • NSAIDs, warm/cold packs, avoidance of exacerbating activities

Abbreviations: GAS, group A streptococci; GBS, group B streptococci; GNC, gram-negative cocci; GNR, gram-negative rods; GPC, gram-positive cocci; IV, intravenous; NSAIDs, nonsteroidal anti-inflammatory drugs; PMNs, polymorphonuclear leukocytes; RA, rheumatoid arthritis; SLE, systemic lupus erythematosus; WBC, white blood cells.

[a] Specific antibiotic regimens should be verified in accordance with the most recent guidelines; consultation with infectious disease and orthopedic specialists is strongly encouraged.

Table 2
Comparison of common infectious causes of arthritis

	Nongonococcal (Bacterial) Arthritis	Gonococcal Arthritis	Acute Rheumatic Fever	Lyme Arthritis
Time of onset	Days to 2 wk	Days to 4 wk	2–3 wk (2–3)	Months
Features of arthritis	Pain; erythema; usually monoarticular	Pain; erythema; usually monoarticular	Pain; polyarticular; self-limited	Oligoarticular; stiffness > pain
Clinical presentation	Fever (60%)	Fever, rash, tenosynovitis, migratory polyarthralgia	Fever, carditis, erythema marginatum, subcutaneous nodules, Sydenham chorea	Antecedent migratory arthralgia, fatigue, occasionally fever
Synovial fluid				
Cell count (WBC/mm³)	2000–>100,000; usually >50,000; >90% PMNs	15,000–>100,000; >75%–90% PMNs	Usually <20,000, >50% PMNs	Average 25,000 (range 500–>100,000); 50%–75% PMNs
Color/transparency	Yellow-green, opaque	Yellow, cloudy – opaque	Yellow, cloudy	Yellow, cloudy
Culture	Positive 60%–90%	Positive < 50%	Negative	Negative
PCR	N/A – variable organisms	Positive (Sn 76%, Sp 96%)	N/A – postinfectious	Positive (80% of untreated); low Sn

Abbreviations: N/A, not applicable; PCR, polymerase chain reaction; PMNs, polymorphonuclear leukocytes; Sn, sensitivity; Sp, specificity; WBC, white blood cells.

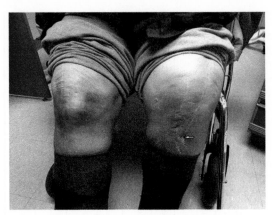

Fig. 1. This 78-year-old man developed a methicillin-resistant *Staphylococcus aureus* (MRSA) infection of his left knee prosthesis with visible draining sinus tract. (*Courtesy of* Christa Eickhoff, MD, Bethesda, MD.)

Gonococcal Arthritis

Gonorrhea remains an important cause of inflammatory arthritis; it is sexually transmitted and caused by the gram negative diplococci *Neisseria gonorrhoeae*. Disseminated gonococcal infection occurs in 0.5% to 3% of patients with untreated mucosal infections.[1,11]

Clinical features

Tenosynovitis is an important clue to the diagnosis, because it occurs rarely with other types of septic arthritis. Other commonly seen features are fever, skin lesions, and polyarthralgias. There are 2 commonly encountered presentations in clinical practice, the arthritis–dermatitis syndrome and septic arthritis. The arthritis–dermatitis subset of patients present with swollen joints and skin lesions; the skin findings usually appear as nonpruritic painless macules, papules, and pustules, often found on the limbs and trunk.[8] Septic arthritis occurs in up to 50% of cases of disseminated gonococcal infection, and is generally monoarticular; most often these patients do not present with skin lesions.[8]

Diagnosis

Diagnosis is based on clinical and laboratory findings (see **Table 2**). In men, Gram staining of urethral exudates has high sensitivity and specificity; there is lower sensitivity for endocervical smears in women. In disseminated gonococcal infection septic arthritis, only about one-fourth of synovial fluid Gram stains will be positive. Therefore, all possible mucosal infectious sites should be tested. Use of nucleic acid amplification tests allows for the noninvasive collection of samples (urine); a main limitation is the inability of nucleic acid amplification tests to provide antibiotic resistance data.[1]

Treatment

Management of disseminated gonococcal infection may require hospitalization, especially if there is a purulent arthritis necessitating serial aspirations. Per the Centers for Disease Control and Prevention 2015 guidelines, a cephalosporin-based regimen plus azithromycin 1 g single dose is generally used for the initial treatment of disseminated gonococcal infection and may be changed after clinical improvement to a susceptible oral regimen.[12]

Osteomyelitis

Osteomyelitis can mimic a number of systemic rheumatic conditions depending on the specific site affected. The incidence increases with age, and is estimated at 2.4 cases per 100,000. Vertebral osteomyelitis most often results from hematogenous spread, direct inoculation (surgery), and extension from contiguous tissues. Hematogenous spread is typically monomicrobial. Posttraumatic osteomyelitis is often polymicrobial. S aureus is the most often cultured infecting organism in both adults and children (see **Table 1**).[13,14]

Clinical features

Osteomyelitis may be either acute (more common in children) or chronic (more common in adults). Acute osteomyelitis is often secondary to hematogenous spread, whereas chronic disease is more commonly associated with fractures and open wounds. Nonspecific constitutional symptoms are common and weight bearing may be limited.[1] Point tenderness and swelling may be appreciated over the affected site, or a draining fistula may be visible. Acute osteomyelitis symptoms may evolve over days, in contrast with chronic osteomyelitis, where there may be insidious symptoms presenting over months to years.[11,12] Vertebral osteomyelitis usually presents with nonspecific back pain and neurologic impairment may be seen; fever is less common.[13]

Diagnosis

The diagnosis of osteomyelitis is based on physical examination, laboratory, and imaging studies. The gold standard is culture and histopathology of the infected bone; however, blood cultures may produce a suspected organism. Wound cultures do not generally correlate with the causative organism and bone biopsies are not always diagnostic. Inflammatory markers (erythrocyte sedimentation rate, C-reactive protein) are neither sensitive nor specific. Conventional radiographs are positive in 90% of patients by 1 month, showing periosteal reaction and focal osteopenia. Among imaging modalities, MRI has the greatest diagnostic accuracy.[13,14]

Treatment

In addition to parenteral antibiotics, surgical drainage and debridement are recommended for abscesses and bone necrosis, which are seen in chronic osteomyelitis. Data showing optimal duration of antibiotics are lacking; a duration of 4 to 6 weeks to 3 months is considered necessary. Culture data are important for antibiotic selection. Bone biopsy should be considered if cultures are negative.[13]

Septic Bursitis

Bursitis may mimic a septic joint. Occupations that result in repetitive trauma to the area are at increased risk, as are alcoholics and diabetics. Bursitis may be septic or aseptic, and these are often difficult to differentiate.[15] See **Table 1** for detailed clinical features and treatment options for bursitis.[1,15]

Clinical features

The most commonly involved sites of septic bursitis are the olecranon in adults and the prepatellar bursa in children. More than 50% will have adjacent cellulitis. The most common causative organism is S aureus (>80%) from a transcutaneous source. In contrast with septic arthritis, joint function is not usually impaired.[15]

Diagnosis

The most important consideration is septic bursitis. The differential diagnosis for septic bursitis includes:

- Traumatic bursitis;
- Cellulitis;
- Crystal-induced disease;
- Hemorrhagic bursitis; and
- Chronic osteomyelitis.

To differentiate, aspiration of the bursa with culture, cell count with differential, and crystal evaluation are required. Imaging may also be necessary if osteomyelitis is suspected.[15]

Treatment

No treatment guidelines exist for septic bursitis. Generally accepted treatment measures include:

- Aspiration;
- Empiric antibiotics while awaiting cultures;
- Avoidance of aggravating activities;
- Cold or warm packs;
- Nonsteroidal antiinflammatory drugsNSAIDs); and
- Bursectomy for treatment failure.[15]

For febrile or immunocompromised patients, IV antibiotics accompanied by serial aspirations are indicated (see **Table 1**).

Other Infection-Related Rheumatic Syndromes

Lyme arthritis

Lyme disease is a multisystem disorder caused by the *Ixodes* tick-born spirochete *Borrelia*. A small subset of patients may go on to develop chronic antibiotic-refractory inflammatory arthritis, which requires NSAIDs or disease-modifying anti-rheumatic drugs.[9]

Epidemiology and pathogenesis *Borrelia* has a worldwide distribution, with most cases reported in Asia, Europe and North America. In the United States *B burgdorferi* is the most common vector.[9] The incidence in the United States in 2015 was 8.9 per 100,000 population. The disease most commonly occurs in the Northeast, upper Midwest, Eastern Seaboard, and northern California, but an increasing case incidence may now be found throughout the United States both owing to human travel and changes in the deer and tick migratory pattern; thus, clinicians in all areas of the country need to be familiar with the common disease manifestations.[16]

Clinical features

Lyme disease presents in early and late phases.

- Early localized phase: The classic erythema migrans (a "bull's-eye") rash occurs 1 to 2 weeks after transmission via tick bite, and is often asymptomatic. Flulike symptoms of fever, headache, arthralgias, myalgias, and fatigue may accompany early infection.[9]
- Early disseminated phase: Weeks to months after infection, neurologic and cardiac manifestations may occur. Features include cranial nerve VII palsy, meningitis, sensory and motor radiculoneuropathies, and carditis.[9]

- Late phase: Inflammatory arthritis presents on average 6 months after infection, occurring in about 60% of untreated patients.[9] Arthritis is usually oligoarticular, inflammatory, and affects large joints; bursitis and tendinitis can be seen. Untreated, Lyme arthritis may wax and wane.[17] Axonal polyneuropathy and encephalomyelitis are rare late neurologic manifestations. See **Table 2** for a comparison of Lyme arthritis with other infectious arthritides.

Diagnosis

Lyme disease should be considered when the patient has potential exposure to borrelia-infected ticks and suggestive clinical features. A 2-tiered approach to serologic assays is used for diagnosis. A serum enzyme-linked immunosorbent assay immunoglobulin (Ig)M and IgG assay is performed first, and if positive or equivocal, is followed by confirmatory IgM and IgG immunoblotting. Sensitivity may be low with early testing (in erythema migrans; 29%–40%), but is higher after 6 to 8 weeks of untreated infection and greater than 95% in late disease.[18] Borrelia IgM may remain positive for years following successful treatment. Synovial fluid polymerase chain reaction should be used for *B burgdorferi* DNA; polymerase chain reaction may also remain positive for months after successful treatment.[9]

Treatment

Treatment for Lyme disease depends on the stage and manifestations of disease. The Infectious Diseases Society of America has published guidelines for the treatment of Lyme disease.[19,20]

Acute Rheumatic Fever

Acute rheumatic fever remains a major problem worldwide, with an annual global incidence of approximately 471,000 cases and more than 230,000 deaths.[21] It is a systemic autoimmune disease caused by a cross-reactive immune response to host tissue epitopes following infection with group A beta-hemolytic streptococci. It most commonly occurs in younger individuals (5–15 years); one-third of these patients will not recall a preceding upper airway infection.[22] The risk of developing acute rheumatic fever after an untreated group A beta-hemolytic streptococci pharyngitis infection is 0.3% to 3.0%.[23]

Clinical features

Clinical features are detailed in **Table 2**. Arthritis is the most common manifestation and usually presents as large joint polyarticular, nonerosive, sterile arthritis in a migratory or additive pattern lasting up to 4 weeks.[22,24]

Diagnosis

By the time symptoms of acute rheumatic fever occur, 75% of patients will have cleared the infection (ie, throat culture will be negative).[25] Rapid streptococcus antigen testing has a high specificity but low sensitivity. Therefore, streptococcal antibody testing is often necessary. Available tests include anti-streptokinase, anti-streptolysin O, anti-DNAse B, antihyaluronidase, and anti-NADase. Titers generally peak 2 to 3 weeks after the initial symptoms of acute rheumatic fever. An initial test and increased titer 2 weeks later confirms recent infection; 95% of patients will have a positive result if 3 antigens are tested.[22] In 2004, the World Health Organization published diagnostic criteria for rheumatic fever and rheumatic heart disease.[25]

Treatment

Treatments include the following.

- Antibiotics to eradicate group A beta-hemolytic streptococci including for household contacts with carriage of streptococcus.
- NSAIDs or aspirin for arthritis and fever.[22]

VIRAL ARTHRITIS

Viral infections are ubiquitous worldwide, and many have been associated with articular and extraarticular rheumatic manifestations. With globalization, novel virus-associated arthritides are becoming apparent in the United States, including Chikungunya and Zika virus. See **Table 3** for rheumatic manifestations of clinically important viral infections.[26-32]

Human Immunodeficiency Virus Infection

Human immunodeficiency virus (HIV) has numerous rheumatic manifestations; certain conditions commonly seen before the advent of combination antiretroviral therapy are now less common in treated patients, and new conditions secondary to treatment side effects have emerged.

Epidemiology

Worldwide, 36.7 million people live with HIV. In 2015, approximately 2.1 million new cases of HIV were diagnosed, with 39,513 of these new diagnoses in the United States.[33]

Clinical features

See **Table 3** for common HIV-associated rheumatic symptoms.[26,27]

Table 3
Virus-associated rheumatic disease, clinical features

HIV	Parvovirus B19	HBV	HCV	Alphaviruses
Pre-cART/ untreated:	Children	• Chronic infection uncommon	• Chronic infection common	Chikungunya, Igo-ora, O'nyong-nyong, Mayaro, Sindbis, Ross River, zika:
• Septic arthritis	• Fever, "slapped cheek" rash, maculopapular rash	• Symmetric arthritis	• Inflammatory arthritis	
• Joint aches/ arthralgia		• Rheumatoid factor positive (25%)	• Cryoglobulins	• Arthritis
• Arthritis	Adults		• Sicca symptoms	• Arthralgias
• Myopathy	• Symmetric arthritis, stiffness	• Medium vessel vasculitis (PAN)	• + RF, ANA	• Myalgias
• Vasculitis			• Low C4 complement	• Conjunctivitis
Post-cART:	• Frequent autoantibody positivity (RF, ANA, anti-DNA, anti-ENA, aPL)		• Cytopenias	• Rash
• IRIS				• Fever
• Drug-induced joint aches				
• Osteoporosis				
At any time				
• Hyperuricemia				
• Gout				

Abbreviations: ANA, antinuclear antibody; aPL, antiphospholipid antibody; cART, combination antiretroviral therapy; ENA, extractable nuclear antibody; HBV, hepatitis B virus; HCV, hepatitis C virus; HIV, human immunodeficiency virus; IRIS, immune reconstitution inflammatory syndrome; PAN, polyarteritis nodosa; RA, rheumatoid arthritis; RF, rheumatoid factor.

Table 4
Common post-antiretroviral therapy rheumatic syndromes

Drug	Manifestation	Treatment
• cART	• Immune reconstitution inflammatory syndrome • New rheumatic disease (RA, reactive arthritis, cutaneous lupus) or exacerbation of preexisting rheumatic disease • Occurs 3–27 mo after cART initiation	• Self-limited
• Zidovudine, didanosine	• Polymyositis-like myopathy	• May require drug discontinuation
• Protease inhibitors	• Rhabdomyolysis • Osteoporosis • Osteonecrosis	• Symptomatic, may require drug discontinuation • Bisphosphonates, calcium/vitamin D
• Indinavir	• Dupuytren contracture • Adhesive capsulitis • de Quervain's Tenosynovitis	• Drug discontinuation
• Tenofovir	• Osteomalacia (Fanconi syndrome)	• May require drug discontinuation

Abbreviations: cART, combination anti-retroviral therapy; RA, rheumatoid arthritis.

Diagnosis and treatment
Treatment is usually symptomatic and includes the initiation of combination antiretroviral therapy when indicated. Generally, HIV patients on combination antiretroviral therapy with good disease control can tolerate immunosuppressive treatments when needed.[27,34] Common antiretroviral drug-associated syndromes are described in **Table 4**.[26,27]

Hepatitis B virus
Hepatitis B virus is a double-stranded DNA virus that can be transmitted sexually, parenterally, or vertically and affects approximately 350 million people worldwide.[29] Rheumatic manifestations are thought to be related to the deposition of immune complexes in the blood vessel walls or synovium, leading to small or medium vessel vasculitis or arthritis. The presence of elevated aminotransferase levels, positive IgM hepatitis B core antibodies and hepatitis B surface antigen is consistent with the diagnosis.[27]

Hepatitis C virus
Hepatitis C virus is an RNA virus, transmitted parenterally, often through injection drug use, sexual contact, or blood transfusions (before 1992). Chronic infection is common and prevalence in the US population is about 1% to 2%.[29,31] Hepatitis C virus-associated inflammatory arthritis may be rheumatoid arthritis-like and require similar treatments.[31]

Parvovirus B19
Parvovirus is a single-stranded DNA virus that is responsible for the childhood exanthem erythema infectiosum (fifth disease). It often presents with fever and the classic "slapped cheek" rash. It is transmitted via respiratory secretions during outbreaks, which typically occur in late winter and spring. Parvovirus is ubiquitous in the general population, and household transmission rates are as high as 50%. The diagnosis is made clinically with the demonstration of a positive parvovirus IgM antibody or via polymerase chain reaction assay. Treatment is supportive.[27,32]

Alphavirus infection Alphaviruses are increasingly recognized in Western Europe and the United States owing to worldwide travel. See **Table 4** for common disease manifestations. No specific therapy is available, and treatment is symptomatic with analgesics and NSAIDs.[28]

MYCOBACTERIAL DISEASE

Infection with mycobacterial organisms may result in musculoskeletal disorders. These infections are most commonly seen in immunocompromised patients.

Mycobacterium tuberculosis

In the United States, 9557 tuberculosis cases were reported in 2015.[35] Musculoskeletal involvement occurs in 9% of infections. Skeletal tuberculosis may manifest as peripheral arthritis, spondylitis, reactive arthritis, osteomyelitis, soft tissue abscesses, bursitis, and tenosynovitis. Peripheral arthritis is inflammatory and destructive, generally monoarticular affecting large joints.[36] The gold standard for diagnosis remains microbiologic identification of *M tuberculosis*. Synovial fluid and biopsy cultures are positive in more than 80% to 90% of cases, and are important to determine drug susceptibility, but generally take 2 to 8 weeks to result; polymerase chain reaction or nucleic acid amplification tests may allow for a more rapid diagnosis.[36,37]

Nontuberculous (atypical) Mycobacterial Infections

Nontuberculous (atypical) mycobacterial infections most commonly cause musculoskeletal infections through penetrating injuries or direct inoculation. Patients present with constitutional symptoms with local pain, soft tissue abscesses, tenosynovitis, and osteomyelitis.[37] In contrast with typical mycobacterial infections, nontuberculous mycobacterial infections often involve the hands, and affect the knees and spine less frequently.[36] More commonly encountered nontuberculous mycobacterial infections in the United States include *M avium* complex, *M marinum*, and *M kansassi*. **Fig. 2** demonstrates an *M marinum* infection of the hand. For diagnosis, histopathologic or bacteriologic samples should demonstrate the causative organism.[37]

FUNGAL DISEASE

A number of potentially pathogenic fungi are endemic to the United States, and may have musculoskeletal manifestations. These infections typically occur in immunocompromised persons, and manifestations such as pulmonary or cutaneous involvement are important clues to the diagnosis. Histoplasmosis, coccidioidomycosis, blastomycosis, and cryptococcosis are the most likely to be seen in clinical practice in the United States; however, infections are relatively uncommon.[38]

Clinical Features

Fungal infections often produce a monoarthritis most commonly affecting the knee or other large joints. See **Table 5** for detailed clinical features, diagnostic clues, and treatment options.[36,38,39]

Diagnosis

Diagnosis requires demonstration of the fungi via tissue biopsy or synovial fluid analysis. The best testing method should be discussed with the local microbiology laboratory.[40]

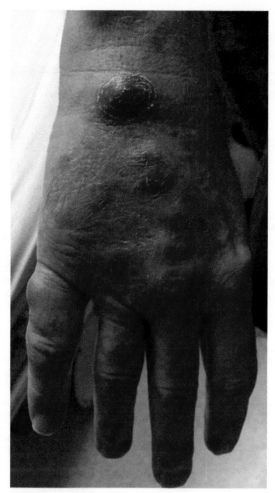

Fig. 2. *Mycobacterium marinum* infection in an aquarium enthusiast. (*Courtesy of* Christa Eickhoff, MD, Bethesda, MD.)

Treatment

See **Table 5** for treatment options. The Infectious Diseases Society of America practice guidelines for specific organisms are available at: http://www.idsociety.org/Organism.

PARASITIC DISEASE

In certain geographic areas of the world, parasitic infections are an important cause of arthritis, sacroiliitis, myositis, and vasculitis. Parasitic rheumatism should be suspected in patients with rheumatic manifestations with poor response to antirheumatic drugs, prior residence or travel in an area of endemic parasitosis, and peripheral blood eosinophilia. The diagnosis is based on clinical history as well as specialized testing and histopathology in consultation with infectious disease specialists.[40]

Table 5
Fungi associated with bone and joint infections

Fungus	Distribution	Transmission	Musculoskeletal Manifestations	Treatment (Osteoarticular)
Histoplasma capsulatum	Worldwide Ohio/Mississippi River valleys	Inhalation Bird/bat feces	Acute polyarthritis Tenosynovitis Erythema nodosum	NSAIDs Itraconazole Amphotericin B Surgical
Blastomyces dermatitidis	Ohio/Mississippi River areas, mid-Atlantic states, Canada, Europe, Africa, South America	Inhalation	Monoarthritis (3%–5%) Osseous (60%) - vertebrae, ribs, tibia, skull, feet	Itraconazole Amphotericin B Surgical Second line: fluconazole
Coccidiodes immitis	Southwestern United States, Central/South America	Inhalation Arid/semiarid regions	Monoarthritis Osteomyelitis Erythema nodosum	Itraconazole Fluconazole Amphotericin B Surgical
Cryptococcus neoformans	Worldwide	Inhalation Urban bird/bat feces, rotten wood	Osteomyelitis Paravertebral abscess Monoarthritis (rare) – knee Muscle	Fluconazole Surgical Amphotericin B
Aspergillus fumigatus	Worldwide	Inhalation Decaying matter	Osteomyelitis (rare) Arthritis (rare)	Voriconazole Surgical Amphotericin B Caspofungin
Candida species	Worldwide	Endogenous to host	Osteomyelitis (rare) – spine (adults) or long bones (children) Monoarthritis or polyarthritis (rare)	Amphotericin B Caspofungin Micafungin Anidulafungin
Sporothrix schenckii	Worldwide	Inhalation (systemic) Scratch/skin prick (cutaneous)	Mono/ oligoarthritis Osteomyelitis Tenosynovitis	Itraconazole Surgical Amphotericin B Fluconazole

Abbreviation: NSAID, nonsteroidal antiinflammatory drug.

MALIGNANCY-ASSOCIATED RHEUMATIC DISORDERS

Musculoskeletal manifestations are common in patients with malignancy. The mechanisms underlying these musculoskeletal symptoms include (1) direct tumor invasion of bones and joints, (2) paraneoplastic effects, and (3) chemotherapeutic adverse effects.

Direct Tumor Invasion

Neoplasms may directly affect the bones, muscles, synovium, articular cartilage, and periarticular structures. In 2016, 3300 primary malignant bone tumors and 172,000

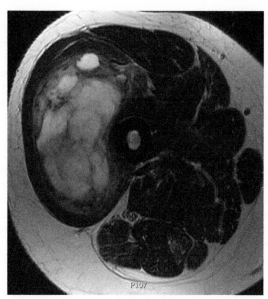

Fig. 3. Soft tissue sarcoma. This 48-year-old man developed the insidious onset of right knee pain. An axial T2-weighted MRI demonstrates a pleomorphic soft tissue sarcoma. (*Courtesy of* Joseph Roswarski, MD, Bethesda, MD.)

hematologic malignancies were diagnosed in the United States.[41] Malignant lesions may present with hypercalcemia and elevated alkaline phosphatase, nonspecific bone pain, joint stiffness or effusion, painless masses, pathologic fractures, or spinal cord compromise. **Fig. 3** demonstrates a soft tissue sarcoma that presented as insidious onset knee pain in a runner. See **Table 6** for examples of important primary and metastatic bone tumors.[42–45]

Table 6
Primary and metastatic bone tumors

Type	Examples
Primary	
Osseous	• *Osteosarcoma*: most common primary malignant bone tumor; most frequently affects the femur, humerus, skull, pelvis; poor survival • *Chondrosarcoma*: second most common primary malignant bone tumor • *Fibrosarcoma*: rare • *Giant cell tumors*
Nonosseous	• *Leukemias*: bone pain common, spinal pain more common in adults, long bone pain more common in children; arthritis • *Multiple myeloma* • *Round cell tumors*: group includes Ewing's sarcoma, primary lymphomas of bone
Metastatic	• Spine/pelvis are common locations of metastatic disease; metastases rarely affect joints, muscles, or adjacent connective tissue
Osteolytic	• *Non-small cell lung cancer, renal cell carcinoma, thyroid cancer, melanoma, non-Hodgkin's lymphoma*
Osteoblastic	• *Prostate, small cell lung cancer, carcinoid, Hodgkin's lymphoma*
Mixed	• *Breast, gastrointestinal, squamous cell carcinoma*

Paraneoplastic syndromes

Numerous malignancy-associated conditions present symptomatically owing to complex interactions of autocrine and paracrine mediators.[42] The strongest data exists for cancer-associated myositis (dermatomyositis, polymyositis, inclusion body myositis), hypertrophic osteoarthropathy, palmar fasciitis and polyarthritis, tumor-induced osteomalacia, and remitting seronegative symmetric synovitis with pitting edema. Classic clinical findings of hypertrophic osteoarthropathy include nail clubbing and periosteal new bone formation.[42,43,46]

SUMMARY

Many factors contribute to the development of musculoskeletal rheumatic syndromes. A plethora of different infectious agents may produce osteoarticular and soft tissue manifestations; likewise, malignancies may manifest rheumatic symptoms via direct invasion or paraneoplastic effects. Awareness of these diseases and their clinical risk factors should result in earlier recognition and intervention, which may improve long-term outcomes and overall patient care.

REFERENCES

1. Balsa A, Martín-Mola E. Infectious arthritis I: bacterial arthritis. In: Hochberg M, Silman A, Smolen J, et al, editors. Rheumatology. 6th edition. Philadelphia: Elsevier; 2015. p. 885–93.

2. Ohl C, Forster D. Infectious arthritis of native joints. In: Bennett J, Dolin R, Blaser M, editors. Mandell, Douglas, and Bennett's principles and practice of infectious diseases. 8th edition. Philadelphia: Elsevier Saunders; 2015. p. 1302–15.

3. Horowitz D, Katzap E, Horowitz S, et al. Approach to septic arthritis. Am Fam Physician 2011;84(6):653–60.

4. Gilliland W. Bacterial septic arthritis, bursitis, and osteomyelitis. In: West S, editor. Rheumatology secrets. 3rd edition. Philadelphia: Elsevier; 2015. p. 291–9.

5. Cook P, Siraj D. Bacterial arthritis. In: Firestein G, editor. Kelley and Firestein's textbook of rheumatology. 10th edition. Philadelphia: Elsevier; 2017. p. 1876–88.

6. Mathews C, Weston V, Jones A. Bacterial septic arthritis in adults. Lancet 2010; 375:846–55.

7. Goldenberg D. Septic arthritis. Lancet 1998;351:197–202.

8. Rice P. Gonococcal arthritis (disseminated gonococcal infection). Infect Dis Clin North Am 2005;19:853–61.

9. Bockenstedt L, Wormser G. Review: unraveling Lyme disease. Arthritis Rheum 2014;66(9):2313–23.

10. Osmon DR, Berbari EF, Berendt AR, et al. Diagnosis and management of prosthetic joint infection: clinical practice guidelines by the Infectious Diseases Society of America. Clin Infect Dis 2013;56(1):e1–25.

11. Bardin T. Gonococcal arthritis. Best Pract Res Clin Rheumatol 2003;17:201–8.

12. Centers for Disease Control and Prevention (CDC)., CDC Gonococcal infections in adolescents and adults. Available at: https://www.cdc.gov/std/tg2015/gonorrhea.htm. Accessed March 11, 2017.

13. Zimmerli W. Vertebral osteomyelitis. N Engl J Med 2010;362:1022–9.

14. Chihara S, Segreti J. Osteomyelitis. Dis Mon 2010;56:5–31.

15. Hanrahan J. Recent developments in septic bursitis. Curr Infect Dis Rep 2013;15:421–5.

16. Centers for Disease Control and Prevention (CDC), CDC reported cases of Lyme disease by state or locality, 2005-2015. Available at: https://www.cdc.gov/lyme/stats/. Accessed March 03, 2017

17. Steere A, Schoen R, Taylor E. The clinical evolution of Lyme arthritis. Ann Intern Med 1987;107:725–31.

18. Aguero-Rosenfeld M, Wang G, Schwartz I, et al. Diagnosis of Lyme borreliosis. Clin Microbiol Rev 2005;18(3):484–509.

19. Arvikar S, Steere A. Diagnosis and treatment of Lyme arthritis. Infect Dis Clin North Am 2015;29(2):269–80.

20. Wormser GP, Dattwyler RJ, Shapiro ED, et al. The clinical assessment, treatment, and prevention of Lyme disease, human granulocytic anaplasmosis, and babesiosis: clinical practice guidelines by the Infectious Diseases Society of America. Clin Infect Dis 2006;43(9):1089–134.

21. Carapetis JR, Steer AC, Mulholland EK, et al. The global burden of group a streptococcal diseases. Lancet Infect Dis 2005;5:685–94.

22. Azevedo P, Rodrigues-Pereira R. Acute rheumatic fever. In: Hochberg M, Silman A, Smolen J, et al, editors. Rheumatology. 6th edition. Philadelphia: Elsevier; 2015. p. 918–27.

23. Guilherme L, Ming P, Kalil J. Rheumatic fever and post-streptococcal arthritis. In: Firestein G, editor. Kelley and Firestein's textbook of rheumatology. 10th edition. Philadelphia: Elsevier; 2017. p. 1956–72.

24. Carapetis J, McDonald M, Wilson N. Acute rheumatic fever. Lancet 2005;366: 155–68.

25. Rheumatic fever and rheumatic heart disease: report of a WHO expert consultation. World Health Organ Tech Rep Ser 2004;923:1–122.

26. Patel N, Patel N, Espinoza L. HIV infection and rheumatic diseases: the changing spectrum of clinical enigma. Rheum Dis Clin North Am 2009;35(1):139–61.

27. Vassilopoulos D, Calabrese L. Rheumatologic aspects of viral infections. In: Hochberg M, et al, editors. Rheumatology. 6th edition. Philadelphia: Elsevier; 2015. p. 912–7.

28. Suhrbier A, Jaffar-Bandjee M, Gasque P. Arthritogenic alphaviruses-an overview. Nat Rev Rheumatol 2012;8:420–9.

29. Vassilopoulos D, Calabrese L. Management of rheumatic disease with comorbid HBV or HCV infection. Nat Rev Rheumatol 2012;8:348–57.

30. Vassilopoulos D, Calabrese L. Rheumatic manifestations of hepatitis C infection. Curr Rheumatol Rep 2003;5:200–4.

31. Rosen H. Clinical practice. Chronic hepatitis C infection. N Engl J Med 2011;364: 2429–38.

32. Young N, Brown K. Parvovirus B19. N Engl J Med 2004;350(6):586–97.

33. Centers for Disease Control and Prevention (CDC), C.D.C. HIV basic statistics. Available at: https://www.cdc.gov/hiv/basics/statistics.html. Accessed March 05, 2017.

34. Adizie T, Moots RJ, Hodkinson B, et al. Inflammatory arthritis in HIV positive patients: a practical guide. BMC Infect Dis 2016;16:100.

35. Centers for Disease Control and Prevention (CDC), C.D.C. Trends in tuberculosis. 2015. Available at: https://www.cdc.gov/tb/publications/factsheets/statistics/tbtrends.htm. Accessed March 04, 2017.

36. Gilliland W. Mycobacterial and fungal joint and bone diseases. In: West S, editor. 3rd edition. Philadelphia: Elsevier; 2015. p. 307–12.

37. Griffith DE, Aksamit T, Brown-Elliott BA, et al. An official ATS/IDSA statement: diagnosis, treatment, and prevention of nontuberculous mycobacterial diseases. Am J Respir Crit Care Med 2007;175:367–416.

38. Limper AH, Knox KS, Sarosi GA, et al. An official American Thoracic Society statement: treatment of fungal infections in adult pulmonary and critical care patients. Am J Respir Crit Care Med 2011;183:96–128.

39. Ruderman E, Flaherty J. Fungal infections of bones and joints. In: Firestein G, editor. Kelley and Firestein's textbook of rheumatology. 10th edition. Philadelphia: Elsevier; 2017. p. 1918–25.

40. Marquez J, Espinoza L. Infectious arthritis II: mycobacterial, brucellar, fungal, and parasitic arthritis. In: Hochberg M, et al, editors. Rheumatology. 6th edition. Philadelphia: Elsevier Mosby; 2015. p. 894–904.

41. Siegel R, Miller K, Jemal A. Cancer statistics, 2016. CA Cancer J Clin 2016;66(1): 7–30.

42. Hashefi M. Rheumatologic manifestations of malignancy. Clin Geriatr Med 2017; 33:73–86.

43. Vaseer S, Chakravarty E. Musculoskeletal syndromes in malignancy. In: Firestein G, editor. Kelley and Firestein's textbook of rheumatology. 10th edition. Philadelphia: Elsevier; 2017. p. 2048–63.

44. Ehrenfeld M, Hanan G, Shoenfeld Y. Rheumatologic features of hematologic disorders. Curr Opin Rheumatol 1999;11:62–7.

45. Gur H, Koren V, Ehrenfeld M, et al. Rheumatic manifestations preceding adult acute leukemia: characteristics and implication in course and prognosis. Acta Haematol 1999;101:1–6.

46. Battafarano D. Malignancy-associated rheumatic disorders. In: West S, editor. Rheumatology secrets. 3rd edition. Philadelphia: Elsevier; 2015. p. 371–7.

Approach to Osteoarthritis Management for the Primary Care Provider

Thomas W. Schmidt, MD*

KEYWORDS

- Osteoarthritis • Management • Treatment • Evaluation • Diagnosis • Primary care
- Review

KEY POINTS

- Osteoarthritis is the most common joint disease affecting patients.
- The pathogenesis of osteoarthritis is complex and involves degenerative, inflammatory, and biomechanical factors.
- Risk factors for the development of osteoarthritis include: age, weight, female sex, genetics, and prior joint injury.
- Diagnosis of osteoarthritis is primarily clinical but radiographs and laboratory data may be used to exclude other conditions.
- Treatment of osteoarthritis primarily focuses on pain relief and includes nonpharmacologic, pharmacologic, and surgical interventions.

INTRODUCTION

Osteoarthritis (OA) is the most common joint disease in the United States affecting more than 27 million Americans, approximately 15% of the population, and contributing to roughly 12 million office visits annually.[1–3] In 2009, it accounted for more than 920,000 hospital admissions, making it the fourth most common diagnosis at discharge.[3] With an aging population, these numbers will continue to rise.[4] Most of this additional care will be handled by primary care providers. Although OA is a joint disease, there is a national shortage and unequal distribution of rheumatologists,[5,6] making an understanding of OA necessary for general practitioners.

Traditional classification has separated OA into primary or secondary. Primary OA is joint damage that occurs without an inciting cause, whereas secondary OA is the result of a proceeding insult: trauma, infection, metabolic, inflammatory, or other

The author has no financial conflicts of interest in the subject matter or materials discussed.
Department of Rheumatology, David Grant Medical Center, 101 Bodin Circle, Travis AFB, CA 94535, USA
* Department of Internal Medicine, 101 Bodin Circle, Travis AFB, CA 94535, USA.
E-mail address: twschmidt1980@gmail.com

Prim Care Clin Office Pract 45 (2018) 361–378
https://doi.org/10.1016/j.pop.2018.02.009
0095-4543/18/Published by Elsevier Inc.

condition (**Box 1**). The classic perspective has been with time joint damage will accrue with everyday living, and primary OA was the natural result of this progression. As our understanding of OA has advanced this perspective has become antiquated. We now understand that aging is just one of many important risk factors.

RISK FACTORS FOR OSTEOARTHRITIS
Age

Age is the greatest risk factor for the development of OA.[7] However, it is not solely the length of time that a joint has been under stress that leads to OA, but a myriad of age-related influences.[7] Atrophied muscle alters biomechanics, and the accompanying redistribution of forces leads to cartilage degradation.[7–10] Cartilage is further altered by age-associated biochemical factors.[11] Protein modifications and the loss of hydrophilic and elastic properties also contribute to cartilage loss.[7,12–15] Additionally, accumulation of reactive oxygen species impact the integrity of protein structures and the extracellular matrix.[16–18] Finally, there has been an observed shift in cellular homeostasis to a proinflammatory milieu and a propensity to develop OA with aging.[19–21]

Genetics

The contribution of genetics in the development of OA has been estimated to range from 40% to 80%, and a subset of early onset OA shows Mendelian inheritance.[22] Evaluating genetic contribution to common OA has identified 17 loci.[23] A summation of genetic influence along with environmental factors likely contributes to OA development. Some heritable contributions include bone shape and surface area in addition to baseline cartilage thickness.[22,24] Other molecular mechanisms that are still being

---

Box 1
Secondary osteoarthritis causes

Inflammatory

Gout

Prior septic arthritis

Rheumatoid arthritis or other systemic inflammatory arthritis

Traumatic

Joint injury: fracture or ligament tear

Prior surgery to joint

Neuropathic arthropathy

Mechanical

Avascular necrosis

Hypermobility syndromes

Congenital/Inherited joint abnormalities

Metabolic

Hemochromatosis

Hyperparathyroidism

Diabetes

Pseudogout (calcium pyrophosphate deposition disease)

evaluated are the role of epigenetics, such as DNA-methylation and the role of non-coding RNAs.[22–24] As we better understand these processes, it may lead to novel gene-directed therapies.

Sex

Women have a higher prevalence and more severe OA than men, in particular post-menopausal women.[25–28] The gender differences and accelerated OA onset of post-menopausal women has led to the consideration that estrogen plays a role in OA development; however, clinical trials have provided conflicting outcomes.[28] Women receiving estrogen supplementation have shown both positive and negative outcomes, suggesting that gender discrepancies in OA development are more complex than solely estrogen concentration. Ongoing research explores estrogen production, the concentration of estrogen receptors, and the use of selective estrogen receptor modulators in altering OA development.[28] Anatomic differences between men and women have also been noted with women having thinner baseline cartilage.[25,26] An additional risk factor is the discordant number of anterior cruciate ligament (ACL) injuries women suffer compared with men.[29–31]

Trauma

Prior joint injury is also a risk factor for OA development. OA following an ACL or meniscal injury is common. Nearly half of patients will suffer some limitation or associated pain 20 years after an initial insult, and approximately 80% of soccer players that suffered an ACL injury showed radiographic evidence of OA 15 years later.[31,32] As previously mentioned, women are at higher risk for OA, and accrue ACL injuries at a rate 2 to 8 times higher than men.[29–31] Not only is a significant joint injury a risk, but repetitive joint stress associated with certain occupations plays a role. Carpenters and dock workers experience more knee OA, whereas professional athletes experience more joint-specific degeneration than their recreational counterparts.[33,34]

Obesity

Obesity has been linked with development of hand and knee OA, but an association with hip OA is less clear.[35–38] Obese individuals reach a 3 times higher risk of knee OA development compared with normal-weight individuals. Subsequently loss of weight is protective. Reducing body mass index by as little as 2 units or 5 kg has reduced the risk of women developing symptomatic knee OA by as much as 50%, and individuals who lose weight tend to have improved pain scores.[39–41] Furthermore, lean mass has been associated with increased cartilage thickness.[35] It is not only the joint forces and trauma of extra weight that can lead to acceleration of OA, but adipose tissue is known to have inflammatory properties.[42–44] Secretion of adiponectin, leptin, and resistin may all contribute to the inflammatory components of OA, and help to explain why obese individuals are more likely to suffer OA in both weight-bearing and non–weight-bearing joints.[35,42–44]

PATHOPHYSIOLOGY

Historically, OA has been defined as a degenerative, noninflammatory arthritis with cartilage loss and joint space narrowing. "Wear-and-tear" arthritis is a phrase commonly used; however, it is a simplification of a complex process.[45] The joint is composed of bone, cartilage, tendons, ligaments, and a synovial lining that function synchronously. A disruption in their interactions can lead to biomechanical and chemical changes triggering the cascade of pathologic events.[45–47]

Articular cartilage is composed of chondrocytes and extracellular matrix that serve to add mechanical support and lubrication to the joint.[47] Normally there is a balance between cartilage degradation and production; however, in OA there is a shift in this homeostasis. Early in the process, cartilage swelling may be seen as chondrocytes increase proteoglycan production.[48] Over time, the proteoglycan levels drop, producing cartilage surface vertical clefts and flaking. Radiographically, this is seen as joint space narrowing.[48] The initial cartilage damage is multifactorial with contributions from aging, trauma, and other biochemical factors altering forces across the articular surface. These disruptions have been implicated in triggering local inflammatory responses.[45,46,49]

Cartilage injury in conjunction with proinflammatory cytokines and metalloproteinases (MMP) propagate the development of OA. When compared with healthy controls, patients with an injured joint have higher levels of proinflammatory cytokines tumor necrosis factor (TNF)-α, interleukin (IL)-1β, and IL-6.[45,49] Furthermore, injured joints have been shown to activate the complement system.[50] Following an injury, these proinflammatory cytokines may remain elevated for several years, leading to further cartilage degradation.[51] The inflammatory, mechanical, and degenerative progression of OA eventually prompts a medical evaluation.

PRESENTATION AND WORKUP
History and Physical Examination

Pain is the most common OA symptom that prompts patients to seek medical care.[52] Weight-bearing joints such as the knees or hips are often affected, but hand involvement of the distal and proximal interphalangeal (DIPs and PIPs) and first carpometacarpal (CMC) joints will commonly be encountered.[53] The pain is typically worse with activity and better with rest. Symptoms progressively get worse over time and sudden onset of pain is not the norm. A review of symptoms accompanied by systemic concerns should raise suspicion for an alternative diagnosis.

When examining the area of concern, keep in mind that where a patient says it hurts and the actual anatomic location of pain may differ. Having the patient point to the area that is the most painful can help differentiate "true joint" pain from soft tissue injuries or periarticular concerns. On examination, an involved joint may show range of motion loss, cracking, or crepitus. The joint is typically cool to touch but an effusion, particularly in the knee, may be present.[54] Associated muscle atrophy, such as in the quadriceps, may be noted.[55,56] Weight bearing may be impaired, but rarely is the patient unable to stand. In OA of the hand, DIPs and PIPs may display Heberden and Bouchard nodes (**Fig. 1**).

Radiographic Studies

After a thorough history and physical examination, radiographic evaluation is common. Radiographic evidence of OA includes joint space narrowing, osteophyte formation, subchondral cysts, and sclerosis (**Fig. 2**). Severity of OA has historically been based on Kellgren and Lawrence (KL) grade values from 0 to 4 with a score of 2 or more consistent with radiographic OA.[57,58] KL grading has been used to evaluate hand, knee, and hip OA.

Although plain radiographs remain the most used imaging technique, additional studies may be beneficial. MRI can add 3-dimensional detail, better evaluate soft tissue defects, uncover synovitis, accurately measure cartilage thickness, and detect effusions. Furthermore, bone marrow lesions can be identified suggesting early OA or associated cartilage or ligament damage (**Fig. 3**).[58] Despite these advantages, MRIs

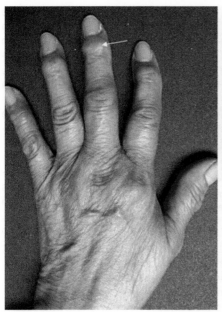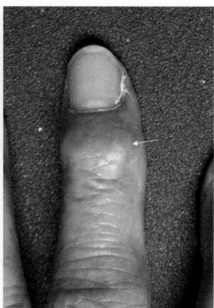

Fig. 1. Hand with osteoarthritis. DIP and PIP involvement will commonly present with nodes. Note the Heberden node at the DIP joint (*white arrow*).

are expensive, time-consuming, and not readily available for routine OA evaluation. Ultrasound is also being incorporated into practice. Advantages of ultrasound are portability, quick examination of several anatomic locations, and low cost, but it remains user dependent and can detect only superficial structures.[58]

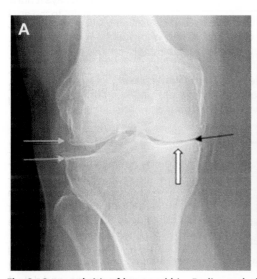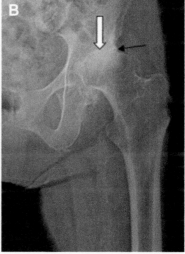

Fig. 2. Osteoarthritis of knee and hip. Radiograph showing a knee (*A*) and hip (*B*) with the classic findings of OA. Note the osteophytes (*yellow arrows*), joint space narrowing (*black arrows*), and sclerosis (*thick white arrows*).

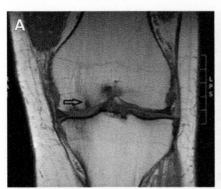 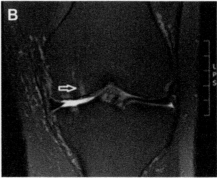

Fig. 3. MRI of knee. T1 (*A*) and T2 (*B*) imaging of the same knee showing bone marrow lesions (BMLs) (*arrows*). On T1 imaging, BMLs are dark, and they appear bright on T2 imaging.

Laboratory Evaluation

If the history, physical examination, and imaging are consistent with OA, additional laboratory testing is not necessary; however, if diagnosis remains in question, laboratory evaluation may be beneficial. Immunologic markers commonly used in the evaluation of other rheumatic diseases are not associated with OA and should be within their normal reference range, but if indiscriminately checked, false positives will be encountered.[59] Nonspecific markers of inflammation such as erythrocyte sedimentation rate and C-reactive protein are generally low, but these markers are influenced by patient age, comorbidities, infections, and recent trauma or surgeries.[59–61] Synovial fluid analysis, when available, is characteristically viscous, clear, noninflammatory (white blood cell count <2 K/μL), and absent of crystals.

Differential Diagnosis

Differentiating characteristics of noninflammatory OA from inflammatory arthritides is crucial (**Box 2**). Inflammatory pain is often associated with prolonged morning stiffness, and joints that are warm, red, and swollen. Inflammatory conditions that should be considered include systemic autoimmune conditions (rheumatoid arthritis, psoriatic arthritis, and spondyloarthropathies), and if monoarticular arthritis: trauma, infectious, and crystalline disease. On examination, redness and warmth are features of inflammatory arthritis; furthermore, swelling of the metacarpophalangeals, nail pitting,

---

Box 2
Differential diagnosis for osteoarthritis

Tendonitis

Rheumatoid arthritis

Seronegative spondyloarthopathy (psoriatic arthritis, reactive arthritis)

Crystalline arthritis (gout and pseudogout)

Septic arthritis or infectious arthritis (bacterial, viral, fungal, and Lyme disease)

Avascular necrosis

Foreign body synovitis

redness around the nail bed, or psoriatic lesions can help to differentiate rheumatoid arthritis and psoriatic arthritis from OA.

PRIMARY PREVENTION OF OSTEOARTHRITIS

Current treatment strategies generally focus on established OA; however, given its known risk factors, primary prevention also should be considered. Two modifiable risk factors are weight and injury. Children who participate in exercise routines are at lower risk for becoming obese and additionally have improved joint development.[29] Identifying at-risk patients and counseling on weight loss is recommended. Preventing joint injuries is another area of ongoing research.

ACL and meniscal injuries have been identified as risk factors for the development of OA, and unfortunately surgical repair may not significantly reduce that risk.[29] Thus, avoiding injuries is desired. During competition, athletes may subject their joints to injury-provoking stresses. Attempts have been made by using knee and ankle braces to prevent injuries, but the results have been mixed.[62–64] Many athletes express concern that braces hinder their performance and compliance is an issue, but as technology improves and braces become more ergonomic, this option may increase in popularity.

Additional interventions have focused on biomechanics. Intrinsic risk factors, including joint kinetics, core and trunk control, landing flat footed, and hip flexion all lend themselves to modification. Prevention programs focusing on neuromuscular training and emphasizing high-intensity plyometrics have shown the most benefit in preventing injury.[29] Thus, along with sport-specific conditioning, athletes and coaches may wish to include injury-prevention strategies to their training regimens.

TREATMENT OF OSTEOARTHRITIS

Most individuals who suffer from OA are most interested in having their pain addressed; however, a treatment plan includes more than just medication. The approach to OA therapy can be simplified into 3 main categories (**Fig. 4**).

Nonpharmacological Treatment of Osteoarthritis

Education
A nonpharmacological treatment approach to OA should begin with patient education. Patients should be familiarized with the type of arthritis they are experiencing, risk factors for the development of OA, available treatment options, and expectations. Appropriate education may improve compliance and efficacy of other treatment modalities,[65] and relieve concerns about their arthritis.

Weight loss
OA commonly involves weight-bearing joints. Weight reduction can off-load the forces of the joint, lessen pain, and slow the progression or disability associated with OA.[39–41] Furthermore, adipose tissue is not inert and has been associated with increased cytokine production.[42–44] Thus, by losing weight, the patient may not only lessen the load the joint is experiencing, but may also counter the proinflammatory mediators associated with adipose tissue. Appropriate weight loss counseling should emphasize these benefits, and avoid judgmental language or blaming the patient to avoid the nocebo effect (unfavorable outcome secondary to a negative patient experience or expectation).[66,67]

Exercise
Physical or occupational therapy should be encouraged and explained to the patient. When a joint hurts, it may be counterintuitive to increase activity.[65,68] By discussing

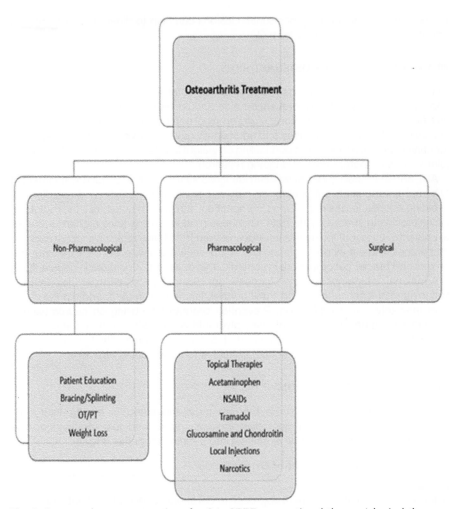

Fig. 4. Suggested treatment options for OA. OT/PT, occupational therapy/physical therapy.

the benefits of exercise, the patient will further understand the complexity of the joint and how strengthening muscles helps to diminish joint forces and improve joint alignment. Ideally, the patient will have a supervised session, but providing home exercises is an alternative option.

Bracing, orthotics, and assistive devices

Joint malalignment is an additional factor contributing to the development and symptoms of OA. Bracing and orthotics to alter joint biomechanics are another popular intervention.[69,70] Efficacy of these interventions is inconclusive; however, they are safe and tolerated.[69–71] Lateral wedge shoe inserts and valgus knee bracing are used to counter medial compartment OA (**Fig. 5**). They may reduce pain, increase function, and have been shown to reduce nonsteroidal anti-inflammatory drug (NSAID) use.[69–71] In osteoarthritis of the CMC joint, use of splints is recommended by the American College of Rheumatology (ACR)[72] (**Fig. 6**). Recommending a cane is another option that may off-load joint forces, and be beneficial in hip OA sufferers.[73]

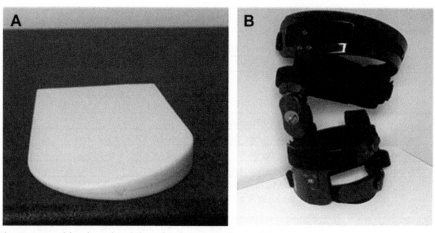

Fig. 5. Lateral heel wedge (*A*) and valgus knee brace (*B*).

Pharmacologic Therapies

Topical agents

Some patients cannot tolerate oral medications secondary to undesired side effects or comorbidities (**Table 1**). Thus, using a topical agent is a more reasonable option. Topical options may include NSAIDs, capsaicin, an anesthetic such as lidocaine, or a compounded agent. Topical NSAIDs have a small to moderate pain reduction when compared with a placebo.[74,75] Capsaicin may improve pain by reducing nociceptive pain through fiber desensitization.[75] Patients tend to be compliant when given

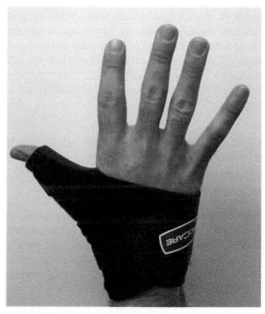

Fig. 6. Thumb soft Spica splint.

Table 1
Common medications and dosing for the treatment of osteoarthritis

Medication	Common Osteoarthritis Dosing	Comments
Acetaminophen	650 mg; 4–6 h	• MAX: 4000 mg/d
NSAIDs		• All NSAIDs carry black box warning for cardiovascular events and serious gastrointestinal events
Celecoxib	200 mg daily or 100 mg BID	
Ibuprofen	400–800 mg; 3–4 times daily	• US MAX: 3200 mg/d
Naproxen	250 mg to 500 mg; BID	
Meloxicam	7.5 mg to 15 mg once daily	• Capsule form: MAX 10 mg/d
Tramadol	50 mg; start at low dose and increase as tolerated every 3 d	• MAX: 400 mg/d. Typical dosing is 50–100 mg every 8–12 h • Warning for serotonin syndrome
Duloxetine	30 mg once daily; can increase to 60 mg daily after 7 d as tolerated	• Doses >60 mg likely of little benefit • Warning for suicidal thoughts

Abbreviations: BID, twice daily; MAX, maximum; NSAID, nonsteroidal anti-inflammatory drug.

these options, and topical therapies tend to be well tolerated, with skin irritation being the most common patient concern.[74]

Acetaminophen

Acetaminophen (paracetamol) is commonly used to treat OA, and is often the first medication a patient may try. It is relatively safe if taken at recommended amounts (<4000 mg/d). Unlike NSAIDs, it has no anti-inflammatory effect and offers only analgesia. The mechanism of action is not fully understood, but likely involves central pain pathways. When compared with placebo, patients taking acetaminophen can anticipate mild improvement in pain. A Cochrane review reported an effect size (ES) of 0.14 (95% confidence interval [CI] 0.05–0.22), which is less beneficial than an earlier meta-analysis that found an ES of 0.21 (95% CI 0.02–0.41).[76,77] Acetaminophen is best used in early or mild OA, or in patients who cannot tolerate NSAIDs. Historically, it has been a safer option for patients with peptic ulcer disease, but doses greater than 3 g per day have been associated with increased gastrointestinal (GI) and liver toxicity, with a hazard ratio of 1.2 (1.03, 1.40).[76]

Nonsteroidal anti-inflammatory drugs

Oral NSAIDs are recommended for the treatment of generalized OA.[72,76] As a class, they are superior to placebo for the treatment of OA pain with an ES of 0.29 (95% CI 0.22–0.35),[76,78] and are more beneficial than acetaminophen. A meta-analysis comparing NSAIDs to acetaminophen found NSAIDs offered more pain reduction (ES 0.20; 95% CI 0.10–0.30).[77] Not all patients will have a similar response to the same NSAID, and switching from one to another may be necessary to get the best response.[79–81] An additional factor influencing NSAID choice is their side-effect profile.

Despite the popularity of NSAIDs to treat OA, the class carries a black box warning. Common concerns include cardiovascular risks, GI bleeding, and acute kidney injury. In terms of cardiovascular risk, naproxen has a lower risk than other NSAIDs, with indomethacin, sulindac, and meloxicam suggested as having higher risks.[78] GI complications are increased in older individuals, those with a history of GI bleed, and concomitant use of aspirin, high-dose acetaminophen, glucocorticoids, or anticoagulation.[76,78]

Administration of a proton pump inhibitor may reduce the GI risk, but the indiscriminate use of proton pump inhibitors carry their own risks. The highest risk of GI complications have been reported with piroxicam and ketorolac, with celecoxib and ibuprofen reportedly having the best GI safety profile.[78] Because of these risks, the ACR recommends using caution when prescribing NSAIDs to patients older than 65.

Tramadol

Tramadol is an additional analgesic to treat OA. It is generally reserved for patients who have not achieved adequate pain relief with acetaminophen or NSAIDs, or cannot tolerate those medications.[72,76] It exerts its pain relief through antagonism of the mu opioid receptor. It also has effects on serotonin and norepinephrine; thus, caution should be taken when using with agents that have been associated with serotonin syndrome. It is available in immediate-release and extended-release formulations. Tolerability may be improved by using extended-release pills.[82] Typical available dosing is 50-mg to 100-mg tablets and maximum daily dosing is 400 mg daily. General prescribing practice is to start at a low dose (50 mg daily) and increase slowly to twice or 3 times a day as tolerated.

Duloxetine

Duloxetine is an option that has been used to treat chronic pain and OA.[72,76,83] Pain is multifactorial and involves nocioceptive, neuropathic, and central components. Local irritation, transmission, perception, and modulation are all factors that determine pain levels.[84] Thus, by using a serotonin and norepinephrine reuptake inhibitor, some patients may achieve benefit through alternative mechanisms. Further benefit may be encountered by treating accompanying depression that often is associated with chronic pain.[85] A recent meta-analysis indicated duloxetine had superiority to both tramadol and hydromorphone, but not other commonly available oral treatments.[86] Most treatment recommendations suggest duloxetine should be used as an adjunctive therapy for OA or as a second-line agent.[72,76]

Opioids

Some patients with severe OA may not be able to tolerate commonly prescribed oral medications or may have contraindications to them. In these cases, opioid pain medications may be needed. Routine use of opioids should be cautioned, given concern for abuse potential. Additional complications of opioid use include nausea, dizziness, constipation, and somnolence. Furthermore, there is evidence that use of opioids is no more effective than NSAIDs, tramadol, or duloxetine with regard to WOMAC scores.[86]

Glucosamine and chondroitin

Glucosamine and chondroitin are popular options for the treatment of OA. In the United States they are commonly found where supplements are sold. Despite their popularity, they are not recommended by the ACR for the treatment of OA.[72] This differs from European guidelines where they are strongly encouraged.[76,87] The primary reason for this discrepancy is that in the United States there is a lack of "prescription"-strength glucosamine and chondroitin, and most of the evidence indicates benefits from once-daily 1500 mg glucosamine sulfate, but not glucosamine hydrochloride.[88] Thus, if recommending glucosamine and chondroitin, specify glucosamine sulfate 1500 mg and chondroitin at 800 mg, and keep in mind supplements are not regulated by the Food and Drug Administration (FDA) in the United States.

Local injections

Given the pathogenesis of OA includes joint inflammation and cartilage defects, localized targeted therapy has been a popular option. The most commonly used modalities include injections of corticosteroids and hyaluronic acid (HA). Corticosteroid therapy takes advantage of the anti-inflammatory properties of these drugs. Total pain relief and length of relief is variable between patients, and despite their anti-inflammatory actions local steroid injections have not been shown to reverse OA progression.[89,90] HA injections take advantage of viscous protein properties to treat OA. The proposed mechanism of action is multifactorial. Initially, the thick supplementation was thought to replace cushioning that was lost with cartilage degeneration. This has been shown to likely play a minor role at best.[91,92] More likely, HA has anti-inflammatory and analgesic properties and may stimulate HA regeneration.[91] Similar to steroid injections, HA injections have variable patient effects. Despite the paucity of clinical data showing a definitive advantage of local injections, they continue to be a commonly used modality, particularly for knee OA, but the ACR recommends against intra-articular steroid injections in the treatment of CMC arthritis.[72]

Surgery

Patients that have failed conservative and medical options may benefit from surgical consultation. Most providers are familiar with surgical options for knee and hip OA; however, CMC joint arthroplasty also is an option that should not be overlooked.[93] Additionally, women are less likely than men to be offered surgery for total knee arthroplasty, and patients with similar pain levels and functional limitations, but less severe radiographic findings, are offered surgery less often.[94] Awareness of these potential biases may prevent delay in surgical referral.

THE FUTURE OF OSTEOARTHRITIS

Despite the expanding comprehension of OA pathogenesis, available therapies are focused on symptom control and, if severe enough, joint replacement. In an age of biologics and small molecule inhibitors for the management of other rheumatic diseases, osteoarthritis sufferers are still limited in their choice of treatments, and the available options are not disease modifying. Current pharmaceutical research is interested in their development, but to date none have shown efficacy to reach FDA approval. Failed options include MMP and cytokine inhibitors (TNF-α, IL-6, IL-1β), bisphosphonates, teriparatide, and calcitonin to name a few.[95] Another area of ongoing research is use of local injections of orthobiologics.[96]

Orthobiologics

Orthobiologics or regenerative injection therapy involves organic substances often harvested or collected from the patient, additionally modified and then injected back into the symptomatic joint. There are several forms and concepts of this therapy. Platelet-rich plasma, autologous conditioned serum, and mesenchymal stem cells are a few examples. Several studies have indicated that they are associated with improved WOMAC scores versus placebo and have sustained pain relief out to 12 months.[96–98] During a discussion on this topic at the ACR meeting in Washington, DC (2016), several questions were raised about lack of long-term safety and efficacy; given these concerns, more studies and experience will be necessary before these modalities are supported by expert consensus.

SUMMARY

OA is a common condition that will be regularly encountered in outpatient clinics. An understanding of its complex pathogenesis that includes local inflammation and biomechanical interactions, along with degenerative changes, will allow for a better approach to its management. Patient education should focus on modifiable risk factors when applicable, and treatment should incorporate medical, surgical, and non-pharmaceutical interventions. Current treatment options focus on symptom control, but future OA treatments may take advantage of genetic, systemic, and local biologic therapies.

REFERENCES

1. Lawrence RC, Felson DT, Helmick CG, et al. Estimates of the prevalence of arthritis and other rheumatic conditions in the United States. Part II. Arthritis Rheum 2008;58:26–35.
2. Johnson VL, Hunter DJ. The epidemiology of osteoarthritis. Best Pract Res Clin Rheumatol 2014;28:5–15.
3. Murphy L, Helmick CG. The impact of osteoarthritis in the United States: a population-health perspective. Am J Nurs 2012;112(3):S13–9.
4. Kontis V, Bennett JE, Mathers CD, et al. Future life expectancy in 35 industrialised countries: projections with a Bayesian model ensemble. Lancet 2017;6736(16): 32381–9.
5. 2015 Workforce Study of Rheumatology Specialists in the United States. 2017. Available at: rheumatology.org/portals/0/files/ACR-Workforce-Study-2015.pdf. Accessed March 1, 2017.
6. Dejaco C, Lackner A, Buttgereit F, et al. Rheumatology workforce planning in western countries: as systematic literature review. Arthritis Care Res 2016; 68(12):1874–82.
7. Shane Anderson A, Loeser RF. Why is osteoarthritis an age-related disease? Best Pract Res Clin Rheumatol 2010;24(1):15–26.
8. Ferrucci L, Cavazzini C, Corsi A, et al. Biomarkers of frailty in older persons. J Endocrinol Invest 2002;25:10–5.
9. Andriacchi TP, Mundermann A, Smith RL, et al. A framework for the in vivo pathomechanics of osteoarthritis at the knee. Ann Biomed Eng 2004;32:447–57.
10. Felson DT, Goggins J, Niu J, et al. The effect of body weight on progression of knee osteoarthritis is dependent on alignment. Arthritis Rheum 2004;50:3904–59.
11. Goldring MB, Goldring SR. Osteoarthritis. J Cell Physiol 2007;213:626–34.
12. Buckwalter JA, Roughley PJ, Rosenberg LC. Age-related changes in cartilage proteoglycans: quantitative electron microscopic studies. Microsc Res Tech 1994;28:398–408.
13. Bayliss MT, Osborne D, Woodhouse S, et al. Sulfation of chondroitin sulfate in human articular cartilage. The effect of age, topographical position, and zone of cartilage on tissue composition. J Biol Chem 1999;274:15892–900.
14. Wells T, Davidson C, Morgelin M, et al. Age-related changes in the composition, the molecular stoichiometry and the stability of proteoglycan aggregates extracted from human articular cartilage. Biochem J 2003;370:69–79.
15. Grushko G, Schneiderman R, Maroudas A. Some biochemical and biophysical parameters for the study of the pathogenesis of osteoarthritis: a comparison between the processes of ageing and degeneration in human hip cartilage. Connect Tissue Res 1989;19:149–76.
16. Del Carlo M Jr, Loeser RF. Increased oxidative stress with aging reduces chondrocyte survival: correlation with intracellular glutathione levels. Arthritis Rheum 2003;48:3419–30.

17. Jallali N, Ridha H, Thrasivoulou C, et al. Vulnerability to ROS-induced cell death in ageing articular cartilage: the role of antioxidant enzyme activity. Osteoarthritis Cartilage 2005;13:614–22.

18. Loeser RF, Carlson CS, Carlo MD, et al. Detection of nitrotyrosine in aging and osteoarthritic cartilage: correlation of oxidative damage with the presence of interleukin-1beta and with chondrocyte resistance to insulin-like growth factor 1. Arthritis Rheum 2002;46:2349–57.

19. Campisi J. Senescent cells, tumor suppression, and organismal aging: good citizens, bad neighbors. Cell 2005;120:513–22.

20. Campisi J, d'Adda di Fagagna F. Cellular senescence: when bad things happen to good cells. Nat Rev Mol Cell Biol 2007;8:729–40.

21. Loeser RF, Shanker G, Carlson CS, et al. Reduction in the chondrocyte response to insulin-like growth factor 1 in aging and osteoarthritis: studies in a non-human primate model of naturally occurring disease. Arthritis Rheum 2000;43:2110–20.

22. Van Meurs JBJ. Osteoarthritis year in review 2016: genetics, genomics, and epigenetics. Osteoarthritis Cartilage 2017;25:181–9.

23. Steinberg J, Zeggini E. Function genomics in osteoarthritis: past, present and future. J Orthop Res 2016;34(7):1105–10.

24. Panoutsopoulou K, Zeggini E. Advances in osteoarthritis genetics. J Med Genet 2013;50:715–24.

25. Pan Q, O'connor MI, Coutts RD, et al. Characterization of osteoarthritic human knees indicates potential sex differences. Biol Sex Differ 2016;7(27):2–15.

26. Boyan BD, Tosi L, Coutts R, et al. Sex differences in osteoarthritis of the knee. J Am Acad Orthop Surg 2012;20:668–9.

27. O'Connor MI. Sex differences in osteoarthritis of the hip and knee. J Am Acad Orthop Surg 2007;15(suppl 1):S22–5.

28. Xiao YP, Tian FM, Dai MW, et al. Are estrogen related drugs new alternatives for the management of osteoarthritis? Arthritis Res Ther 2016;18(151):1–15.

29. Ratzlaff CR, Liang MH. Prevention of injury-related knee osteoarthritis: opportunities for the primary and secondary prevention of knee osteoarthritis. Arthritis Res Ther 2010;12:1–8.

30. Lohmander LS, Englund PM, Dahl LL, et al. The long-term consequence of anterior cruciate ligament and meniscus injuries: osteoarthritis. Am J Sports Med 2007;35:1756–69.

31. Lohmander LS, Ostenberg A, Englund M, et al. High prevalence of knee osteoarthritis, pain, and functional limitations in female soccer players twelve years after anterior cruciate ligament injury. Arthritis Rheum 2004;50:3145–52.

32. von Porat A, Roos EM, Roos H. High prevalence of osteoarthritis 14 years after an anterior cruciate ligament tear in male soccer players: a study of radiographic and patient relevant outcomes. Ann Rheum Dis 2004;63:269–73.

33. Cooper C, McAlindon T, Coggon D, et al. Occupational activity and osteoarthritis of the knee. Ann Rheum Dis 1994;53(2):90–3.

34. Panush RS. Does exercise cause arthritis? Long-term consequences of exercise on the musculoskeletal system. Rheum Dis Clin North Am 1990;16(4):827–36.

35. Wen L, Kang JH, Yim YR, et al. Associations between body composition measurements of obesity and radiographic osteoarthritis in older adults: data from Dong-gu study. BMC Musculoskelet Disord 2016;17:1–7.

36. Gelber AC, Hochberg MC, Mead LA, et al. Body mass index in young men and the risk of subsequent knee and hip osteoarthritis. Am J Med 1999;107(6):542–8.

37. Heliovaara M, Makela M, Impivaara O, et al. Association of overweight, trauma and workload with coxarthrosis. A healthy survey of 7,217 persons. Acta Orthop Scand 1993;64(5):513–8.
38. Vingard E. Overweight predisposes to coxarthrosis. Body-mass index studied in 239 males with hip arthroplasty. Acta Orthop Scand 1991;62(2):106–9.
39. Bliddal H, Christensen R. The management of osteoarthritis in the obese patient: practical considerations and guidelines for therapy. Obes Rev 2006;7:323–31.
40. Messier SP, Loeser RF, Mitchell MN, et al. Exercise and weight loss in obese older adults with knee osteoarthritis: a preliminary study. J Am Geriatr Soc 2000;48: 1062–72.
41. Felson DT, Zhang Y, Anthony JM, et al. Weight loss reduces the risk for symptomatic knee osteoarthritis in women. Ann Intern Med 1992;116:535–9.
42. Richter M, Trzeciak T, Owecki M, et al. The role of adipocytokines in the pathogenesis of knee joint osteoarthritis. Int Orthop 2015;39:1211–7.
43. Clockaerts S, Bastiaansen-Jenniskens YM, Runhaar J, et al. The infrapatellar fat pad should be considered as an active osteoarthritic join tissue: a narrative review. Osteoarthritis Cartilage 2010;18:876–82.
44. Conde J, Scotece M, Abella V, et al. Identification of novel adipokines in the joint. Differential expression in healthy and osteoarthritis tissues. PLoS One 2015;10: e0123601.
45. Berenbaum F. Osteoarthritis as an inflammatory disease (osteoarthritis is not osteoarthrosis!). Osteoarthritis Cartilage 2013;21:16–21.
46. Kapoor M, Martel-Pelletier J, Lajeunesse D, et al. Role of proinflammatory cytokines in the pathophysiology of osteoarthritis. Nat Rev Rheumatol 2011;7(1): 33e42.
47. Chu CR, Williams AA, Coyle CH, et al. Early diagnosis to enable early treatment of pre-osteoarthritis. Arthritis Res Ther 2012;14:2–10.
48. Charlier E, Biserka R, Deroyer C, et al. Insights on the molecular mechanisms of chondrocytes death in osteoarthritis. Int J Mol Sci 2016;17:1–36.
49. Greene A, Loeser R. Aging-related inflammation in osteoarthritis. Osteoarthritis Cartilage 2015;23(11):1966–71.
50. Struglics A, Okroj M, Sward P, et al. The complement system is activated in synovial fluid from subjects with knee injury and from patients with osteoarthritis. Arthritis Res Ther 2016;18:1–11.
51. Liu-Bryan R. Synovium and the innate inflammatory network in osteoarthritis progression. Curr Rheumatol Rep 2013;15(5):1–12.
52. Smelter E, Hochenberg MC. New treatments for osteoarthritis. Curr Opin Rheumatol 2013;25:310–6.
53. Pereira D, Peleteiro B, Araujo J, et al. The effect of osteoarthritis definition on prevalence and incidence estimates: a systemic review. Osteoarthritis Cartilage 2011;19:1270–85.
54. Hunter DJ, Lo GH. The management of osteoarthritis an overview and call to appropriate conservative treatment. Rheum Dis Clin North Am 2008;34:689–712.
55. Slemenda C, Brandt KD, Hellman DK, et al. Quadriceps weakness and osteoarthritis of the knee. Ann Intern Med 1997;127:97–104.
56. Ikeda S, Tsumura H, Torisu T. Age-related quadriceps-dominant muscle atrophy and incident radiographic knee osteoarthritis. J Orthop Sci 2005;10:121–6.
57. Kellgren JH, Lawrence JS. Atlas of standard radiographs. Oxford (United Kingdom): Oxford University Press; 1963.
58. Mathiessen A, Cimmino MA, Hammer HB, et al. Imaging of osteoarthritis (OA): what is new? Best Pract Res Clin Rheumatol 2016;30:653–69.

59. Colglazier CL, Sutej PG. Laboratory testing in the rheumatic diseases: a practical review. South Med J 2005;98(2):185–91.

60. Morley JJ, Kushner I. Serum C-reactive protein levels in disease. Ann N Y Acad Sci 1982;389:406–18.

61. Sox HC Jr, Liang MH. The erythrocyte sedimentation rate: guidelines for rational use. Ann Intern Med 1986;104:515–23.

62. Sitler M, Ryan J, Hopkinson W, et al. The efficacy of a prophylactic knee brace to reduce knee injuries in football. A prospective, randomized study at West Point. Am J Sports Med 1990;18:310–5.

63. Rovere GD, Haupt HA, Yates CS. Prophylactic knee bracing in college football. Am J Sports Med 1987;15:111–6.

64. Rishiraj N, Taunton JE, Lloyd-Smith R, et al. The potential role of prophylactic/functional knee bracing in preventing knee ligament injury. Sports Med 2009; 39:937–60.

65. Chang RW, Semanik PA, Lee J, et al. Improving physical activity in arthritis clinical trial (IMPAACT): study design, rationale, recruitment, and baseline data. Contemp Clin Trials 2014;39(2):224–35.

66. Sanderson C, Hardy J, Spruyt O, et al. Placebo and nocebo effects in randomized controlled trials: the implications for research and practice. J Pain Symptom Manage 2013;46(5):722–30.

67. Dieppe P, Goldingay S, Greville-Harris M. The power of placebo and nocebo in painful osteoarthritis. Osteoarthritis Cartilage 2016;24:1850–7.

68. Franek J. Self-management support interventions for persons with chronic disease: an evidence based analysis. Ont Health Technol Assess Ser 2013;13(9): 1–60.

69. Duivenoorden T, Brouwer RW, van Raaij TM, et al. Braces and orthoses for treating osteoarthritis of the knee (review). Cochrane Database Syst Rev 2015;3:1–4.

70. van Raaij TM, Reijman M, Brouwer RW, et al. Medial knee osteoarthritis treated by insoles or braces: a randomized control trial. Clin Orthop Relat Res 2010;468: 1926–32.

71. Pham T, Maillefert JF, Hurdy C, et al. Laterally elevated wedged insoles in the treatment of medial knee osteoarthritis: a two-year prospective randomized controlled study. Osteoarthritis Cartilage 2004;12:46–55.

72. Hochberg MC, Altman RD, Toupin April K, et al. American College of Rheumatology 2012 recommendations for the use of nonpharmacologic and pharmacologic therapies in osteoarthritis of the hand, hip, and knee. Arthritis Care Res 2012;64(4):465–74.

73. Brand RA, Crowninshield RD. The effect of cane use on hip contact force. Clin Orthop 1980;147:181–4.

74. Argoff CE. Topical analgesics in the management of acute and chronic pain. Mayo Clin Proc 2013;88(2):195–205.

75. Persson MS, Fu Y, Bhattacharya A, et al. Relative efficacy of topical non-steroidal anti-inflammatory drugs and topical capsaicin in osteoarthritis: protocol for an individual patient data meta-analysis. Syst Rev 2016;5(165):1–8.

76. Zhang W, Nuki G, Moskowitz RW, et al. OARSI recommendations for the management of hip and knee osteoarthritis part III: changes in evidence following systematic cumulative update of research published through January 2009. Osteoarthritis Cartilage 2010;18:476–99.

77. Zhang W, Jones A, Doherty M. Does paracetamol (acetaminophen) reduce the pain of osteoarthritis? A meta-analysis of randomised controlled trials. Ann Rheum Dis 2004;63:901–7.

78. Pelletier JP, Martel-Pelletier J, Rannou F, et al. Efficacy and safety of oral NSAIDs and analgesics in the management of osteoarthritis: evidence from real-life setting trials and surveys. Semin Arthritis Rheum 2016;45:S22–7.

79. Essex MN, O'Connell MA, Bhadra BP. Response to non-steroidal anti-inflammatory drugs in African Americans with osteoarthritis of the knee. J Int Med Res 2014;40:2251–66.

80. Essex MN, Behar R, O'Connell MA, et al. Efficacy and tolerability of celecoxib and naproxen versus placebo in Hispanic patients with knee osteoarthritis. Int J Gen Med 2014;7:227–35.

81. Bruno A, Tacconelli S, Patrignani P. Variability in the response to non-steroidal anti-inflammatory drugs: mechanisms and perspectives. Basic Clin Pharmacol Toxicol 2014;114(1):56–63.

82. Gana TJ, Pascual ML, Fleming RR, et al. Extended release tramadol in the treatment of osteoarthritis: a multicenter randomized, double-blind, placebo-controlled trial. Curr Med Res Opin 2006;22:1391–401.

83. Lunn MP, Hughes RA, Wiffen PJ. Duloxetine for treating painful neuropathy, chronic pain, or fibromyalgia. Cochrane Database Syst Rev 2014;(1):CD007115.

84. Perrot S. Osteoarthritis pain. Best Pract Res Clin Rheumatol 2015;29:90–7.

85. Jesus C, Jesus I, Aquis M. Treatment of depression in patients with osteoarthritis: the importance of an early diagnosis and the role of duloxetine. Psychiatr Danub 2016;28(S1):149–53.

86. Myers J, Wielage RC, Han B, et al. The efficacy of duloxetine, non-steroidal anti-inflammatory drugs, and opioids in osteoarthritis: a systematic literature review and meta-analysis. BMC Musculoskelet Disord 2014;15(76):1–16.

87. Jordan KM, Arden NK, Doherty M, et al. EULAR recommendations 2003: an evidence based approach to the management of knee osteoarthritis: report of a task force of the standing committee for international clinical studies including therapeutic trials. Ann Rheum Dis 2003;62:1145–55.

88. Bruyere O, Altman RD, Reginster JY. Efficacy and safety of glucosamine sulfate in the management of osteoarthritis: evidence from real-life setting trials and surveys. Semin Arthritis Rheum 2016;45:S12–7.

89. Bjordal JM, Klovning A, Ljunggren AE, et al. Short-term efficacy of pharmacotherapeutic interventions in osteoarthritic knee pain: a meta-analysis of randomised placebo-controlled trials. Eur J Pain 2007;369:1621–6.

90. Bellamy N, Capbell J, Robinson V, et al. Intraarticular corticosteroids for treatment of osteoarthritis or the knee. Cochrane Database Syst Rev 2006;(2):CD005328.

91. Moreland LW. Intra-articular hyaluronan (hyaluronic acid) and hylans for the treatment of osteoarthritis: mechanisms of action. Arthritis Res Ther 2003;5(2):54.

92. Aggarwal A, Sempowski IP. Hyaluronic acid injections for knee osteoarthritis. Systemic review of the literature. Can Fam Physician 2004;50:249–56.

93. Melville DM, Taljanovic MS, Scalcione LR, et al. Imaging and management of thumb carpometacarpal joint osteoarthritis. Skeletal Radiol 2015;44(2):165–77.

94. Fraenkel L, Suter L, Weis L, et al. Variability in recommendations for total knee arthroplasty among rheumatologists and orthopedic surgeons. J Rhueumatol 2014;41(1):47–52.

95. Karsdal MA, Michaeilis M, Ladel C, et al. Disease-modifying treatments for osteoarthritis (DMOADs) of the knee and hip: lessons learned from failures and opportunities for the future. Osteoarthritis Cartilage 2016;24:2013–21.

96. Crane DM, Oliver KS, Bayes MC. Orthobiologics and knee osteoarthritis: a recent literature review, treatment algorithim, and pathophysiology discussion. Phys Med Rehabil Clin N Am 2016;27:985–1002.

97. Kawamura Demange M, Sisto M, Rodeo S. Future trends for unicompartmental arthritis of the knee: injectable and stem cells. Clin Sports Med 2014;33:161–74.

98. Lai LP, Stitik TP, Foye PM, et al. Use of platelet-rich plasma in intra-articular knee injections for osteoarthritis: a systematic review. PM R 2015;7:637–48.

Printed and bound by CPI Group (UK) Ltd, Croydon, CR0 4YY

07/10/2024

01040502-0003